Principles of
MANUAL THERAPY

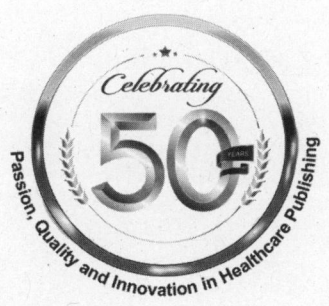

Principles of MANUAL THERAPY

THIRD EDITION

Deepak Sebastian
DPT DO ND PhD Fellow AAOMPT CES Cert DN Cert MSKUS
AB Orthopaedic Physical Therapy, Manual Osteopath
and Musculoskeletal Naturopath
Clinical Instructor and Director
Institute of Therapeutic Sciences
Certification and Clinical Residency in Orthopedic Physical Therapy
Fellowship in Orthopedic Manual Physical Therapy
Alternative Rehab Inc
Livonia, Michigan, USA

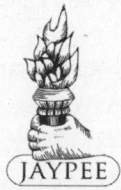

JAYPEE BROTHERS MEDICAL PUBLISHERS
The Health Sciences Publisher
New Delhi | London | Panama

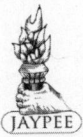
Jaypee Brothers Medical Publishers (P) Ltd

Headquarters
Jaypee Brothers Medical Publishers (P) Ltd
4838/24, Ansari Road, Daryaganj
New Delhi 110 002, India
Phone: +91-11-43574357
Fax: +91-11-43574314
Email: jaypee@jaypeebrothers.com

Overseas Offices

J.P. Medical Ltd
83 Victoria Street, London
SW1H 0HW (UK)
Phone: +44 20 3170 8910
Fax: +44 (0)20 3008 6180
Email: info@jpmedpub.com

Jaypee-Highlights Medical Publishers Inc
City of Knowledge, Bld. 235, 2nd Floor
Clayton, Panama City, Panama
Phone: +1 507-301-0496
Fax: +1 507-301-0499
Email: cservice@jphmedical.com

Jaypee Brothers Medical Publishers (P) Ltd
Bhotahity, Kathmandu, Nepal
Phone: +977-9741283608
Email: kathmandu@jaypeebrothers.com

Website: www.jaypeebrothers.com
Website: www.jaypeedigital.com

© 2019, Jaypee Brothers Medical Publishers

The views and opinions expressed in this book are solely those of the original contributor(s)/author(s) and do not necessarily represent those of editor(s) of the book.

All rights reserved. No part of this publication may be reproduced, stored or transmitted in any form or by any means, electronic, mechanical, photocopying, recording or otherwise, without the prior permission in writing of the publishers.

All brand names and product names used in this book are trade names, service marks, trademarks or registered trademarks of their respective owners. The publisher is not associated with any product or vendor mentioned in this book.

Medical knowledge and practice change constantly. This book is designed to provide accurate, authoritative information about the subject matter in question. However, readers are advised to check the most current information available on procedures included and check information from the manufacturer of each product to be administered, to verify the recommended dose, formula, method and duration of administration, adverse effects and contraindications. It is the responsibility of the practitioner to take all appropriate safety precautions. Neither the publisher nor the author(s)/editor(s) assume any liability for any injury and/or damage to persons or property arising from or related to use of material in this book.

This book is sold on the understanding that the publisher is not engaged in providing professional medical services. If such advice or services are required, the services of a competent medical professional should be sought.

Every effort has been made where necessary to contact holders of copyright to obtain permission to reproduce copyright material. If any have been inadvertently overlooked, the publisher will be pleased to make the necessary arrangements at the first opportunity. The **CD/DVD-ROM** (if any) provided in the sealed envelope with this book is complimentary and free of cost. **Not meant for sale.**

Inquiries for bulk sales may be solicited at: jaypee@jaypeebrothers.com

Principles of Manual Therapy

First Edition: 2009

Second Edition: 2013

Third Edition: **2019**

ISBN: 978-93-5270-301-2

Printed at Rajkamal Electric Press, Plot No. 2, Phase-IV, Kundli, Haryana.

Dedicated to

*My parents, Mr R Sebastian and Dr Mrs S Snehalatha
The Almighty
My wife, Anupama Gopalakrishnan
My son, Taneesh
and my profession, my very
reasons for being.
Prof Mary Chidambaram
my first impression of a physiotherapist
All my teachers in India and
the United States
and
All my patients and students*

Preface

Principles of Manual Therapy is ready for another update. Reviews suggest that it has been a valuable guide for the novice clinician, to have a good basic overview of the principles underlying manual therapy. Some of the methodology has been modified and updated and continues to be in a clinically applicable format. Manual therapy management of musculoskeletal dysfunction has been enhanced to add the neural component of somatic dysfunction. In this section, complementary to joint mobilization principles, terms like neurokinematics and interface mobilization have been described. Further, manual therapy interventions for specific conditions have been added as a section which gives the practitioner an idea as to how hands on interventions influence the primary musculoskeletal clinical diagnosis. A new section described the 'neglected zones' of the somatic chain outlines the need for addressing musculoskeletal dysfunction as a kinematic chain and offers as basic insight as to how adjacent joints can influence the primary dysfunction. Lastly, a new section has been added to the Thoracic Spine section describing the prevalence of rib related pain and dysfunction and their management.

Deepak Sebastian

Acknowledgments

Behind every endeavor stand able and enthusiastic minds and sources of inspiration, I wish to thank Prof Mary Chidambaram, formerly Chief Physiotherapist, College of Physiotherapy, Chennai, Tamil Nadu, India, for her dynamism as a clinician and teacher which was indeed a great source of inspiration and her constant emphasis on the character of a clinician. I express my gratitude to Prof IS Shanmugam, MBBS, D Ortho, DPhys Med, retired Director, Government Institute of Rehabilitation Medicine, Chennai, for giving me an opportunity in this profession and for his guidance and encouragement. My deepest gratitude to Prof PVA Mohandas, MBBS, D Ortho, MS, MCh (Orth), Professor, Department of Orthopedic Surgery, Madras Institute of Orthopaedics and Traumatology (MIOT), Chennai, for giving me an exposure for new work cultures his dynamic mentorship and emphasis on innovation. His ideology is followed and shared to this day. My heartfelt thanks to my teachers Dr George Ibrahim, PT, DO, Consultant, St Joseph Mercy Health System, Ann Arbor, Michigan, USA and Dr Stanley V Paris, PhD, PT, FAPTA, FAAOMPT, Professor, Department of Manipulative Therapy and President, University of St Augustine for Health Sciences, St Augustine, Florida, USA, my very sources of motivation to specialize in manual therapy. I wish to thank Helen Smith, MSA, PT, Systems Manager, Department of Physical Therapy, St Joseph Mercy Health System, Ann Arbor, Michigan, for her friendship and support through the early days of my career in United States. We pray that her soul rests in peace. My sincere thanks to Dr Peter Loubert, PhD, PT, ATC, Professor, Department of Physical Therapy, Central Michigan University, Mount Pleasant, Michigan, and President of the Michigan Physical Therapy Association, for his valuable academic advice over the last decade. My immense gratitude to *late* Dr MG Mokashi, PhD, PT, formerly Head, Department of Physical Therapy, All India Institute of Physical Medicine and Rehabilitation, Mumbai, Maharashtra, India, my first exposure to controlled research and critical enquiry. We pray his soul rests in peace.

Much is owed to my colleagues Raghu Chovvath, PT, DPT, OCS, FAAOMPT; Ramesh Malladi, PT, DPT, FAAOMPT, and Toby Manimalethu, PT, Alternative Rehab Inc, Livonia, Michigan, for their dedication and zealous enthusiasm despite their hectic work and family responsibilities. Their clinical and technical support has indeed made this book a possibility.

I wish to recognize and thank Nazir VM Ahmed, PT, MSc, Consultant, Henry Ford Health System, Detroit, Michigan, a friend and colleague who dedicates most of his valuable time caring for patients who to him stand as his biggest priority.

Words cannot express the moral support that I received from my friends Salil Raje, BSc, MBA, MS; Kshitija Raje, PT, MSc, MS, GCS, DPT; Suvarna Aphale, PT; Sanjay Kulkarni, MD, PhD; Amit Mehta, PT, MBA, Smita Mehta, PT; Sachin Desai, PT, MSc, and Swapna Desai, PhD, whose genuine love and affection saw me through some very hard phases of my life as I began writing this book.

I wish to thank my residents and fellows whom I refer to as the 'new generation' of clinicians, for their passion for the craft and unceasing desire to improve. You most certainly keep me going.

Lastly, *but truly firstly*, my parents, Dr S Snehalatha, MD, Professor, Department of Pathology and formerly Vice-Principal/Acting Dean of Madras Medical College, and Mr R Sugumar Sebastian, retired Abrasive Consultant, Chennai (now in heaven), who set an example and constantly instilled in me the value of education and the importance of persistent hard work. They, to this day, motivate me to move on. I would, but fail, if I did not mention my wife, Anupama Gopalakrishnan, BA, MA, MS, Product Development and Web Consultant, Michigan, and my son, Taneesh Sebastian, for giving me a new meaning to my current existence. I thank them for their genuine love and support throughout the making of this book.

Contents

PART 1: A Manual Therapy Approach to Musculoskeletal Dysfunction

Section 1: Introduction and Principles

1. Introduction — 5
2. The Evolution of the Practice of Manual Therapy — 8
3. Manipulation: Definition and Types — 14
4. Understanding Mechanical Dysfunction — 17
5. Principles of Management of Mechanical Dysfunction — 21
6. Palpation — 25
7. Principles of Diagnosis — 34

Section 2: Spinal Manipulation

8. Cervical Spine — 51
9. Thoracic Spine and Ribs — 77
10. Lumbar Spine — 96
11. The Pelvic Complex — 105

Section 3: Extremity Manipulation

12. Ankle and Foot — 129
13. Knee — 146
14. Hip — 157
15. Shoulder — 167
16. Elbow — 186
17. Wrist and Hand — 197

PART 2: A Manual Therapy Approach to Mechanical Peripheral Nerve Entrapment Dysfunction

18. Introduction — 215
19. Relevant Anatomy — 217
20. Understanding Mechanical Nerve Dysfunction — 232
21. Examination — 237
22. Treatment — 245

PART 3: Regional Conditions and Relevant Manual Therapy Intervention

23. Cervical Region — 253
24. Thoracic Region — 262
25. Lumbopelvic Region — 269

26. Hip Region	283
27. Knee Region	290
28. Ankle and Foot Region	297
29. Shoulder Region	306
30. Elbow, Wrist and Hand Region	316

PART 4: The Critical and Neglected Zones of the Upper and Lower Quarter in the Management of Regional Conditions

31. The Upper Quarter	327
32. The Lower Quarter	342
Index	*353*

PART 1

A Manual Therapy Approach to Musculoskeletal Dysfunction

Sections

Section 1: Introduction and Principles
Section 2: Spinal Manipulation
Section 3: Extremity Manipulation

Section 1

Introduction and Principles

Chapter 1: Introduction
Chapter 2: The Evolution of the Practice of Manual Therapy
Chapter 3: Manipulation: Definition and Types
Chapter 4: Understanding Mechanical Dysfunction
Chapter 5: Principles of Management of Mechanical Dysfunction
Chapter 6: Palpation
Chapter 7: Principles of Diagnosis

CHAPTER 1

Introduction

Manual therapy is a skilled, specific hands on approach used by clinicians including physical therapists to diagnose and treat soft tissue and joint structures for the purpose of decreasing pain, improving joint range and alignment, improving contractile and noncontractile tissue repair, extensibility and stability and facilitating function. Assisted therapeutic exercise and passive movement most definitely encompass the practice of manual therapy, but manual therapy today has evolved as a science with a greater degree of specificity and broader area of application. Most importantly in the diagnosis of musculoskeletal dysfunction which are usually not visualized by complex imaging procedures.

Management of musculoskeletal dysfunction is often symptom-based. The pain is often treated as opposed to the cause of the pain.[1] The reason being, ignorance of the intricacy of the cause or time constraints. When the cause is detected, the chronicity of the problem is minimized and the need for complicated procedures, including surgery probably avoided.

The musculoskeletal system is a system of chains and links united in function and enveloped by fascia. No part of the body functions independently. In which case no injury that is cumulative in nature occurs secondary to a single entity. The reverse is true as in when injury occurs secondary an outside force or trauma (falls, motor vehicle accidents) that recovery, especially normal functional recovery, does not occur due to restoration of functional integrity in a single entity. A whole chain or functional chain is usually involved and its integrity is essential for normal function. This functional chain consists of the osseous component (bone and joint), the soft tissue component (muscle, fascia and ligaments) and the neural component (central and peripheral). Infrequently, the autonomic component may be of relevance to the physical therapist. The detection of aberrant function of this functional chain as a whole and correlating it to the existing pathology is the essence of the art and science of manual therapy.[2]

Hence, manual therapy as is traditionally viewed as a technique-based treatment mode is in reality, a diagnostic tool. The diagnosis is made by sensitive feel and astute clinical observation of the functional chain, both requiring a great deal of practice.[3] The treatment 'technique' is often the smallest component of the management strategy and truly the diagnosis, or detection of the dysfunction is where a lot of the mental energy is exercised.

The health care arena is now headed towards what is known as evidence-based practice. This implication is felt significantly by the profession of physical therapy, especially physical therapist's practicing manual therapy. Quantification[4] of favorable outcomes or hard facts denoting efficacy of treatment procedures is often times stressed upon. It is unfortunate if there is a monetary implication to this, however, effective documentation and representation of examination and intervention procedures, is the direction to clinical growth. If this can be combined with an understanding that every individual is unique, with a baggage, and represents parameters that cannot be quantified (that may have a favorable effect on the outcome), management becomes more realistic.

In manual therapy the gray zone is reproducibility. Since most diagnostic procedures are by 'feel', two or more examiners are expected to feel the same finding which is to be statistically significant. This is called inter-rater reliability.[5] The efficacy of examination procedures is undoubted from an empirical perspective, however, interrater reliability has not been found to be good overall, with a few exceptions.[6] One should know that reproducibility within the same examiner has been found to be fair to good. Research would term this intra-rater reliability. This is indeed a consolation, however, the clinician should also know that a similar dilemma exists in other health professions that incorporate palpatory examination in their respective practices. The point to be made is, clinicians, especially manual therapists, should constantly strive to structure and improve consistency in their philosophy. Extensive practice with a sound background of bio and pathomechanics combined with meaningful research, should always be stressed upon.

While manual therapy is viewed as a treatment tool it is in reality a philosophy, combining aspects of clinical reasoning and diagnosis. The diagnosis is based on feel and movement possibly leading to a special test. Subsequent chapters will reveal much of the treatment decisions are based on mobility or other special tests. Contemporary research questions the validity of these tests based on certain criteria and establishes a 'Utility Score' for each of these tests.[7] The criteria is based on the following:
1. Reliability (as mentioned above)
2. Sensitivity/specificity
3. Likelihood ratios
4. Diagnostic odds ratio
5. QUADAS (Quality Assessment of Diagnostic Accuracy Studies).

Specificity: The probability of a positive test result in someone with the pathology.

Sensitivity: The probability of a negative test result in someone without the pathology.

Positive likelihood ratio: The ratio of a positive test result in people with the pathology to a positive test result in people without the pathology.

Negative likelihood ratio: The ratio of a negative test result in people with the pathology to a negative test result in people without the pathology.

Diagnostic odds ratio: A single measure of diagnostic test accuracy combining positive likelihood ratio and negative likelihood ratio.

The above is inferred from critically evaluating literature that studies the diagnostic utility of a test and the findings are summarized in a questionnaire. The QUADAS is a 14 point questionnaire that yield a score based on the number of 'yes' responses. The result is a utility score of 1, 2 or 3.
1. Which strongly supports the test
2. Which moderately supports the test
3. Which minimally supports the test.

The tests described in this literature review, however, are not adequately evaluated for diagnostic utility. Their empirical clinical value has been strengthened as a theory which proposes that most mechanical musculoskeletal dysfunction have a somatic cause which manifest as a positive finding via these tests. Manual therapy treatment interventions for these somatic causes however, have been shown to be effective via randomized controlled trials.[8] This book combines traditional osteopathy with traditional physical therapy principles to establish what is known as a somatic diagnosis based on empirically valuable tests. As much as structure would govern function, the harmonius movement interplay of this structure that is influenced by neuromuscular integrity, would also govern function. When an aberrance in this unity occurs, mechanical neuro-musculoskeletal dysfunction may result. Hence, the clinician should remember that manual therapy, or orthopedic manual physical therapy (OMPT) is a science and a philosophy that encompasses a methodology of reasoning and management.

Just like any other treatment philosophy, manual therapy is not a cure all. It has to be combined with other philosophies as appropriate. When addressing each single component of the neuromusculoskeletal apparatus all appropriate tests and most importantly all standard precautions and contraindications should be considered to avoid unfavorable outcomes.

This book hence intends to enlighten the physical therapy clinician, not only the techniques of application, but also the conceptual basis of why such techniques are incorporated with an emphasis on detection or diagnosis of the dysfunction. It also intends to reinforce the fact ever so often to..... *"treat the cause not the symptom".*

REFERENCES

1. Paris SV. Manual therapy: Treat function not pain. In: Michel TH (ed). Pain Churchill Livingston, 1985.
2. Greenman PE. Principles of Manual Medicine. 1996, Lippincott William and Wilkins, Baltimore
3. Sahrmann SA. Diagnosis by the physical therapist—A prerequisite for treatment. Phys Ther. 1988;68:1703-6.
4. Van Dillen LR, Sahrmann SA, Norton BJ, Caldwell CA, Fleming DA, McDonnel MK, et al Reliability of physical examination items used for classification of patients with low back pain. Phys Ther. 1998; 78:979-88.
5. Gonella C, Paris SV, Kutner M. Reliability in evaluating passive intervertebral motion. Phys Ther. 1982; 62: 436-44.
6. Sebastian D, Chovvath R. Reliability of palpation assessment in non neutral dysfunctions of the lumbar spine. Orthopedic Physical Therapy Practice. 2003;16:23-6.
7. Cook CE Hegedus EJ. Orthopaedic physical examination tests: An evidence-based Approach. New Jersey: Prentice Hill, 2008.
8. Bronfort G, Haas M, Evans R, Leininger B, Triano J. Effectiveness of manual therapies: the UK evidence report. Chiropr Osteopat. 2010;18:3.

CHAPTER 2

The Evolution of the Practice of Manual Therapy

THE BEGINNING

The earliest records of hands on treatments date back to 3000 BC. The oldest known book written about hands on treatments is Cong-Fu of the Toa-Tse. Literature on hands on healing is available in Chinese textbooks as far back as the Nei Jing (2760 BC) period. The Chinese practiced hands on treatments that are similar in principles to the current trigger point and acupuncture treatments. They are known as the Amno, Press and Rub, Tui na Push and Grasp and the Dian Xue point press. They were widely used to treat joint, muscle and internal disorders.

In 2500 BC, the Egyptians created reflexology. It is a focused pressure technique directed on the feet or hands to stimulate reflexes that correspond to organs and glands in the body. The pressure claims to activate corresponding electrical energy to maintain homeostasis.

The earliest records of medical practice dates back to 1000 BC, with Ayurveda being considered the mother of all practice forms. Dhanvantri, Charaka and Sushruta,[1] in ancient India, being considered the pioneers of medicine and modern surgery have described forms of manual treatment in their works Charaka Samhita and Sushruta Samhita. Their forms were called Panchkarma and Marma therapy. Panchkarma includes Snehana and Abhyanga. They refer to internal and external oleation which are done to cause superficial and deep tissues to become supple. This process nourishes the nervous system and loosens and facilitates the removal of accumulated doshas from the body. In addition Sushruta described points on the body where contractile and noncontractile structures meet and named them marma points. He describes detecting them with fingers units (anguli) and treating them with pressure. He has mentioned 107 such points.

The 'hands on' approach of healing dates back to the old testament, however, some of the recorded but the so-called modern manual medicine had its birth with *Hippocrates (460-355 BC)*.[2] Hippocrates was a physician of great skill and recognized as the father of medicine. He has described a number of manipulation techniques, including traction. He has also described the use of steam heat prior to manual therapy procedures which is a concept that is still being followed. His famous successor *Galen (131-202 AD)* also preached the use of manual medicine and has described manual therapy procedures for the extremities and the cervical vertebrae.

The Middle Ages and Renaissance

In the middle ages, a written summary of medicine that survived as an authoritative text until the 17th century was the work done by an Arabian physician Abu' Ali ibn Sina (1980–1037 AD). It included manual medicine techniques advocated by Hippocrates. Chang Chung King, referred to as the Chinese Hippocrates also advocated treating patients with manual medicine during the middle ages.

The renaissance (new learning) in medicine began with *Andreus Versalius*, who in 1543 described the detailed anatomy of the human body. He also outlined the anatomy of the intervertebral disk, and differentiated the annulus and the nucleus. A little more than 30 years hence, *Ambrose Pare*, a famous surgeon to four successive French kings did much to raise the standard of orthopedic surgery and also used a considerable amount of manipulation. The use of spinal traction, as well as medieval Turkish manipulation during traction were recorded in the leading textbooks of the renaissance. Ambrose Pare wrote, "When a vertebra dislocates posteriorly and protrudes, the patient should be tied down prone with ropes under the armpits, waist and thighs. He should then be pulled and stretched as much as possible from up and below, but not violently".[3] This concept is still being followed as lumbar traction for discogenic pain.

Dawn of Modern Manual Medicine/Therapy

John Hunter (1728-1793) in his teachings emphasized the value of moving joints after injury in order to prevent stiffness and adhesions. He recommended the need for stretching, to breakdown adhesions that are end products of inflammation. A concept that is the basis for mobilization practiced by physical therapists. However, in the 17th and 18th centuries, the treatment by manual means lost favor in the medical profession but manual treatments were being practiced outside of the medical community by who were known as "Bone Setters".

Bone Setting

A practice called "bone setting"[4] flourished in Britain in the 17th and 18th centuries. It was based on the belief that little bones were out of place and the click that followed manipulation was that of little bones going back in place. Bone setting is practiced in India to this day in places like Puthur for more serious conditions sometimes with good results often times with consequences. Bone setting as in India, was not favored by the medical community in Britain, however, in 1867, Sir James Paget (1814-1899) lectured on "Cases That Bone-Setters Cure". He advocated that too long a rest is by far the most frequent cause of delayed recovery after injury of joints and not only to injured joints but to those that are kept at rest because parts near them have been injured.[2] He emphasized early movement to prevent delayed recovery, which is a concept being followed to this day by physical therapists. Bone-setters were dying out in the middle of the 20th century when osteopathy, chiropractic and physical therapy assumed its place.

Osteopathy

The roots of manipulative therapy in the United States began with Andrew Taylor Still (1828-1917), who founded osteopathic medicine in 1874. He was a physician from Kansas city and was an eccentric, non-conformist. He pursued his beliefs with intensity and devoted himself to the philosophy of medicine and the study of man as a total unit. Perhaps the loss of his three children to a meningitis epidemic in 1864 intensified his pursuits as he felt that the status of medicine was inadequate.

Andrew Still focused mainly on restricted joints. He theorized that as long as a joint was restricted it favored congestion and diminished arterial blood flow to the area. This deprived the muscle, ligament, nerve and the artery of nourishment leading to disease. He observed that when some of these restrictions were freed, certain disease conditions improved. Thus was enunciated what was to be known in osteopathy as *The Law of the Artery*.

The osteopathic concept has been briefly stated as:[5]
- The body is a unit
- Structure and function are reciprocally interrelated; and
- The body possesses self-regulatory mechanisms for rational therapies based on an

understanding of body unity, self-regulatory mechanisms and the interrelation of structure and function.

Osteopathy continued to grow but also embraced the advances made by medicine as it was not a stand alone cure-all. Hence it was losing some of its appeal. In the United States, few osteopaths manipulate while a majority of them practice traditional medicine (which is not the case in Europe). A lot of what they have left behind are being practiced in physical therapy clinics, but of course for neuromusculoskeletal dysfunction only and not for disease, that osteopathy originally claimed to cure. It is inferred that Still, during his period of research had adopted many of his techniques from that of bone setters in India, a fact that might lead us to believe that manual therapy was practiced in India long before, however with no strong scientific basis.

Chiropractic

The founder of the chiropractic (from the Greek words *cheir,* meaning *hand* and *praxis*, meaning *done by hand*) profession was *Daniel David Palmer*, a grocer and a practicing magnetic healer. He asserted his philosophy in 1895. Although proponents of chiropractic attribute the discovery to Palmer, he himself admits in his writings that it was learnt from a medical practitioner.

The theoretical basis of chiropractic defined by chiropractors Janse, Houser and Wells is as follows:
- That a vertebra may become subluxed.
- That this subluxation tends to impinge other structures (nerves, blood vessels and lymphatics passing through the intervertebral foramen).
- That, as a result of impingement, the function of the corresponding segment of the spinal cord and its connecting spinal and autonomic nerves is interfered with and the function of the nerve impulse impaired.
- That as a result thereof, the innervation to certain parts of the organism is abnormally altered and such parts become functionally or organically diseased or predisposed to disease.
- That adjustment of a subluxed vertebra removes the impingement of the structure passing through the intervertebral foramen, thereby restoring to diseased parts their normal innervation and rehabilitating them functionally and organically.

This philosophy in chiropractic came to be known as the *Law of the Nerve*. Chiropractors who follow the above traditional philosophy are known as "straights" and are losing appeal. Most chiropractors today are known as "mixers" who mix traditional chiropractic and physical therapy rehabilitation techniques like electro and exercise therapy.

Both osteopathy and chiropractic are similar in their philosophies in two aspects, they advocate the release of an obstruction or an impingement and their assessment is based on positional faults of anatomic structures.

Contribution to Manual Therapy by Physicians

Notably, the biggest contribution to manual therapy by a physician is coining the word 'manual therapy', as it minimized some of the confusion in terminology. The credit goes to James Mennel, who along with his son John Mennel contributed much to the field of manual therapy.[6] The other very important and credible name that offered much to scientifically enhance the diagnostic aspect of manual therapy was James Cyriax,[7] whose father Edgar Cyriax, laid a foundation for his work.

In 1907, James Mennel[6] associated himself with the Chartered Society of Physiotherapy, and instructed joint and soft tissue manipulation techniques. He encouraged his medical colleagues to send patients to physical therapists by prescription. He authored a book called 'Manual Therapy' in which he exclusively addressed topics of massage, passive, assisted and resisted movement, and joint manipulation. His son John Mennel published his book 'Joint Pain', in 1960, and described that the principal cause for joint pain and pathology was the synovial joint and not the intervertebral disk.

He may also have been the first to use the term 'joint play' to describe the quality of motion within a joint. He, like his father instructed techniques principally to physical therapists.

Edgar Cyriax, in 1917, published a paper 'Manual Treatment of the Cervical Sympathetics', in which he outlined the technique of palpating the cervical sympathetic ganglions and treating them by transverse friction in order to stimulate their function. His son James published the 'Textbook of Orthopedic Medicine' in two volumes which has become a classic and is valuable to this day for its detail in differentiating between soft tissues on examination. He also popularized the terms like end feel, capsular pattern, close and open packed position, contractile and non-contractile structures, etc. He strongly emphasized on evaluation and identification of the problem rather than treatment which is the best piece of instruction for any manual therapist. He trained physical therapists and advocated that they, more than the physician, were the appropriate clinicians, to perform manipulation.

1940's marked some valuable contributions to the specialty of manual therapy. Herman Kabat MD, felt that he should offer his neurologically challenged patients, more than range of motion exercises and assistive devices. He extensively reviewed literature on work done by pioneers in neurophysiology like Sherrington, Gessel, etc. and discovered the fact that a muscle can be influenced by proprioceptive stimuli like stretch and resistance. He finally structured his principles which laid the foundation for proprioceptive neuromuscular facilitation (PNF), an effective form of manual therapy for the neurologically and orthopedically challenged.

Fred Mitchell DO, an osteopathic physician, hypothesized and developed a manual therapy approach where a specific restriction in a joint can be loosened by a specifically and precisely execute counterforce on a corresponding muscle. The initial location of application was the spine, where contractions of the multifidus muscle was used to pull the vertebra through restrictions. This was called the muscle energy technique (MET).[8]

Janet Travell MD, developed the trigger point concept in the 1940's. She described trigger points as tender points on the muscle secondary to prolonged contraction and trauma and described manual and injection techniques to manage them.[9]

Lawrence Jones DO, osteopathic physician, developed a system of manual treatments in the 1960's called strain counterstrain.[10] The underlying basis is that, the activity that causes a muscle to strain places it in a contracted position. According to Irvin Korr's muscle spindle theory, the gamma motor neuron activity to the spindle of the shortened muscle is increased and remains contracted. There hence is a distinctly palpable tender area in the contracted muscle. Appropriate positioning can minimize this aberrant activity.

Dr. Alf Breig, of Söderhamn, Sweden, in the 1960's developed the concept of adverse mechanical tension in the nervous system. He demonstrated on fresh cadavers how the nervous system behaves with spinal and limb movements. He published 'Biomechanics of the Central Nervous System' in 1960 where he described the dynamics of cranial nerves, brain tissue and ventricles. In 1978 he published another book 'Adverse Mechanical Tension in the Central Nervous System' where he described the clinical ramification of adverse neural tension.

Contribution to Manual Therapy by Physical Therapists

The early physiotherapists in England and reconstructive aides in the United States were well-versed in massage, joint manipulation and exercises. Most of their knowledge base came from the medical model, however a structured form of manipulation arose in the 1930's owing to the emergence of arthrokinematics. Movement had been traditionally described from an osteokinematic perspective, as gross ranges of motion in the 3 planes. Hence, joint movement was described as flexion, extension, etc. In 1927, Walmsley[11] began using a new terminology called arthrokinematics which was later adopted by Gray's Anatomy, where he described movements taking place within the joint such as roll, glide and spin. Freddy Kaltenborn, a physical therapist saw the significance of the emerging field of arthrokinematics and applied it to joint manipulation. He hence developed a whole new approach to manipulation unique to physical therapy and also propounded the 'concave convex rule'. In 1955, Steindler,[12] in his work "Kinesiology of the Human Body under Normal and Pathologic Conditions", summarized earlier research and added a great deal of additional arthrokinematic knowledge. Kaltenborn[13] was the first to relate manipulation to this new knowledge of arthrokinematics and in 1961 he published 'Extremity Joint Manipulation'.

Stanley V Paris[3,5] did much to promote manipulation by physical therapists in the United States. He was originally from New Zealand and is known for his dynamism as an instructor, teacher and visionary. While he was on the faculty of the New Zealand school of Physiotherapy in 1963, he published "The Theory and Technique of Specific Spinal Manipulation" in the New Zealand Medical Journal. He wrote "degeneration will commence in any joint in which there is loss of movement and while this is happening other joints above and below will suffer injury, degeneration and pain". He called the restriction as a 'dysfunction' and advocated treating the restriction which is the cause, rather than pain which is the symptom of the persisting dysfunction.[1] His philosophy was hence aimed at treating movement faults and had a functional emphasis. He has been an avid educator, clinician, entrepreneur, researcher, swimmer, and sailor. He is probably the only physical therapist in the world credited to have established a university for physical therapy education, the University of St. Augustine for Health Sciences, in Florida, USA.

Geoffery Maitland[14] is a name familiar to most physical therapists around the world. His techniques of oscillatory manipulation has been popularized and taught worldwide. In 1964 he published his work in his classic textbook 'Vertebral Manipulation'. His philosophy was based exclusively in the treatment of reproducible signs. His focus was to gate pain and to improve articular mobility.

The British Association of Manual Medicine was formed in the sixties, however, a formal organization of that capacity was lacking in the profession of physical therapy. The genesis of such an endeavor was following a meeting on October 26, 1966, when physical therapists Maitland, Grieve, Kaltenborn and Paris met for the first time in London and discussed setting up an international body to exchange educational ideas and to maintain standards in manual therapy. As an outgrowth in 1974, the International Federation of Orthopedic Manual Therapy (IFOMPT) was founded in Montreal, Canada, during the meeting of the World Confederation of Physical Therapy under the chairmanship of Paris. Erhard from the United States was elected president.

In the late 1970's McKenzie[15] began to popularize the concept where he described spinal extension for the treatment of low back pain. He described that the posterior bulging of the disk was aggravated by flexion due to the hydrodynamics of the disk which was compressed anteriorly by the vertebral bodies. He felt that extension hence compressed the posterior elements, which minimized the risk of the disk moving further posterior towards the pain sensitive structures. His methods have gained worldwide acceptance and his school conducts training programs all over the world.

Elvey,[16] Butler in the 1980's and 1990's revitalized Dr Alf Breig's work into developing a new method of testing adverse neural tension in the peripheral nerves and subsequently treatment methods for the same. Their methods are now being used worldwide by physical therapists.

In the 1990's Brian Mulligan a physical therapist from New Zealand developed mobilization with movement. All form of manual therapy described earlier were passive as in with the patient resting and the clinician performing the procedure. However, with the Mulligan concept, the joint was mobilized while the patient performed the function that the joint was originally intended to do. His methods have gained popularity throughout the world.

In 1991, the American Academy of Orthopedic Manual Physical Therapy (AAOMPT) was founded with Farrel as the first president, which later gained membership in IFOMPT. The AAOMPT decided that manual therapy was a hands on subject and that theoretical knowledge should be combined with mentored hands on training. It realized the need for residency training and hence established residency standards for manual therapy training in the United States.

The practice of manipulation by physical therapy is quite eclectic or a mixture of philosophies. Most clinicians examine both positional and movement faults and use mechanical, isometric, oscillatory, direct and indirect techniques. Hence, the focus of this book will be to combine all philosophies taking the most appropriate from each to be able to provide the best of available care. This book has been written as a unique contemporary philosophy with a base formed by four existing philosophies, namely Paris, Kaltenborn, Alf Breig and Osteopathy. Somatic causes are outlined with a correlation to existing, conventional orthopedic diagnosis. A better understanding of appropriate choice of intervention may be the result. Additionally, this literature review also describes the need for a more eclectic approach with other physiotherapeutic intervention to enhance the effect of manual intervention. The mandates being, stabilization exercises and care during function.

REFERENCES

1. Raju VK. Susruta of ancient India. Indian J Ophthalmol. 2003;51:119-22.
2. Ventegodt S, Kandel I, Merrick J. A short history of clinical holistic medicine. Scientific World Journal. 2007;7:1622-30.
3. Paris SV. A history of manipulative therapy through the ages and up to the current controversy in the United States. Journal of Manual and Manipulative Therapy. 2000;8:66-7.
4. Hood W. On so called "bone setting", its nature and results. Lancet. 1871;1:336-8, 372-4, 441-3.
5. Paris SV, Loubert PV. Foundations of clinical orthopaedics, 1990. Institute press, Division of Patris Inc, St. Augustine, FL.
6. Mennel J. Rationale for joint manipulation. Physical Therapy. 1970;50:181-6.
7. Cyriax J. The pros and cons of manipulation. Lancet. 1964;1:571-3
8. Wilson E, Payton O, Donegan-Shoaf L, Dec K. Muscle energy technique in patients with acute low back pain: A pilot clinical trial. J Orthop Sports Phys Ther. 2003;33:502-12.
9. Kuan TS, Hong CZ, Chen JT, Chen SM, Chien CH. The spinal cord connections of the myofascial trigger spots. Eur J Pain. 2007;11:624-34.
10. Woolbright JL. An alternative method of teaching strain/counterstrain manipulation. J Am Osteopath Assoc. 1991;91:370, 373-6.
11. Walmsley T. Articular mechanism of diarthrosis. J Bone J Surg. 1927;10:40-5.
12. Steindler A. Kinesiology of the human body under normal and pathological conditions. Thomas, Springfield, IL: 1955.
13. Kaltenborn F. Mobilization of the extremity joints: Examination and basic techniques. 3rd edn, 1980. Olaf Noris Bokhandel A/S, Oslo, Norway.
14. Maitland GD. Manipulation—Mobilisation. Physiotherapy. 1966;52:382-5.
15. McKenzie RA. Comments on a systematic review of the McKenzie method. Spine. 2006 5;31:2639; author reply 2639-40.
16. Hall TM, Elvey RL. Nerve trunk pain: physical diagnosis and treatment. Man Ther. 1999;4:63-73. Review.

CHAPTER 3

Manipulation: Definition and Types

The discrepancy in terminology in manual therapy literature may be secondary to the need for philosophies to be original. So this chapter aims to simplify the types for easier understanding, especially for the novice practitioner. 'Manual Therapy' is a broad term and comprises terms such as articulation, mobilization and manipulation. Some of the manual therapy gurus have a preference to one more than the other. For example, Kaltenborn uses the term mobilization while Paris uses the word manipulation in his courses. Some describe manipulation only for high velocity thrust techniques that results in a 'pop' or a 'crack',[1] while mobilization[2] is a term used for non-thrust techniques. The reason why manipulation is a term often avoided is because of the apprehension of the medical community towards chiropractors and the possible adverse effects of a manipulation, (as it was considered a forceful movement) especially on the spine. Thus physical therapists used less controversial terms such as mobilization. But how often have we heard the term soft tissue manipulation for massage, which is almost never very forceful or manipulation under anesthesia done by physicians, which is not always a high velocity thrust type of a procedure. So manipulation by definition is:

A skilled passive movement to a joint.[3]

A skilled passive movement with a therapeutic intent (2004)

The passive movement thus executed may be of different types, it may be a sustained stretch or range of motion or an oscillation or a high velocity procedure. It may be over the joint or on a soft tissue. So for purpose of simplification since all skilled passive movements are considered manipulations, it can be broadly classified as Non-thrust (which comprises mobilization and articulation) and thrust (which comprises high velocity procedures).

Whether the type of manipulation is thrust or non-thrust, the area where it is applied is of relevance. It can be applied to a very specific area like an individual vertebra or a specific soft tissue, or a general area like several vertebra or a wider area of soft tissue. Hence, the next differentiation to make is between a general (*regional*) and a specific (*localized*) manipulation (Table 3.1).

TABLE 3.1: Manipulation.

Thrust	(General or Specific)	Non-thrust

High velocity		• Mobilization/Articulation comprising
		• Graded oscillations
		• Progressive or sustained stretch or loading
		• Soft tissue mobilization Myofascial release
		• Neuromuscular therapies
		  – Neural mobilization
		  – PNF
		  – MET
		  – SCS

(PNF: Proprioceptive neuromuscular facilitation; MET: Muscle energy technique; SCS: Strain counter strain)

MANIPULATION

The skilled passive movement to a joint.

Thrust

When a sudden, high velocity short amplitude motion is delivered at the restricted physiological limit of a joint's range of motion.[1]

Non-thrust

When a joint or soft tissue is taken within or to the limit of the available active or passive range (within physiological limits), and stretched or oscillated. Neuromuscular therapies also comprise non-thrust manipulation.

Graded Oscillation

Graded oscillation is a form of cyclic loading whereby alternative pressure, on and off, are delivered at different parts of the available range. Graded oscillation techniques have been widely promoted by Maitland[4] and he describes four grades.

Grade 1: Small amplitude movement performed at the beginning of the range.

Grade 2: Large amplitude movement performed within the range but not reaching the limit of range.

Grade 3: Large amplitude movement performed up to the limit of the range.

Grade 4: Small amplitude movement performed at the limit of the range.

Progressive Loading/Stretch

Progressive loading mobilization involves a successive series of short amplitude, spring type pressures. The pressure is imparted at progressive increments of the range and is defined on a 1-4 scale as in a graded oscillation. Progressive loading is utilized for mechanical, joint and soft tissue restrictions. Brian Mulligan has incorporated this principle with movements in the direction of physiological joint motion. He has termed it mobilization with movement (MWM).[5]

Sustained Loading/Stretch

Sustained loading is continuous, uninterrupted pressure or force which may remain the same in intensity, increase or decrease depending on the patient reaction. The viscoelastic properties of adaptively shortened soft tissues can be influenced by the use of sustained loading. Sustained loading mobilization, however, may not be sufficient to mobilize a joint that possesses an intra-articular restriction.

Soft Tissue Mobilization

The manual manipulation of soft tissues done for producing effects on the nervous, muscular, lymph and circulatory systems. Massage, rolfing are examples. The characteristics influenced are tone or tension status and extensibility or the ability to elongate.

Myofascial Release

It is a form of soft tissue therapy which is based on neuroreflexive responses that reduce tissue tension. The key is location of the best point of entry into the musculoskeletal system, application of the most suitable type of stress to induce inhibition, and sensitivity in palpation to react properly to tissue response. The result is a relaxation of tissue tension and decrease in myofascial tightness, leading to improved tissue extensibility and reduction of pain.

Neuromuscular Therapies

Neural Mobilization

Elvey and Butler revitalized Dr. Alf Breig's work into developing a new method of testing adverse neural tension in the peripheral nerves and subsequently treatment methods for the same. The concept being that a nerve moves like any other structure and their inability to move creates dysfunction. The key to diagnosis is identifying their inability to move, which is termed adverse neural tension which is a compensation for the lack of mobility. Subsequent restoration of movement is the treatment.[6]

Proprioceptive Neuromuscular Facilitation

Proprioceptive neuromuscular facilitation (PNF) is developed by Herman Kabat MD, and

Margarett Knott PT. It is a method of promoting the response of the neuromuscular mechanism through stimulation of proprioceptors. It describes that all movements in the body occur in diagonal patterns and the application of manual stimulus specific in direction, timing and resistance helps to elicit the desired neuromuscular response.[7]

Muscle Energy Technique

Muscle energy technique (MET) is developed by Fred Mitchell Sr DO (Doctor of Osteopathy). It is a form of manipulative treatment where an active muscle contraction (usually isometric) is used to induce movement in a bony element by virtue of its insertion, and subsequently mobilize joint restrictions. The key is to localize the contraction to the desired area. While avulsion fractures occur by displacement of bony elements due to violent contractions of the inserting tendon, a similar concept may be applied beneficially to move bony elements by moderate contractions of the tendon.[8]

Strain Counterstrain

Strain counterstrain (SCS) is developed by Lawrence Jones DO. The underlying basis is that, the activity that causes a muscle to strain places it in a contracted position. According to Irvin Korr's muscle spindle theory, the gamma motor neuron activity to the spindle of the shortened muscle is increased and remains contracted. There hence is a distinctly palpable tender area in the contracted muscle.

By the passive placement of the strained muscle in a shortened or contracted position for 90 seconds (which can be further confirmed by a marked decrease in local muscle tenderness) the aberrant gamma motor activity in the muscle spindle is decreased restoring the muscle to its normal length and decreasing pain.[9]

This simplified classification may help the novice practitioner to be able to interpret the existing discrepancies in classification, when he or she pursues further reading. The treatment techniques described in this book is a combination of the components of this classification. However, the neuromuscular therapies are not elaborated on as they are beyond the scope of this book and the reader is suggested alternate reading.[10]

REFERENCES

1. Cleland JA, Flynn TW, Childs JD, Eberhart S. The audible pop from thoracic spine thrust manipulation and its relation to short-term outcomes in patients with neck pain. J Man Manip Ther. 2007;15:143-54.
2. Landrum EL, Kelln CB, Parente WR, Ingersoll CD, Hertel J. Immediate Effects of anterior-to-posterior talocrural joint mobilization after prolonged ankle immobilization: a preliminary study. J Man Manip Ther. 2008;16:100-5.
3. Paris SV. Mobilization of the spine. Phys Ther. 1979;59: 988-95.
4. Maitland GD. Manipulation—Mobilisation. Physiotherapy. 1966;52:382-5.
5. Exelby L. The Mulligan concept: its application in the management of spinal conditions. Man Ther. 2002;7:64-70.
6. Hall TM, Elvey RL. Nerve trunk pain: physical diagnosis and treatment. Man Ther. 1999;4: 63-73. Review.
7. Rees SS, Murphy AJ, Watsford ML, McLachlan KA, Coutts AJ. Effects of proprioceptive neuromuscular facilitation stretching on stiffness and force-producing characteristics of the ankle in active women. J Strength Cond Res. 2007;21:572-7.
8. Wilson E, Payton O, Donegan-Shoaf L, Dec K. Muscle energy technique in patients with acute low back pain: a pilot clinical trial. J Orthop Sports Phys Ther. 2003;33:502-12.
9. Dardzinski JA, Ostrov BE, Hamann LS. Myofascial pain unresponsive to standard treatment: successful use of a strain and counterstrain technique with physical therapy. J Clin Rheumatol. 2000;6:169-74.
10. Nyberg R, Basmajian JV. Rational manual therapies. 1993, Lippincott Williams and Wilkins, Baltimore.

CHAPTER 4

Understanding Mechanical Dysfunction

The novice clinician should understand the basic terminology that underlie movement. Often, the word 'restriction' is used, and may be described as one of the main causes for a dysfunction, but where this restriction occurs is understood better if the basic terminology is understood.

Movement as we know is primarily described as spatial relationships of the limbs to the axis of the body and are termed as flexion, extension, abduction, etc. These are called 'osteokinematic' movements and these are gross movements of the limbs. A restriction of these movements can be visually observed and measured with a goniometer. However, as these movements occur outside of the joint, simultaneous movement occurs within the joint as well. The best analogy would be a moving door. As the door moves to open or close the hinges by which the door is fixed also moves. If the hinge is restricted, then the movement of the door is restricted as well. The door can be compared to the limbs or the long bones of the body and the hinge can be compared to the joints. Hence as the limbs move there should be relative movement 'within' the joint as well. This movement that occurs within the joint surface is described as 'arthrokinematic' movement (Fig. 4.1). Arthrokinematic movement cannot be visualized. They have to be passively elicited and are small in range, hence making their examination is difficult.[1,2]

In manual therapy, when the term 'joint restriction leading to a dysfunction' is used, it is a restriction in the arthrokinematic motion that is being referred to. The skill in detecting a restriction in arthrokinematic motion is a strong essential basis for diagnosing a dysfunction. Gross range of motion is described in degrees of movement, whereas arthrokinematic movement is not described so for each joint, and would be difficult to measure as well.

Hence, a manual therapist will make an assessment of arthrokinematic restriction by the following means[3]:
- The amount of restriction of the gross range of motion.
- Detecting an asymmetry by comparing arthrokinematic movement with the other normal joint.
- Detecting an asymmetry or faulty position of bony landmarks during motion.

A more detail description of detecting an arthrokinematic restriction or asymmetry, is covered in the chapter titled *'Principles of Diagnosis'*. However, the reader should understand that whether the goal is to diagnose a dysfunction, or treat a dysfunction, the concept of movement 'within' the joint or arthrokinematic motion should be understood.

A consult or a referral to a musculoskeletal physical therapy clinician is a patient whose symptoms are commonly pain, some type of restriction causing a change in mobility, or weakness.

They usually have a diagnosis or a diagnosis is made in the physical therapy clinic.

Assume the referral is a cricketer with shoulder pain, the onset being after a bout of bowling practice. A medical cause is ruled out

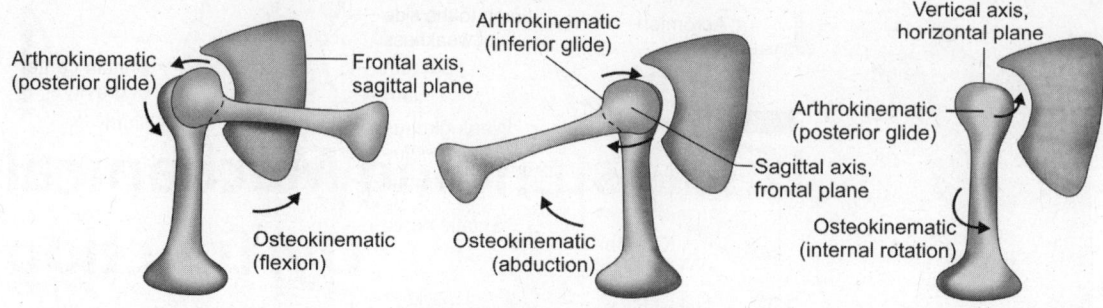

Fig. 4.1: Planes of motion.

and you make a diagnosis of a supraspinatus impingement tendonitis. You begin to address the pain with appropriate electrotherapy, modalities and exercise therapy including mobilization to restore gross range of motion. He is an active cricketer and a bowler and he does obtain relief of symptoms, resumes playing cricket and the pain recurs. We should hence, question ourselves as follows:

The cause for the pain..... bowling, but is that the real cause ?

The diagnosis..... supraspinatus tendonitits, but is that an appropriate physical therapy diagnosis?

Consider two common objective findings in your day-to-day examination—joint restriction and muscle weakness. This is to bring about a conceptual idea and simple as they may sound, the implication may be significant. They will be dealt with more specific detail in subsequent chapters.

JOINT RESTRICTION

Consider a ball and socket joint.

A gross motion occurs by the ball of the joint effectively gliding over the socket. The supporting cartilage is minimally stressed as the ball moves over the entire area of the socket and the forces of loading are evenly distributed (Fig. 4.2). Consider a restricted situation. The arc of movement of the ball over the socket decreases. Hence, the forces of loading are not distributed over a wider area but rather are focused on a smaller area. This may

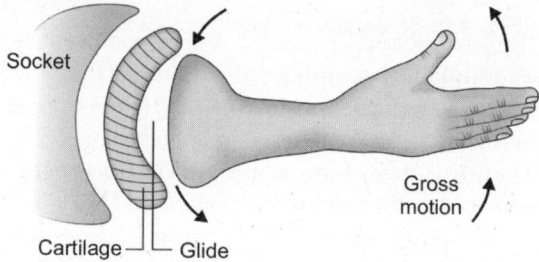

Fig. 4.2: Movement in a ball and socket joint.

result greater local stress resulting in cartilage wear, osteoarthritis, irritation of the surrounding soft tissue and pain.[4]

Now consider a clinical situation. The shoulder, being a ball and socket joint can be an example. During abduction the head of the humerus glides inferiorly and externally rotates on the glenoid. When this occurs the space between the greater tuberosity and the acromion is adequate and the supraspinatus tendon is not impinged. If a restriction prevails then the inferior glide of the humeral head decreases and the greater tuberosity may pinch the tendon against the acromion as it rides up on forceful abduction. If the thoracic segments are restricted in flexion it can disturb the mechanics of the trapezius and the rhomboids which in turn attach to the scapula. A resulting downwardly rotated and protracted scapula[5] may disturb the scapulohumeral rhythm, bring the acromion closer to the greater tuberosity and cause an impingement of the tendon between it (Fig. 4.3). Routine local injections or medication

Understanding Mechanical Dysfunction

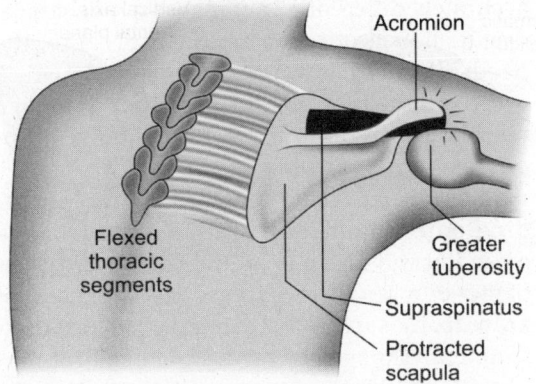

Fig. 4.3: Sequence of events in a dysfunction.

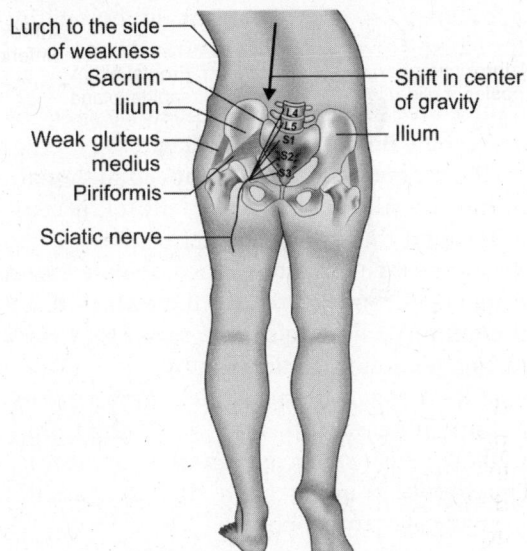

Fig. 4.4: Pathomechanics in muscle weakness of left gluteus medius.

may provide symptomatic relief but to obtain a more functional outcome the inferior glide of the humeral head has to be restored, backward bending of the thoracic segments have to be achieved, efficiency of the trapezius, rhomboids and shoulder rotators has to be restored, then the cause for the problem is addressed. Your physical therapy diagnosis will be a flexed rotated sidebent thoracic segment, weak lower trapezius, or a decreased inferior and posterior glide of the humeral head. This results in a supraspinatus tendonitis. Range of motion may be restored by forceful mobilization maneuver but may be at the risk of overstretching the ligaments or associated soft tissue structures and further impinging the tendon.

MUSCLE WEAKNESS

There is undoubtedly no dispute that normal musculature move and attenuate or absorb shock in a joint, on loading. In many instances the reason why strengthening exercises are prescribed for pain is to support the joint and attenuate shock. Consider a weightbearing joint supported by weak musculature. Chronic overuse or loading can result in excessive stress on the cartilage, ligament and other soft tissue structures including the muscle, due to decreased shock absorption resulting in wear and tear and subsequently pain.

Now consider a clinical situation. The gluteus medius runs from the gluteal surface of the ilium to the greater trochanter of the femur and functions to abduct the hip and stabilize the pelvis during one legged stance. It is well known that weakness of the gluteus medius[6] results in what is called a 'Trendelenburg Sign' (Fig. 4.4). (The following scenario can occur even if a classical trendelenburg sign is not present but just a mild weakness of the gluteus medius). As the patient continues to weight bear on a hip supported by a weak gluteus medius the sacroiliac joints can be strained due to the pelvic asymmetry on weightbearing. A restriction of the sacrum results as the mechanics is affected resulting in a sacral dysfunction. The piriformis muscle can be involved by virtue of its attachment to the sacrum, and, as it runs very close to the posterior aspect of the hip joint it causes pain in the hip area and may be mistaken for a hip pathology. The bursa can become irritated due to faulty mechanics resulting in a bursitis. The sciatic nerve that runs close to the sacroiliac joint and sometimes through the piriformis can be irritated resulting in a radiculopathy and can be mistaken for a disc pathology.

Hence, when the physical therapist is looking at a so-called diagnosis like hip pain, bursitis, sacroiliac pain, sciatic pain or radiculopathy, the cause for the problem may be a sacral dysfunction (restricted torsion) or weakness of the gluteus medius and hence would be the appropriate physical therapy diagnosis.

The list goes on but the conceptual thought is that the physical therapy clinician must understand that faulty skeletal alignment and mechanics including soft tissue imbalances can result in joint and soft tissue injury which result in common pathologies like sprains, strains, bursitis, tendonitis, radiculopathy, etc. These are what are known as 'mechanical dysfunctions' and not diseases. If the pain is arising from a medical cause say a malignancy, a vascular compromise or an infection, then they are not mechanical dysfunctions.

Thus mechanical dysfunctions manifest as either increases or decreases of motion usually due to restriction, faulty mechanics weakness, and present as aberrant motion.

This aberrant motion continues to stress the pain sensitive supporting structures resulting in pain. Treatment should hence focus on the cause for the abnormal movement and not just medications or therapeutic modalities for pain caused by the abnormal movement.[7]

The cause(s) for a certain symptom, say sciatic pain may be different. It may be mechanical as in a restricted sacroiliac joint, or medical, like a tumor in the pelvic area compressing the sciatic nerve, but the symptoms may be the same as they can both produce sciatic pain. Hence, it is important for the physical therapy clinician to combine traditional knowledge in addition to a thorough understanding of functional anatomy and relevant mechanics to be able to accurately differentially diagnose a mechanical dysfunction as opposed to a medical cause. The need, obviously, is to not diagnose the medical cause but to know that the symptom is not of a mechanical origin and thence execute an appropriate referral.

Appropriate therapeutic modalities including pain medication still have their place provided the cause is addressed. As a matter of fact they very well address the soreness that accompanies manual treatments besides their actual physiological effects. Hence their use as an adjunct or in conjunction can be continually encouraged.

REFERENCES

1. Walmsley T. The articular mechanism of diarthrosis. J Bone and J Surg. 1928;10:40-5.
2. Steindler A. Kinesiology of the human body under normal and pathological conditions. Charles Thomas, Springfield, IL, 1955.
3. Snider KT, Johnson JC, Snider EJ, et al. Increased incidence and severity of somatic dysfunction in subjects with chronic low back pain. J Am Osteopath Assoc. 2008;108:372-8.
4. Birrell F, Afzal C, Nahit E, et al. Predictors of hip joint replacement in new attenders in primary care with hip pain. Br J Gen Pract. 2003;53:26-30.
5. Ludewig PM, Reynolds JE. The association of scapular kinematics and glenohumeral joint pathologies. J Orthop Sports Phys Ther. 2009;39:90-104.
6. Nelson-Wong E, Gregory DE, Winter DA, et al. Gluteus medius muscle activation patterns as a predictor of low back pain during standing. Clin Biomech (Bristol, Avon). 2008;23:545-53.
7. Paris SV. The Spinal Lesion. New Zealand Medical Journal. 1965, Penguin press.

CHAPTER 5

Principles of Management of Mechanical Dysfunction

ALIGNMENT

It is obvious that there is an inseparable interdependence between structure and function. Structural integrity brings about harmonious motion with minimal stress on the supporting structures. Movement can still be achieved with abnormal structure, but only by increasing stress on supporting structures resulting in further pain and dysfunction. In other words, normalcy of 'alignment' is the key for normal musculoskeletal function. As a manual therapy clinician it is the skill in detection of a specific cause for faulty alignment that is of importance.

Consider this example quoted by Dr SV Paris, in his teachings.[1] The 'atlas' or the first cervical vertebra always follows the occiput or the head in all movements of the occiput. The joints of the atlas may sustain an injury for various reasons, say a sudden jerky movement of the head as in a whiplash injury or a hit on the head, etc. This may favor holding the region in a certain direction due to muscle guarding. Assume the direction of guarding is in right rotation of the atlas. If untreated it may remain stuck in right rotation due to formation of adhesions from the serofibrinous exudate of the joint injury and adaptive shortening of the soft tissues. Since the occiput and the atlas work together, a right rotation of the atlas may favor a right rotation of the head (occiput). The patient obviously would prefer to turn the head and face level and hence a compensatory left rotation should occur elsewhere to compensate. This left rotation occurs at a lower level in the midcervical region. The joint orientation of the midcervical region however is such that the left rotation occurs with left side bending which unlevels the eyes. To level the eyes a compensatory right side bending occurs in the midthoracic region. The result is a structural scoliosis of a minimal degree and the resultant faulty mechanics may stress the supporting soft tissues resulting in head, neck, radicular and thoracic pain (Fig. 5.1).

Symptomatic treatment may temporarily relieve pain but resumption of activity may continue to stress the supporting structures as the cause for the dysfunction remains untreated.

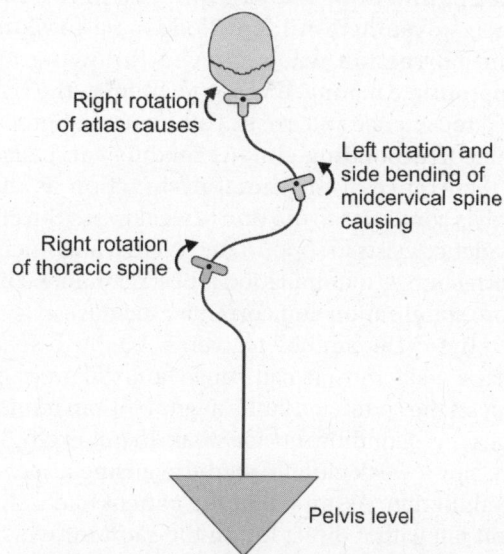

Fig. 5.1: To maintain head and eyes level sequence of events in a dysfunction.

The cause obviously is the atlas stuck in right rotation. This is the so-called specific cause for the faulty alignment. Conceptually this segment-specific alignment rather than gross alignment forms the basis for the diagnosis of a mechanical dysfunction.[2,3]

STRENGTH/STABILITY/LENGTH: (RELEVANT TO ALIGNMENT)

In the previous chapter under the subtitle muscle strength, the relevance of muscle strength to mechanical dysfunction was discussed. In this chapter, however, the relevance of muscle strength to alignment will be discussed. Although same, conceptually, it is just a matter of specificity.

'Alignment' continues to form the basis for management of mechanical dysfunction. Nondysfunctional states are achieved as long as normal alignment is maintained. As the skeletal system is a functional unit, the risk of stress on the alignment can occur with varying intensities of function. The key to maintaining nondysfunctional alignment is by adequate supporting musculature. Consider the previous example of the gluteus medius and its effect on alignment of the sacrum. Assuming the sacral dysfunction identified was a torsion, and correction was achieved following an appropriate manual therapy technique, the risk of a recurrence still exists. Failure to strengthen the corresponding gluteus medius can cause a recurrence of the sacral dysfunction as the pelvis continues to dip due to weakness.[4] Strong evidence exists to support the fact that alignment correction by manipulation is best maintained by core stabilization and corrective exercises.[5]

The cycle can be vice versa. We have seen that a weak muscle can cause faulty alignment but on the contrary a faulty alignment can render the corresponding muscle weak. In this example we saw a weak gluteus medius causing a sacral dysfunction. Assume that the patient had a slip and fall with a direct hit on the sacrum (which is very common in colder countries due to icy conditions) then the impact of the fall can cause a sacral dysfunction which can restrict the sacroiliac joint on the corresponding side and cause a change in the normal pelvic mechanics. When the original range is decreased the corresponding muscle does not function in its full range or capacity and over a period of time can weaken. This further adds to the dysfunction and the vicious cycle continues.

Hence, it is important to know the exact history and duration of the problem to make an effective mechanical diagnosis.

Muscle tightness or the length of excursion is of equal importance as muscle strength with relevance to a mechanical dysfunction. All muscles have a certain length which helps to achieve optimal function. Activity that is in conflict with the length of a muscle can cause injury. How often have we heard of hamstring strains in individuals who do not stretch adequately prior to activity? Remember that all muscles with a few exceptions have insertions into the bony skeleton by way of which they move the joints. They not only move a joint but also help to support the bones. Hence, if the length is inadequate then the possibility of stressing the alignment exists.

Consider a tent which has a pole in the center held by two ropes on either sides. Assume the lengths of the ropes are the same then the pole is in neutral alignment. However, if one rope is shorter in length then the alignment of the pole is altered. A similar analogy can be applied to the body with the spine as the pole and the spinal musculature as the ropes. The importance however, is the specificity as one should consider that each vertebra has muscle attachments on either sides. Consider the levator scapulae as an example. It attaches into the transverse processes of the first four cervical vertebrae on either sides. If one side is tighter than the other it can pull a specific segment into side bending and rotation to the same side and if it persists it can cause a restriction in that position causing faulty alignment (Fig. 5.2). Hence, even if the dysfunction is detected at a later date and corrected using a manual technique, the corresponding levator scapulae

Principles of Management of Mechanical Dysfunction

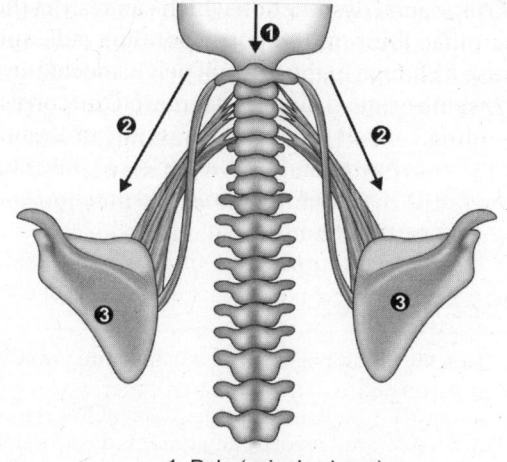

1. Pole (spinal column)
2. Ropes (levator scapulae)
3. Scapula

Fig. 5.2: Posterior view.

should be stretched to minimize recurrence of the dysfunction.[6]

CARE DURING FUNCTION

In principles of management we inferred two important aspects, alignment and soft tissue integrity. Once this is addressed, the most important component emerges and that is care during function, or proper body mechanics.[7] A dysfunction starts with a particular function and can be viewed regionally. Consider the neck and a computer professional. Constant viewing of the computer in a forward head position can cause the anterior and posterior neck and thoracic muscles to fatigue as they have to work harder to support the head which is in their perspective a little further away. If the strength in the musculature is adequate, then the fatigue component can be minimized. However, in weak situations which is common a prolonged forward head and rounded shoulders position can fatigue the anterior and posterior neck muscles and posterior thoracic muscles. The response to fatigue is a contraction. As the contraction progresses, it alters the length of the muscle which by virtue of its attachment to the vertebra can cause a faulty alignment by pulling on it. If the faulty activity is continued the muscle continues to be stressed, contracted, and the dysfunction can persist.[6]

Hence, in the management of musculoskeletal dysfunction, all three components should be addressed—alignment, muscle strength/length, and care during function. When management in the clinic is completed the patient must be instructed home exercises to maintain proper alignment and instructed on proper function (proper body mechanics, proper footwear, etc.) as appropriate. Failing which the probability of a recurring dysfunction is high.

Chronic pain is a term to denote pain that persists for an extended period of time. Routine and conventional treatments offer temporary relief but the pain continues to recur. If the pain is secondary to a mechanical dysfunction it may persist to a chronic state as long as the dysfunction persists. Hence, often times the reason why mechanical pain is rendered chronic is because the underlying cause remains undetected. Consider the example of the stuck atlas. The resulting dysfunction can cause significant headaches.

The greater occipital nerve and the auricular nerves supply the superficial occipital and temporal areas respectively. A restriction of the atlas and the axis (C1 and C2) can irritate the suboccipital musculature which can subsequently irritate these nerves and cause significant occipital and temporal headaches. This patient may be continually treated for headaches of a neurological or vascular origin with medications, etc. with no significant relief and the pain may persist to a chronic state. The bigger implication is that an investigative procedure like an X-ray or a CT scan may be ruled normal. The reason being that they may not reveal the restriction as there is no disruption in the anatomy as in a soft tissue tear or fracture. However, a skilled manual exam of the C1 and C2 for mobility, position and palpatory tenderness may indicate a dysfunction and the physical therapy clinician can relate the headaches to a 'myogenic' or muscular origin rather than vascular or neurologic origin. Manual treatment of the first and second cervical vertebra and the suboccipital musculature can minimize these headaches.

A similar example, the lateral ligament of the ankle is commonly strained, and in many instances recurrent strains are seen especially in athletes. Symptomatic treatment like local injections, or ultrasound may still heal the ligament but recurrences can occur with resumption of vigorous activity. Hence, the clinician should consider that the reason why recurrent strains occur is due faulty alignment of the subtalar joint and midtarsal joints or an external rotation of the tibia or the femoral neck. These are causes for the dysfunction which predisposes the foot to buckle into forced inversion and subsequently straining the lateral ligament. Appropriate manual treatment to mobilize the involved joints and prescription of exercises to strengthen the evertors in addition to an orthotic, to maintain neutral alignment, will address the cause. If the cause is not addressed then the result is a 'chronic', recurrent ankle strain.

The point here is, a skilled mechanical diagnosis can often times help to detect an underlying unidentified cause for a medical diagnosis.[3] In the first example, the medical diagnosis of a migraine headache may in actuality be muscular rather than vascular (and hence a myogenic headache).

The consequences may be frustrating if the cause is not identified as the pain does not resolve and the patient may be considered to be faking the pain. The pain continues to persist, eventually to a chronic state limiting the patient of his/her functional ability. It may hence be concluded that treating the cause may prevent chronic dysfunctional and painful states.

REFERENCES

1. Paris SV. S3 course notes. 1988, Institute press, St Augustine, FL.
2. Snider KT, Johnson JC, Snider EJ, et al. Increased incidence and severity of somatic dysfunction in subjects with chronic low back pain. J Am Osteopath Assoc. 2008;108:372-8.
3. Jull G, Bogduk N, Marsland A. The accuracy of manual diagnosis for cervical zygoapophyseal joint pain syndromes. Med J Aust. 1988;148: 233-6.
4. Lamoth CJ, Meijer OG, Daffertshofer A, et al. Effects of chronic low back pain on trunk coordination and back muscle activity during walking: changes in motor control. Eur Spine J. 2006;15:23-40.
5. Greenman PE. Principles of Manual Medicine. 2nd edn, 1996, Lippincott Williams and Wilkins, Baltimore.
6. Travell JG, Simons DG, Simons LS. Myofascial pain and dysfunction: the trigger point manual.Volume 1:Upper half of the body. 1999, Lippincott Williams and Wilkins,. Baltimore.
7. Hanson H, Wagner M, Monopoli V, et al. Low back pain in physical therapists: a cultural approach to analysis and intervention. Work. 2007;28:145-51.

CHAPTER 6

Palpation

INTRODUCTION

Palpation is the key tool used for examination procedures in manual therapy. The hand is an extremely sensitive tool considering the fact that 25% of the pacinian corpuscles in the human body are in the hand. A trained manual therapist may claim that he or she feels something that is difficult to see or even feel. Do not doubt him or her until you have practiced hard enough, and that word cannot be emphasized enough...... hard.

Technology today has rendered a situation where clinicians rarely touch or palpate their patients. This may be a tragic situation and we as physical therapists should consider our position favorable as we continue to feel and touch our patients. A well read mind and a trained pair of hands can detect clinical situations that complex imaging procedures do not. It may be of benefit to always remember that a compassionate and caring touch, for reasons that cannot be described or quantified, can also have a healing effect.[1]

As the famous words by Alan Stoddard would describe....

"By continuous practice and thinking hard through the fingers, in other words concentrating upon the senses observed through the fingertips, it is possible to develop that elusive quality of the manipulative skill- tissue tension sense."

PRINCIPLES

The first question, when we palpate to identify musculoskeletal dysfunction what, are we looking for? The word to bear in mind is **ART** and comprise the following:[2]

A: Alignment deviation of landmarks or unilateral weakness and tightness of soft tissue
R: Restricted joint or tissue mobility
T: Tenderness locally.

ALIGNMENT DEVIATION OF LANDMARKS OR UNILATERAL WEAKNESS AND TIGHTNESS OF SOFT TISSUE

It helps that most musculoskeletal landmarks come in pairs. This helps to aid in making a mechanical diagnosis. Asymmetry may not be synonymous to alignment, but rather we can say that by detecting an asymmetry we confirm faulty alignment. Unilateral hypertrophy or wasting of muscles, unilateral weakness, unilateral muscle or tissue tightness can be considered an asymmetry. An elevated scapula on one side can be considered an asymmetry. Such changes can usually be visualized, however, a more intricate method of detecting asymmetry is one that cannot be visualized but rather palpated. As an example, often times pelvic asymmetries arise and to detect them by palpation will be to place both hands over the iliac crests to detect a difference in heights. This obviously is an easier example, as undergraduate students perform evaluations of this type on polio patients. Still a good precursor for palpatory skills.

More intricate situations occur with palpation of vertebral asymmetries. Knowing the levels of the segments or knowledge of anatomy is a prerequisite. The bony landmark that is easiest to palpate in a vertebra is the spinous process. These are the projections we see (in a lean individual) or feel, in the center of the back. By knowing the levels and how many vertebra in each level the correct segment can be identified.[3,4] Similar methods are adopted by knowing bony landmarks for extremity joints.[5,6]

RESTRICTED JOINT OR TISSUE MOBILITY

Restriction of mobility is the most common component of mechanical dysfunction.

The resulting dysfunction that can occur because of restriction in a joint was described in earlier chapters. Hence the ability to detect a restriction by palpation is mandatory in a manual therapy examination as it has to be treated. Technically restriction of mobility is also an asymmetry if it occurs unilaterally. For example, each vertebra has two facet joints on either sides. A restriction on one side can cause an asymmetry in vertebral segment movement causing faulty alignment. Hence, a restriction can cause an asymmetry that results in faulty alignment.

As described earlier, the arthrokinematic component of motion is what is palpated, as gross range of motion can be visualized. Hence, a manual therapist will make an assessment of an arthrokinematic restriction by palpating the appropriate bony landmark and inducing a passive motion. A relatively easier example will be the patella. By palpating the lateral borders of the patella and inducing knee flexion, one can feel the patella moving laterally. Similar methods are adopted, however with increasing difficulty, to detect arthrokinematic motion in other joints. Again restricted tissue mobility should also be considered.

TENDERNESS LOCALLY

This aspect of palpation can be made elaborate but to simplify it to the essential aspect, the one finding in a soft tissue in conjunction with a mechanical dysfunction is tenderness with soft tissue thickening. Tenderness in a muscle can lead to an assumption that the muscle is the source of the dysfunction. This may be the case but not always. Every joint or motion segment has a corresponding muscle that helps to effect movement. Dysfunctional states of the joint can cause additional stress on the supporting soft tissue and result in muscle guarding. This can lead to an accumulation of metabolites in the involved muscle and result in local tenderness, with hypertrophy due to guarding.

Tissue texture abnormality comprises yet another component which will be described in the chapter chapter titled 'principles of diagnosis'. This is the soft tissue pain elicited with contraction. A concept called selective tissue tension will help assess pain in the contractile elements of the soft tissue component of a dysfunction. Palpation for local tenderness has yet another important aspect which is reproduction of the symptom at hand. This is called a 'comparable sign'. When this is done, with caution to not increase irritability, it adds diagnostic value and assures the patient of your ability to identify his problem.

PALPATION LAB

The bony skeleton is the framework of the body, hence identifying bony landmarks by palpation can help provide a baseline for identifying a dysfunction. They are described in a descending order with an emphasis on the more obvious and clinically relevant landmarks. Additional references are suggested.[7,8]

CERVICAL SPINE

External Occipital Protuberance and Nuchal Line

Found on the midline of the skull, posteriorly, at the level where the posterior neck muscles attach to the skull.

The nuchal line is palpated just below the external occipital protuberance and can be felt as a dip at the base of the skull.

Mastoid Process

The mastoid process is palpated just behind the ear as bony prominences.

Transverse Process of C1

This is palpated just below the mastoid, deep to the soft tissue, and is tender on palpation.

Spinous Process of C2

With the neck in mild flexion, the nuchal line is palpated as a bony rim. The first bony prominence below it is the spinous process of C2 (as C1 does not have a spinous process).

Spinous Process of C7

At the level of the shoulders the prominent spinous process which dips on neck extension. Also called the vertebra prominens.

Transverse Processes/Articular Pillars of C3 to C7

Approaching the neck laterally, the bony landmarks immediately palpable beyond the muscle tissue are the articular pillars and the facet joints of C3 to C7. Remember that the midcervical spine does not have prominent transverse processes. The articular pillars can be palpated in line with the mastoid process, behind the SCM.

Hyoid

The hyoid is the palpated as the most superior landmark of the Adam's apple. It lies immediately above the prominent hyoid bone. It corresponds to C3.

Thyroid Gland and Cartilage

The thyroid cartilage is the most prominent bone in the Adam's apple. The thyroid gland is a smooth structure on either sides. It is palpable more easily when enlarged in dysfunctional states. It corresponds to C4,5.

Cricoid

This is palpated as a ring-shaped structure just below the hyoid. It corresponds to C6.

Trapezius, Scalenes, SCM, Longi, Suboccipitals

Refer to myofascial tender points chart.

Lymph Nodes

There are multiple lymph nodes around the cervical region but the most common area to palpate are under the mandible and the lateral cervical area. Enlarged or tender lymph nodes indicate inflammation or disease.

Common Carotid or Temporal Artery

The carotid artery is palpated on the lateral cervical area anterior to the sternomastoid bulk. The temporal artery is palpable in the region of the temple just posterior to the orbital area.

THORACIC SPINE

Angle of First Rib

This is palpated above the clavicle just below the superficial contour of the upper fibers of trapezius.

Spinous Process of Third Thoracic Spine (T3)

This can be palpated approximately at the level of the medial end of the spine of the scapula.

Spinous Process of Seventh Thoracic Spine (T7)

This can be palpated approximately at the level of the inferior angle of the scapula.

Spinous Process of T12/ Thoracolumbar Junction

This can be palpated approximately at the level of the last rib angle laterally which is rib number 10.

Thoracic Outlet

The costoclavicular space is palpated by tracing the clavicle to its medial end and palpating the inferior aspect of the clavicle.

SHOULDER

Spine of Scapula

This is palpated as an obvious bony prominence in the upper part of the posterior thoracic cage.

Inferior Angle of Scapula

On palpating the medial border of the spine of scapula and tracing downward and medially to the tip of the inferior end, the angle can be palpated. Alternately, by placing the base of the palm on the inferior aspect of the scapula and pushing upwards, the inferior angle can be felt.

ACROMION

By tracing laterally over the spine of scapula, the acromion can be palpated on the lateral and superior surface of the shoulder joint.

Greater Tuberosity of Humerus

This is palpated slightly below and anterior to the lateral rim of the acromion.

Coracoid Process

This is palpated anterior and medial to the acromion and the medial aspect of the head of the humerus, and is a deeply placed bony landmark.

Long Head Biceps

This is palpated deep in the anterior deltoid bulk.

Acromioclavicular Joint

Trace the clavicle laterally and the joint can be palpated where the clavicle meets the acromion.

Sternoclavicular Joint

This is palpated at the medial end of the clavicle.

Spinoglenoid Area

The spine of the scapula is palpated and moved till the lateral end. The inferior aspect of the lateral end is the spinoglenoid area.

Teres Major and Minor

This is palpated over the lateral border of the scapula.

Pectoralis Major and Minor

The pectoralis major is the thick palpable bulk over the medial axillary area. The pectoralis minor is deep to the pectoralis major underlying its lateral bulk.

Quadrilateral Space and Triangular Interval

The quadrilateral space is palpated under the posterior axillary area deep to the superior lateral border of the scapula. The triangular interval is where the triceps bulk meets the teres major over the superior lateral border of the scapula.

Deltoid Tuberosity and Radial Groove

This can be palpated over the posterolateral aspect of the midhumeral area.

Coracobrachialis

This can be palpated over the inferior aspect of the anterior deltoid bulk where it meets the biceps.

ELBOW

Olecranon

This is palpated as a bony projection on the posterior aspect of the elbow joint.

Radial Head

With the elbow flexed to 90° the lateral epicondyle is palpated. Just distal to the lateral epicondyle, the radial head is palpated. To confirm, the radial head can be felt moving with pronation and supination of the forearm.

Brachioradialis/Supinator

With the elbow extended, it is palpated as a prominent bulk over the lateral border of the cubital fossa, one inch distally.

Pronator Teres

This is palpated on inch distal to the cubital fossa anteriorly.

Cubital Tunnel/Flexor Carpi Ulnaris

This is palpated immediately distal to the medial epicondyle.

Ulnar Nerve

This is palpated immediately proximal to the medial epicondyle slightly posteriorly.

Extensor Carpi Radialis Longus/Brevis

The tendinous origin can be palpated distal to the radial head. It becomes more obvious on middle finger extension.

WRIST AND HAND

Radial Styloid

This is palpated as a bony prominence on the lateral side of the wrist.

Ulnar Styloid

This is palpated as a bony prominence on the medial side of the wrist.

Capitate

This is the standard landmark of the carpal bones and is palpated at the base of the third metacarpal. There is a slight palpable depression on the capitate.

Lunate

This is palpated immediately proximal and lateral to the capitate next to the scaphoid.

Scaphoid

This is palpated as a depression just distal to the radial styloid. It protrudes with ulnar deviation.

Trapezium

This is palpated just distal to the scaphoid as an immediate elevation.

Triquetrium

This is palpated immediately distal to the ulnar styloid. It protrudes on radial deviation.

Pisiform

On the palmar surface of the hand, the ulnar styloid is first palpated. If you move slightly distally and medially, the first bony prominence is the pisiform.

Hook of Hamate

Moving slightly medially and distally from the pisiform, the hook of the hamate is palpated deeply (it is slightly more difficult to palpate).

Abductor Pollicis Longus/Extensor Pollicis Brevis

This can be palpated by resisting thumb extension. The tendon that stands out prominently is the abductor pollicis longus. The tendon lateral to the abductor pollicis longus at the level of the radial styloid is the extensor pollicis brevis.

LUMBAR SPINE, PELVIS AND HIP

Iliac Crest

At the level of the pelvis, lateral to the abdomen, the obvious bony prominences are the iliac crests.

Anterior Superior Iliac Spine

The anterior most portion of the iliac crest is palpated as a prominence which are the anterior superior iliac spine (ASIS).

Posterior Superior Iliac Spine

The posterior most part of the iliac crests are seen as dimples and inferior aspect of these dimples are palpated as the posterior superior iliac spines (PSIS).

Ischial Tuberosity

This landmark is palpated just at the inferior gluteal line and is very obvious as we sit on it.

Spinous Process of L4

This is palpated in the midline at the level of the iliac crests.

Spinous Process of L5

The PSIS is first palpated, and moving 30° superiorly and medially, the spinous process of L5 is palpated. This is the least prominent of the lumbar spinous processes.

Spinous Process of S2

This is palpated in the midline at the level of the PSIS.

Base of the Sacrum

Just immediately medial to the PSIS, the base of the sacrum is palpated. This is a difficult landmark to palpate and requires practice.

Inferior Lateral Angle of the Sacrum

By placing the base of the palm on the buttock and pushing upwards, the sacrococcygeal joint can be felt. On palpating the sacrococcygeal joint, moving slightly upwards and laterally the sacrum just begins to flare out. Just at the out-flare, moving to the superior surface, the inferior lateral angle (ILA) can be palpated.

Pubic Tubercle

This can be palpated on either sides of the genital area, lateral to the midline. It is slightly higher in males and lower in females.

Sciatic Notch/Piriformis

The piriformis can be palpated just lateral to the sacrum in the center of the gluteal mass.

Deep to the piriformis, the sciatic notch is palpated as a bony ring in a superomedial direction.

Gluteus Medius

The gluteus medius is palpated midway and slightly posterior to the greater trochanter and iliac crest.

Sacroiliac Joint and Posterior Sacroiliac Ligament

The PSIS is seen as a dimple below the L5 region on either sides. It is palpated as a bony rim running superioinferior. Just medial and inferior to it is the sacral base and lateral to the sacral base is the sacroiliac joint. The posterior sacroiliac ligament lies over the sacral base.

Greater Trochanter

With the hip flexed to 90° the greater trochanter can be palpated on the lateral sides of the hip.

Sartorius

The sartorius muscle can be palpated just below the ASIS and traced anteromedial and inferior along the thigh.

Tension Fasciae Latae

The tension fasciae latae (TFL) is palpated midway and slightly anterior to the greater trochanter and iliac crest.

Iliotibial Band

The iliotibial (ITB) is palpated as a thick chord below the greater trochanter and can be traced down to the lateral knee. It gets thicker and more palpable inferiorly.

Gracilis and Adductors/Inguinal Lymph Nodes

The gracilis and adductors can be palpated on the superomedial aspect of the thigh.

The inguinal lymph nodes can be palpated in the groin area slightly anterior to the medial adductor bulk. Enlargement or tenderness indicates dysfunction.

KNEE

Lateral Condyle and Medial Condyle of Femur

The two obvious bony landmarks palpated on the superior medial and lateral surfaces of the knee joint are the medial and lateral condyles, respectively.

Head of Fibula

This can be palpated postero-laterally and just below the lateral condyle of femur.

Lateral Tibial Condyle

This is palpated just medial to the head of fibula.

Medial Tibial Condyle

This is palpated inferior to the medial condyle of femur.

Hamstrings

The medial and lateral hamstring tendons are palpated just above and to either sides of the popliteal fossa posteriorly. The lateral hamstrings are palpated along the lateral and posterior aspect of the thigh. The biceps femoris is lateral and the semimembranosus and semitendinosus are medial.

Popliteus

This is palpated just below the popliteal fossa centrally.

Peroneus

This is palpated just below the fibular head and slightly posterior.

Medial Patellofemoral Joint

This is palpated just inferomedial to the patella. This area is often irritable in patellofemoral compression.

Lateral Retinaculum

This is palpated immediately over the superior lateral edge of the patella.

Medial Joint Line and Meniscus

With the knee in flexion the medial joint line is palpated just medial to the central part of the patella. On internal and external rotation of the tibia, the meniscus is felt to move in and out.

Lateral Collateral Ligament

This structure is palpated above the fibular head with the patient sitting cross-legged.

Patellar Tendon

This is palpated just inferior to the patella.

Pes Anserine Area

This area is palpated over the posterior and medial border of the superior aspect of the tibia.

Anterior Tibial and Shin Area

This area is palpated over the anterior tibial area slightly lateral to the tibial prominence.

ANKLE AND FOOT

Tibialis Posterior

This structure can be palpated posterior and inferior to the medial malleolus. The tendon can be further enhanced by resisting plantarflexion and inversion. The tendon can also be palpated medial to the calf bulk.

Achille's Tendon

This is palpated as a thick tendon posterior to the ankle. At the level of the posterior ankle palpate the medial and lateral aspect of the tendon to localize pain. Typically the medial aspect is more tender than the lateral aspect.

Sinus Tarsi/Anterior Talofibular Ligament

This area is palpated just superior and lateral to the lateral malleolus.

Superficial Peroneal Nerve

This can be palpated slightly anterior to the lateral malleolus in full plantarflexion and inversion.

Tibialis Anterior Tendon

This tendon can be palpated over the superomedial aspect of the ankle joint and is accentuated by dorsiflexion with inversion.

Peroneal Tendon

The conjoint tendons of the peroneus longus and brevis can be palpated above the lateral malleolus as a thick chord. Tenderness can also be elicited posterior and inferior to the lateral malleous where the tendon passes through the peroneal retinaculum.

Talus

This is palpated immediately anterior to the inferior and anterior surface of tibia.

Navicular

This is palpated as a bony prominence immediately anterior and inferior to the medial malleolus.

Medial Cueniform

This is palpated immediately anterior to the navicular.

Cuboid

This is palpated immediately posterior to the base of the fifth metatarsal.

Plantar Fascia

With the great toe in full extension the plantar fascia can be palpated as a thick chord on the inferior and medial aspect of the sole of foot.

Abductor Hallucis

This is palpated on the medial aspect of the heel pad at the junction of the rearfoot to the midfoot.

Metatarsal Heads

These can be palpated inferiorly just proximal to the metatarsophalangeal joint.

REFERENCES

1. Montagu A. Touching: The human significance of the skin. 1971, Columbia University Press, New York.
2. Adams T, Steinmetz MA, Heisey SR, et al. Physiological basis for skin properties in palpatory physical diagnosis. J Am Osteopath Assoc. 1982;81:366-77.
3. Robinson R, Robinson HS, Bjørke G, et al. Reliability and validity of a palpation technique for identifying the spinous processes of C7 and L5. Man Ther, 2009;14:409-14.
4. Schneider M, Erhard R, Brach J, Tellin W, Imbarlina F, Delitto A. Spinal palpation for lumbar segmental mobility and pain provocation: an interexaminer reliability study. J Manipulative Physiol Ther. 2008;31:465-73.
5. Bron C, Franssen J, Wensing M, et al. Interrater reliability of palpation of myofascial trigger points in three shoulder muscles. J Man Manip Ther. 2007;15:203-15.
6. McKenna L, Straker L, Smith A. The validity and intra-tester reliability of a clinical measure of humeral head position. Man Ther. 2008;14:397-403.
7. Hoppenfield S. Physical Examination of the Spine and Extremities. 1976, Appleton-century-crofts, Connecticut, Norwalk.
8. Byfield D, Kinsinger S. A Manual therapists guide to surface anatomy and palpatory skills. 2002, Butterworth Heinemann Oxford.

CHAPTER 7

Principles of Diagnosis

The reader is advised to not misinterpret the aspect of 'diagnosis'. The principles described in this chapter apply to the concept of a 'somatic' diagnosis. The hypothesis being, it is the 'cause' for the conventional diagnoses we see in daily practice. A more detail description is available in part 3 of this book. Diagnosis of a musculoskeletal dysfunction essentially applies the three parameters described earlier, alignment deviation of landmarks or unilateral weakness and tightness of soft tissue, restricted joint or tissue mobility, tenderness locally.[1,2] How, when and where is essentially the application of principles.

The two important factors that the clinician needs to consider is that any musculoskeletal dysfunction has a structural component and a movement component. Take the ankle for example. Assume the presentation is in equinus, the restriction of mobility hence, is dorsiflexion, as the foot is restricted in plantarflexion. Thus when you assess this structure without movement the ankle is in equinus and hence would be the abnormal position of the ankle. This is what is known as the structural or positional fault. On moving this ankle, since it is restricted in plantarflexion preventing dorsiflexion, it would be the abnormal movement of the ankle. This is what is known as a movement fault. To review:

Positional Fault

Ankle restricted in equinus.

Movement Fault

Prevents dorsiflexion as it is restricted or 'stuck' in plantarflexion.

The alignment deviation here is the equinus foot and tight gastroc-soleus in comparison to the other neutral, normal foot.

The restriction joint or tissue mobility is dorsiflexion.

The tenderness locally would be a tender gastrocsoleus tendon, if present, being constantly stretched and overworked as it does not effectively decelerate pronation.

This is a simplified example for purpose of understanding the basic concept as the level of complexity increases. From what we recollect from the earlier chapters this would be a gross motion and hence an example form an 'osteokinematic' standpoint. An exactly similar principle is applied from an arthrokinematic perspective for a more intricate manual diagnosis.

The regional application in most manual therapy schools are categorized as 'spine' and 'extremities' and is hence being followed in this book. Their principles of diagnosis vary as well, due to the variation in anatomy and joint mechanics. Hence they will be described separately.

SPINE

Prior to discussing the principles, the clinician must understand where mobility occurs in the spine and subsequently the areas of probable restriction. The spine like any other synovial joint is a functional unit for the fact that it is mobile and effects motion. The spine as we know are blocks of skeletal structures arranged over each other. Hence they require an articulation for mobility and stability. These articulations that hold the vertebrae together and effect movement, are what are known as 'facet joints'. They are paired structures and lie laterally in each vertebral body. Each vertebral body has a pair of superior and inferior articulating facets. The inferior articulating facets of one vertebra articulates with the superior articulating facets of the vertebra below it to form a vertebral motion segment. Vertebral movement is described as the superior segment moving over an inferior segment and not vice versa. For example, L4 is described as moving over L5 and never L5 over L4. Hence when a segment is described as being restricted or moving excessively, it is with relevance to the segment below it. Three movements occur in a vertebral motion segment and during function they invariably occur together. The three movements are flexion (forward bending), extension (backward bending) and rotation (with side bending).

Assume as shown here:
L4°
L5•

The circles denote the articulating surfaces of the facet joints of inferior L4 and superior L5.

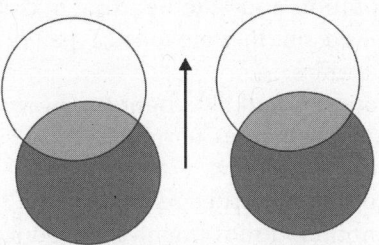

Fig. 7.1: Forward bending.

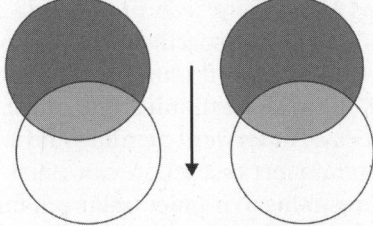

Fig. 7.2: Backward bending.

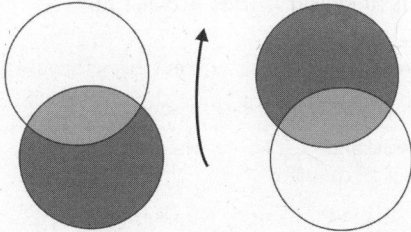

Fig. 7.3: Right rotation.

FORWARD BENDING

During forward bending, the superior facets on either sides of the vertebral segment slide equally forward over the inferior facets. This is termed as a flexed or 'open' position of the facet (Fig. 7.1).

BACKWARD BENDING

During backward bending, the superior facets on either sides slide equally backward over the inferior facets. This is termed as an extended or 'closed' position of the facet (Fig. 7.2).

ROTATION AND SIDE BENDING

Rotation is one movement where the facets do not slide equally in the same direction, but rather opposite. For example, in right rotation, the right facet slides backward and the left facet slides forward. Hence, the right facet has 'closed' and the left facet has 'opened' (Fig. 7.3).

The exact opposite occurs during left rotation.

Since rotation and side bending do not occur individually, they are called coupled movements. However, depending on the curvature of the spine, they occur either to the same side or to opposite sides. Three situation's can occur and they are termed as 'Fryettes rules,'[1] and are as follows:

- If rotation and side bending occur to the opposite side they are called Type 1 or neutral mechanics.
- If rotation and side bending occur to the same side they are termed as Type 2 or non-neutral mechanics.
- A third situation occurs when in the 3 planes of motion, if movement is introduced in 1 plane, the movement in the other 2 planes is reduced. This is termed as Type 3 mechanics.

Types 1 and 2 are seen in vertebral motion dysfunctions and are specific to the regions of the spine. As an example, the lumbar spine normally exhibits neutral mechanics,[3] however, faulty mechanics as in forward bending and twisting, or unilateral facet restriction can cause this to change, resulting in nonneutral mechanics and will require correction. Hence knowledge of the type of mechanics in the different regions of the spine is necessary. They are as follows:

Subcranial spine	Neutral
Midcervical spine	Nonneutral
Subcranial and midcervical coupled	Neutral[4]
Thoracic spine	Upper-neutral
	Lower-nonneutral
Lumbar spine	Neutral[3]
Sacrum and pelvis	Neutral

This requires explanation from a movement perspective. All movements in the human body occur as triplanar motion, hence, diagonal. Therefore, walking is a diagonal activity. One may then argue that the individual should be headed in a diagonal direction and purposive walking along a straight line may not be possible. Recall PNF principles of reciprocal diagonals. In function, if one has to throw a ball the opposite hand is automatically in the opposite diagonal. The examples are numerous, as in during walking, forward movement of the opposite arm and leg occur followed by the other arm and leg. Reciprocal diagonals convert diagonal motion into straight purposive motion. The concept of neutral mechanics is the same. The coupled motion in opposition maintains neutral mechanics. If one observes the spine collectively, the entire spine moves in reciprocal diagonals. For example, although the midcervical spine is nonneutral, the combined mechanics of the upper and midcervical spines are still neutral.

Type 3 mechanics is incorporated to localize motion during manipulation techniques. Interestingly, the normal motion segment seeks neutral mechanics. As an example, although the midcervical spine exhibits nonneutral mechanics, collectively in combination with the upper cervical spine, it exhibits neutral mechanics.

POSITIONAL FAULTS

Palpation

The bony landmarks that are palpable in a vertebral body are the spinous processes which is one in number for each vertebra and is the posterior projection of the spine. On observing a skinny individual, the bony projections in the middle of the back are the spinous processes. They are arranged in a straight line one above each other with equal distances between them. They can be palpated by pinching (gently) their lateral borders and determining their position (Fig. 7.4).

Dysfunction

The position of the spinous process can determine the faulty position of that individual segment and is done by observing:

a. The distance between each spinous process.
b. The position of the spinous process with relevance to the one above and below it in their vertical arrangement.

T12 ☐

L1 ☐

L2 ☐   L3 is forward bent on L4

Principles of Diagnosis

L3
L4
L5

Spinous process position and resulting dysfunction

Observe the arrangement of the spinous process above. There is equal distance between L1 and L2 and subsequently L4 and L5. However, L3 has moved forward and is closer to L2 with relevance to L4. It can be presumed that the L3 segment is in a forward bent position.

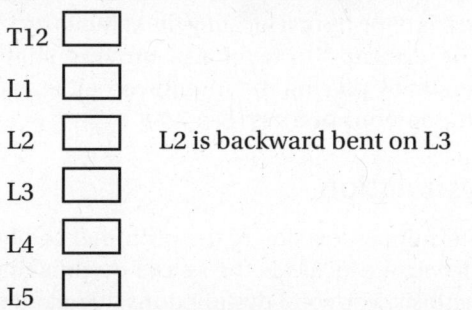

L2 is backward bent on L3

Spinous process position and resulting dysfunction

In the above arrangement the distance between T12 and L1 is equal and so are the distances between L3,4 and L4,5. However, L2 has moved backwards and is closer to L3 with relevance to L1. It can be presumed that L2 is in a backward bent position.

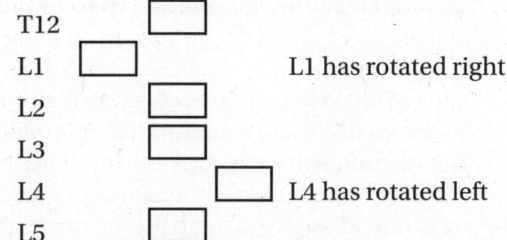

L1 has rotated right

L4 has rotated left

Spinous process position and resulting dysfunction

Here, T12, L2, L3 and L5 are in a straight line, however, L1 has moved slightly left and L4 has moved slightly right. This could mean that the segments are rotated but the direction of rotation is important to understand.

Figure 7.5 observing the segment from above, note that the spinous process is placed posteriorly. Since the vertebra is a circular structure, rotation to one side will move the spinous process to the other side, so if the spinous process has moved left, technically the segment has rotated right and vice versa. Hence in the above arrangement, since the spinous

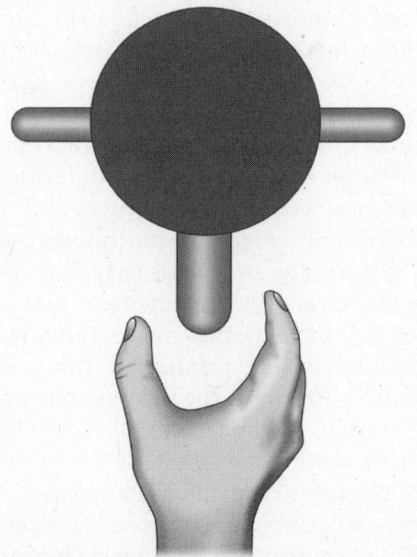

Fig. 7.4: Palpation of spinous process.

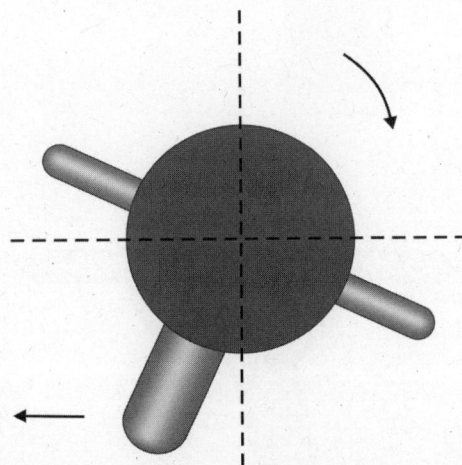

Fig. 7.5: Right rotation results in spinous process deviating to the left.

process of L1 has moved left, it has rotated right with relevance to T12 and L2.

Similarly, since the spinous process of L4 has moved right with relevance to L3 and L5, it has rotated to the left. Hence in the above arrangement, L1 is in right rotation and L4 is in left rotation.

The validity of a positional diagnosis should be questioned[5] because anatomical anomalies of the spinous process can be misleading. This is due to the fact that the spinous process of a vertebral segment can be abnormally deviated in a faulty position, As an example, in the above illustration (Fig. 7.6) the spinous process is shown to have deviated left due to an anatomical anomaly, but the vertebral segment is neutral. Since the position of the spinous process is anomalous, it cannot be assumed that the segment is rotated to the right. Hence the clinician should exercise caution and not make a diagnosis based on positional faults alone.

MOVEMENT FAULTS

Palpation

On observing the body of a vertebra the two lateral projections of the vertebral body are the transverse processes. They are placed about an inch lateral to the spinous process and their

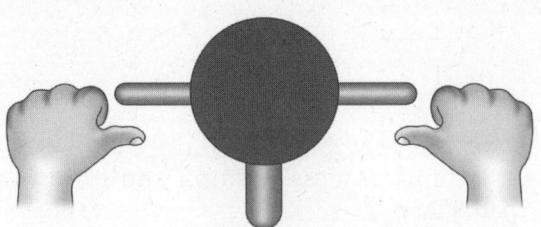

Fig. 7.7: Palpation of transverse processes.

levels with relation to the spinous process vary with the different levels of the vertebral column. They will be discussed in the regional application chapters. These are difficult structures to palpate and it is done by first locating the spinous process to determine the level and moving slightly laterally by placing the thumbs on either sides of the spinous process (Fig. 7.7).

Dysfunction

Determining the side of the prominence of the transverse process is the key to establishing a diagnosis. Vertebral dysfunctions do not always occur in isolation. It is usually a combination of movements occurring in three planes of motion. This is owing to:
1. The nature of normal movement
2. The orientation of the facet joints.

Normal movements occur in patterns or diagonals. It is usually a combination of movements in all three cardinal planes (flexion/extension, side bending, and rotation) and the key movement is rotation. The reason being that it is the rotation that will determine the prominence of the transverse process.

For example, on placing the thumbs on either sides of the spinous process (which is over the transverse process), a greater prominence on the left will indicate that the segment is in left rotation because a rotation of the vertebral segment will move the transverse process posteriorly on the side of the rotation (Fig. 7.8).

This prominence is called a 'posteriority' and is the key to making a diagnosis of spinal movement dysfunction. It appears as a posterior projection on forward and backward bending owing to the layers of muscle that it pushes outward adding to the prominence.[1,2,5,6]

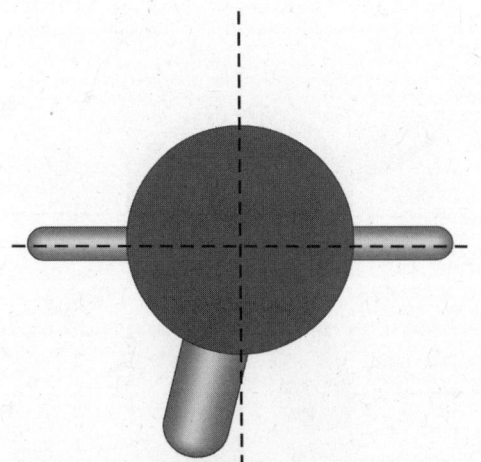

Fig. 7.6: Spinous process deviation as a congenital anomaly.

Principles of Diagnosis

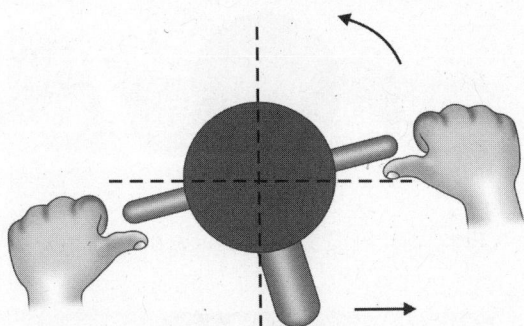

Fig. 7.8: Left rotation with posteriority of left transverse process.

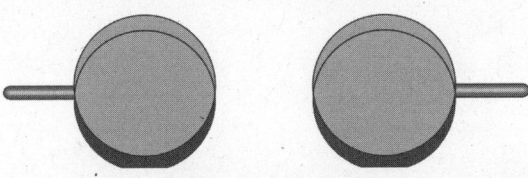

Fig. 7.9: Neutral.

The movements of the vertebral column occur in diagonal patterns and two possibilities can exist as far as dysfunctions are concerned.[1,2] They are as follows:

Extension, rotation, side bending (ERS) (stuck in a closed position and not opening). Flexion, rotation, side bending (FRS) (stuck in an open position and not closing).

ERS (Stuck in a Closed Position and not Opening)

On reviewing spinal joint motion we inferred that during flexion the facets slide equally forward and the exact opposite during extension. Let us consider two segments, L4 and L5. Assume the right facet of L4 is restricted, or stuck in extension (closing). In the neutral position, the transverse processes are neutral and hence will appear neutral (Fig. 7.9).

L4°
L5•

In backward bending, the right facet is already stuck in extension and hence will appear posterior. The left facet also moves posteriorly as it is not stuck and is moving freely. Since both are posterior they will technically appear neutral in backward bending (Fig. 7.10).

However, in forward bending, since the left facet is moving freely it slides forward but since the right facet is stuck in extension it remains where it is (in extension). This will appear as a prominence of the L4 transverse process on the right (Fig. 7.11). Hence your diagnosis will be an ERS right of L4 (not opening), as the segment is stuck in extension and the rotation and side bending go with it. Remember, the 'side' of your diagnosis is always the side of the posteriority (Fig. 7.12).

FRS (Stuck in an Open Position and not Closing)

Assume that the right L4 facet is stuck in flexion (not closing). In neutral they invariably appear neutral (Fig. 7.13).

L4°
L5•

During forward bending, the right facet is already stuck in flexion and hence has slide forward. The left facet is freely moving and will also slide forward. On palpation of the transverse processes, in forward bending there will be no evidence of a posteriority as both facets have slide forward and are neutral (Fig. 7.14).

However, during backward bending the left facet moves freely and hence slides backward.

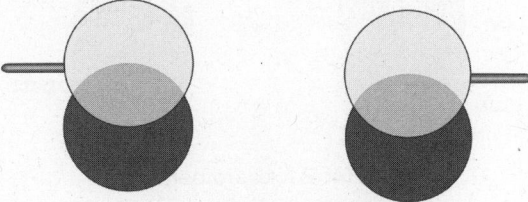

Fig. 7.10: Forward bending.

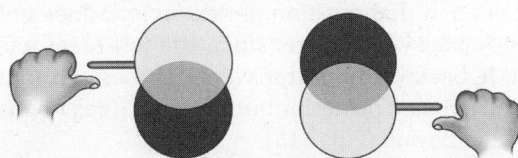

Fig. 7.11: ERS right/right facet not opening.

Principles of Manual Therapy

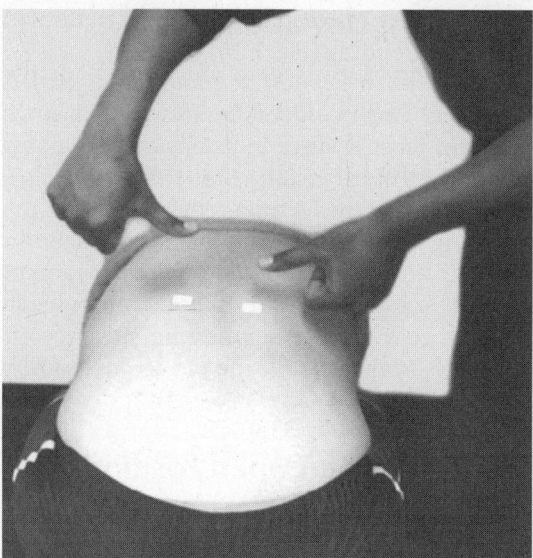

Fig. 7.12: ERS left (individual sitting and forward bending).

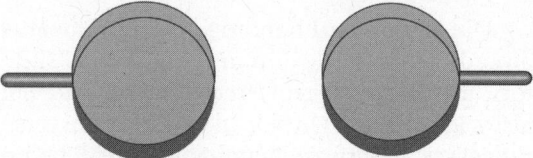

Fig. 7.13: Neutral.

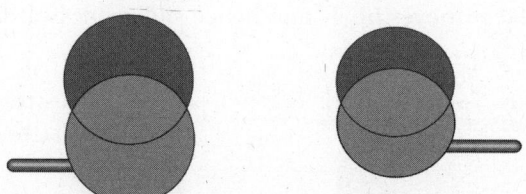

Fig. 7.14: Backward bending.

The right facet however is stuck in flexion. Hence, it stays in that position of flexion and does not slide backward. Here, since the left facet has slide backward the transverse process on that side appears posterior but the right does not as it is in flexion (Fig. 7.15).

The restriction is on the right as it is the right facet that is stuck in flexion, but the posteriority is

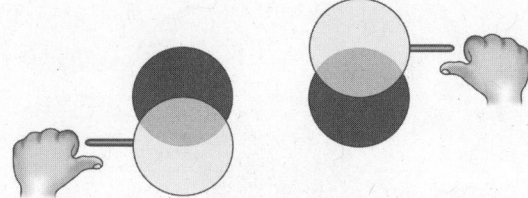

Fig. 7.15: FRS left /right facet not closing.

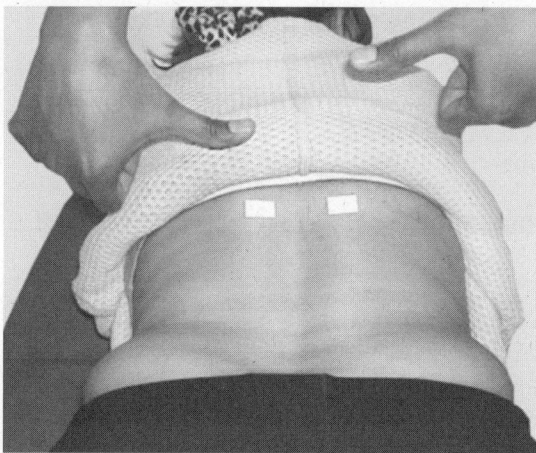

Fig. 7.16: FRS right (Individual in a prone prop up position).

on the left as the freely moving left facet has slide backward. Hence, the diagnosis will be FRS left of L4 (right not closing) as the diagnosis is always by the side of the posteriority and not by the side of the restriction (Fig. 7.16). However, to make the situation simple, this scenario indicates the right L4 not closing.

CLINICAL IMPLICATION

Abnormal alignment/mechanics, be it an ERS or a FRS can produce clinical scenarios we see in our day-to-day practice. The dysfunction that was discussed earlier of the L4 segment is depicted in the Figure 7.17. Note that L4 is restricted in extension and would hence be an ERS. If movement continues to occur in this abnormal position it can significantly shear the disc (which is part of the motion segment) and may result in a disc pathology. The size or

Principles of Diagnosis

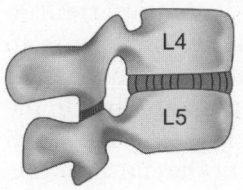 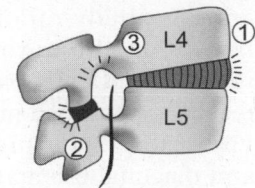

Fig. 7.17: Consequences of facet restriction 1. Disc shearing; 2. Facet shearing; 3. Foraminal narrowing.

the patency of the foramen is altered and as the nerve exits through the foramen it can be pinched resulting in a radiculopathy. The facet, due to abnormal weightbearing stresses of faulty alignment can be susceptible to cartilage and facet capsule shearing. The effusion that occurs due to this can be poured into the foramen increasing nerve root symptoms. Hence, by freeing the facet restriction and correcting the alignment, the patency of the foramen is restored, the shearing of the disc is reduced and the facet joints are rendered less susceptible to loading stresses. This can significantly minimize symptoms.

The large muscle groups that effect movement in this motion segment can be stressed due to faulty mechanics. Hence, correcting vertebral alignment can reduce the workload of these large spinal and pelvic muscles which can later be effectively stabilized to maintain alignment.

Mechanical traction may temporarily open the foramen. Facet injections may temporarily relieve facet and nerve root pain so do other aspects of management including medication. They most definitely have their place as acute pain has to be addressed by these means, but in combination, if the mechanics and alignment are addressed, it may address the 'cause' of the dysfunction.

To summarize, in the above scenario, the:

Positional Fault

Deviation of spinous process.

Movement Fault

L4 not sliding forward or backward (FRS, ERS).

Alignment Deviation

Posteriority of transverse processes or faulty position of spinous process.

Restricted Joint or Tissue Mobility

L4 stuck in flexion or extension and side bending/rotation.

Tenderness Locally

Local tenderness over the transverse processes and dysfunctional states of large and local small supporting musculature. While a large emphasis has been laid on the facet joint and vertebral motion segment, the soft tissue cannot be overlooked. Local tenderness over the supporting musculature, or weakness may be the first and best adjunct. Ligamentous tenderness may also be excellent indicators, a good example being the posterior sacroiliac and sacrospinous/sacrotuberous ligaments in sacral dysfunctions. Detail examination of the supporting soft tissue is hence recommended.

EXTREMITIES

From a manual therapy and a physical therapy perspective, the functional outcome is the bigger concern. Joint classification based on morphology is indeed of importance to us, however, it is important to know what type of (bone) movement occurs in each joint. MacConail's classification of joints reflects this theory.[7] He describes joint surfaces as either ovoid or sellar (Fig. 7.18).

Ovoid

This can be either convex or concave in all directions and are similar to a piece of egg shell in that their surfaces are of a continually changing angular value.

Sellar (Saddle)

These are inversely curved with convex and concave surfaces situated at right angles to each other.

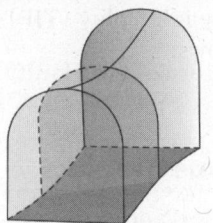 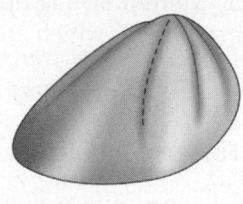

Fig. 7.18: Sellar and ovoid.

MacConail's Classification of Joints

1. Unmodified ovoid (ball and socket), triaxial, e.g. hip and shoulder.
2. Modified ovoid (ellipsoid), biaxial, e.g. Metacarpophalangeal (MCP) joints.
3. Unmodified sellar (saddle), biaxial, e.g. Carpometacarpal (CMC) joints.
4. Modified sellar (hinge) uniaxial, e.g. interphalangeal joints.

It would be of importance to know that in most joint positions, the articular surfaces are not fully congruent. This may be because the convex partner may be more curved than the concave partner.

It was been described earlier that the manual therapist is more concerned about arthrokinematic movement rather than osteokinematic movement. In manual therapy jargon, osteokinematic movements are termed as bone movements. Joint movements are what we traditional learn in our introductory anatomy occurring in the three cardinal planes as flexion/extension, abduction/adduction and internal/external rotation.

However, bone movements are ones that occur within the joint and are as follows:[7]
1. Rotation
2. Translation.

The principal difference between the two movements is that rotation is under voluntary control and translation is not.

Rotation

All active movements are essentially rotations because they occur around an axis. Hence the normal movements of flexion, extension, etc. occurring in the three cardinal planes are essentially rotations. It is important to know that the normal function occurs in rotatory and diagonal patterns, if one could recollect, patterned motion is described in the PNF texts. This is probably due to the spiral and diagonal orientation of the musculature. Coincidingly, it is interesting to note that as much as osteokinematic movement occurs in rotatory diagonals, arthrokinematic or bone movements occur in the same fashion. For example, during knee extension there is an anterior glide and an external rotation of tibia.

Roll and Gliding

All bone rotations produce a combination of roll and gliding. Rolling occurs when new points of equal distances in one surface comes into contact with new points of equal distances in another surface (Fig. 7.19).

Gliding occurs when one point on a joint surface contacts new and different points in another joint surface (Fig. 7.20).

Gliding and rolling occur together in all bone movements. Gliding with rolling can only occur on flat or curved/congruent surfaces. There are no entirely flat or curved/congruent surfaces and hence pure gliding does not occur in the

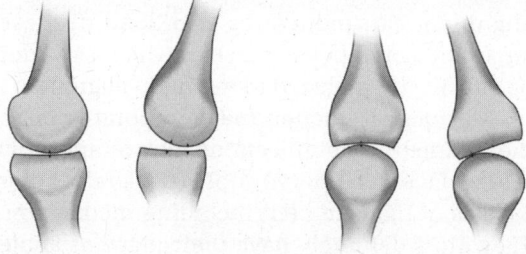

Fig. 7.19: Roll.

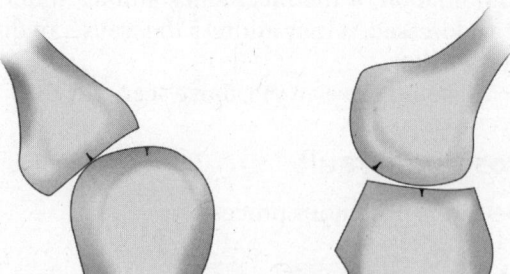

Fig. 7.20: Glide.

human body. Hence a joint surface need to roll and glide to be able to negotiate surfaces as a purely flat surfaces do not exist. The direction of gliding depends on whether a convex or concave surface is moving. When a concave surface moves, joint gliding is in the same direction, e.g. knee (Fig. 7.21).

When a convex surface moves, joint gliding is in the opposite direction, e.g. shoulder (Fig. 7.22).

This is what is known as the *Kaltenborn concave-covex rule* and has an universal principle applied during joint mobilization.[7] While this has been universally accepted as a theory, its application to treatment is being critically evaluated. Critics argue gliding and rolling to be already programed and that if there is adequate capsular freedom, gliding and rolling may resume.

TRANSLATION

Translation is a bone movement that is not under voluntary control, however, they are essential for free painless motion. Bone translation produce isolated traction, compression or gliding joint play movements. These are described by Kaltenborn as translatory joint play (TJP) movements which are as follows:

Traction

Traction is a TJP movement that results in separation of joint surfaces.

Compression

Compression is a TJP movement that results in approximation of joint surfaces.

Passive Gliding

Passive gliding is a TJP movement that results in a sliding movement of joint surfaces. They are possible in small proportions over short distances. Passive gliding is different from the normal roll-gliding that happens during active movement. This passive gliding is induced by the manual therapist in a loose packed position to restore normal active roll-gliding. A traction movement usually precedes a passive gliding movement for ease and safety of performance. Additionally, traction may assist in effectively lengthening the capsule, for programed roll-gliding to resume.

To summarize, the gross motions of our limbs in normal conditions are a result of rotations (roll-gliding) that occur within the joint. The TJP movements normalize the roll-gliding that is essential for active movement. During dysfunction this mechanism is lost due to restriction of TJP movements. This affects the normal mechanics of the joint and abnormally loads the contractile and non-contractile elements of the joints resulting in pathology. Hence, from a manual therapy diagnosis perspective, it is the TJP movements that needs to be examined with the corresponding soft tissue irritability, tenderness, weakness, and tightness. The most clinically relevant TJP movements would be the passive gliding both for examination and treatment. Moreover, restoring passive gliding may restore normal roll-gliding that occurs in joints. At times restriction in TJP movements may be more

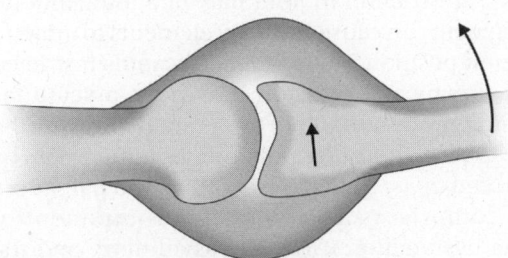

Fig. 7.21: Concave on convex.

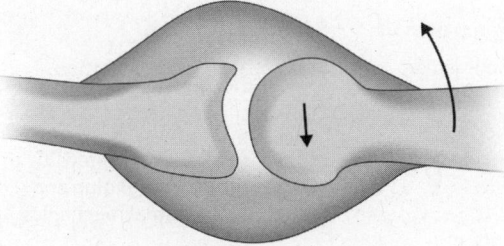

Fig. 7.22: Convex on concave.

obvious. A good example being a rearfoot varus resulting in restricted calcaneal eversion with weak evertors, causing a lateral ligament strain.

Consider the following example[8] which is the normal mechanics (roll-gliding) that occurs during the osteokinematic movement of wrist extension.

The distal row of carpal bones glides dorsal and the proximal row volar.

The primary joint that effects movement is the radially placed radiocarpal joint. This with the activity of the extensor carpi radialis longus (ECRL) and extensor carpi radialis brevis (ECRB) causes radial deviation of the wrist.

Radius Moves Cephalad

Common extensors are contracting.

When a blow is received on the extended hand, the force is taken via the 3rd metacarpal to the lunate, scaphoid and thence to the radius and to the common extensor origin.

Consider a clinical situation. Assume a tennis player or a typist that does periodic extension of the wrist either repetitively overtime or against a resistance as in tennis. If the above mentioned mechanics is intact with good muscle strength, the forces are evenly distributed and the risk of injury is lesser. If the mechanics is altered for various reasons, say a restriction of superior glide of radius or dorsal glide of the distal row of carpal bones (or for that matter weakness of the wrist extensors). This can affect the normal excursion of the wrist extensors and the stresses on the muscle may be higher as it is subjected to more loading to compensate for the altered mechanics. The stresses may be felt greatest at the tendon insertion resulting in a tennis elbow or lateral epicondylitis.

Symptomatic treatments are essential, no doubt, as in local ultrasound or injections or a rest cuff, but if the alignment and mechanics including strength is not addressed the problem can recur with resumption of activities. Similarly, ligament strains, nerve entrapments and tendon injuries can occur due to altered mechanics.

A manual therapy diagnosis will assess the restriction of passive-gliding movements that comprise the mechanics, that lead to a pathology. Every joint in the human body has a similar clinical implication. This example is merely to bring to light what the focus of a manual therapy diagnosis is.

The evaluation of this altered passive gliding movement requires firstly a thorough knowledge of normal roll-gliding and passive-gliding that occurs with each joint of the human body during normal motion. The normal roll-gliding is described in the section on mechanics and the passive-gliding is described in the section for improving overall joint range of motion.

They will be described when describing each joint in subsequent chapters. The passive-gliding movements are evaluated passively by feel, position, movement and to make an accurate finding requires a great deal of practice. The novice clinician may compare findings with the opposite normal joint to arrive at a sense of what he or she is looking for. The one aspect that makes the whole process less complicated is that the evaluation method comprises the treatment technique as well. For example, in the above scenario, while testing for a superior glide of the radius, the same procedure (with some modification) is the treatment technique as well, to restore that motion.

A restriction in joint play in a joint/motion segment can cause the bony elements to move to a new position. For example, a scapula restricted in downward rotation may have a scapular spine more horizontal in comparison with the scapula on the other side. This asymmetry can be picked up by skilled observation and palpation. It comprises the asymmetry component of the dysfunction triad. The asymmetry and the restricted roll-gliding, together interfere with the normal mechanics of the joint. To summarize:

Bone rotation	Bone translation
Roll-gliding	Passive-gliding (with traction, seldom compression)
Normal mechanics	To be passively induced when normal mechanics is altered. It restores normal roll-gliding and subsequently normal mechanics

There is an obvious emphasis on joint restriction, however, the soft tissue cannot be undermined in its notoriety in causing dysfunction.[9-11] Soft tissue mobilization is an absolute necessity and a science by itself. Its description is beyond the scope of this literature review. However, the location of possible areas of soft tissue irritability, are outlined at the end of each chapter.

When abnormal mechanics occur continually in the presence of dysfunction, they render the pain sensitive supporting structures vulnerable. When irritated, these vulnerable structures present as conventional diagnosis in our day-to-day practice such as bursitis, tendonitis, etc. The pain sensitive/vulnerable supporting structures of a joint motion segment are:
1. Muscle and tendon
2. Capsule
3. Bursa
4. Ligament
5. Nerve.

Muscle and Tendon

It is hypothesized that just as a muscle can be rendered tight due to disuse or injury a joint can, as well. When this occurs inside the joint, it is detected by clinical examination as a restriction in the passive gliding movements. A restricted position from neutral can change the position of the bony elements of the joint and result as an asymmetry. With the knowledge of bony landmarks around a joint, this asymmetry can be detected in comparison with the other normal joint. This positional diagnosis in correlation with the movement restriction (passive gliding) can strengthen the diagnosis of a mechanical dysfunction.

Taking this concept one step further, the diagnosis of mechanical dysfunction unique to this philosophy is that it is made with relevance to the dysfunction leading to the pathology rather than a routine motion restriction.

For example, the traditional physical therapy clinician will evaluate a certain motion restriction and upon sensing it will apply a technique to restore that motion for an overall increase in motion and thence function. As an example, consider a patient who has had say, ankle surgery and was immobilized for a certain period of time, resulting in joint restriction. The physical therapy clinician will incorporate treatment techniques to restore this restricted osteokinematic mobility. A more informed clinician especially one that is trained in manual therapy will approach it a step further and work at an arthrokinematic level to restore motion. However, remember that all orthopedic dyfunctions in the clinic are not postsurgical, or postimmobilization situations. For example, the mechanical neuromusculoskeletal pathologies that are described as in, say, a tibialis posterior tendonitis or iliotibial band friction or pain are not postsurgical situations or postimmobility situations. They may present with functional osteokinematic mobility, but they still present with restriction at an arthrokinematic level. That restriction hence is very unique to the dysfunction in question. Identifying the restriction (by both abnormal position and movement) that predisposes to the dysfunction is what a somatic diagnosis is all about, rather that identifying overall motion dysfunction. If one happens to read texts or literature on extremity joint mobilization or manipulation, an angular or osteokinematic motion is described and all the arthrokinematic components necessary to restore that motion is described, in addition to the type of joint (ball and socket, hinge, concave over convex) and their mechanical rules. Although this knowledge is required to restore the motion, the direction of restriction of motion most relevant to the pathology being treated is important and an absolute necessity. The philosophy on which this textbook is written aims to address this component. A bicipital tendonitis will be described with relevance to identifying and diagnosing an internally rotated humerus. A tibialis posterior tendonitis will be described with relevance to the diagnosis of an everted calcaneus or an internally rotated navicular.

In addition, the overall functional mobility and their relevant arthrokinematics/joint play will also be addressed like other philosophies. This is still a valuable tool to address overall restriction that is seen in a postimmobility

situation. Hence, treatment of mechanical dysfunction in the extremity joints will be described in two categories:
1. Treatment for specific somatic dysfunction.
2. Treatment for overall improvement of range of motion.

Selective Tissue Tension Testing

Muscles work together in a synergy to produce a movement. As in the 'tennis elbow' scenario, the movement of wrist extension is the result of a group of muscles working together. Routine manual muscle testing of wrist extension may hence not be reliable in eliciting pain in a selective musculotendinous unit. Hence, selective tissue tension testing (STT) is used. A concept originated by Cyriax,[12] it helps localize the contractile soft tissue involved in the dysfunction.

Wrist extension in the above scenario may elicit pain, but localizing extension to the middle finger may selectively test the ECRB confirming the diagnosis. Hence to maintain normal alignment/mechanics, knowledge of STT may help address selected structures to localize the dysfunction. Although this is a valuable tool for a mechanical diagnosis, another component that might be included is detection of the presence of tender points. This will encompass the tissue texture abnormality component of the ART triad. Most mechanical dysfunctions indicate hyperactivity of the soft tissue components of the lesion which might be the pathology itself and may present as tender points. Knowledge of the presence of tender points may aid the clinician to arrive at the resulting pathology and pain and when elicited may be a psychologically enhancing for the patient that the clinician has an idea as to where the pain or discomfort lies.

Several theories exist as to why such a persistent soft tissue lesion can occur secondary to overuse. The three most common theories are as follows:
1. Prolonged and excessive contraction as would occur with overuse may induce fatigue in a muscle. The muscle contracts in response to fatigue and persists to create a local soft tissue dysfunction with localized tender point called 'trigger points'.[13] Prolonged and excessive actin and myosin cross bridging is hence the precedent.
2. Excessive and faulty muscle contraction can cause injury to the myofibrils of the muscle bulk which may heal with scarring. This scarring can inhibit normal physiological contraction and deprive the area of nutrition and encourage chemical accumulation causing pain. In addition, possible nerve endings in the healed scar may also be pain sensitive.
3. Faulty activity can influence the muscle at an intrafusal level creating constant aberrant gamma motor activity which renders the soft tissue dysfunctional.[14]

Soft tissue irritability can aid in the diagnosis as it is obvious as palpable tender points. These tender points are seen in muscles, musculotendinous and tenoperiosteal junctions. Breaking down the scar or transverse friction compression of trigger points are suggested forms of manual therapy in addition to restoring normal arthrokinematics. This is effective both for the spine and extremity joints and hence will be described in the regional application chapters. The neuromuscular component suggests further reading. At the end of each regional chapter is a body chart of commonly dysfunctional myofascial points. The clinician is suggested, in the absence of contraindication, to apply deep frictions to these points as a management strategy.

Capsule

This structure envelopes the joint and protects it. It contains synovial fluid and lubricates the joint allowing the bones to glide smoothly against each other. Tightness in the capsule is seen as a primary cause, however, faulty mechanics in the joint can also render the capsule tight causing specific patterns of restriction. This can decrease the ability of the joint surfaces to glide smoothly resulting in dysfunction.

Bursa

These are pouches of fluid that help prevent friction between two moving surfaces. In the presence of mechanical dysfunction (asymmetry or restricted passive gliding), the intervening bursa can be vulnerable to stress. Repetitive motion causing prolonged and excessive pressure on the bursa can irritate the bursa resulting in bursitis.

Ligament

In the presence of mechanical dysfunction (asymmetry or restricted passive gliding), the supporting ligament can be subjected to increased tensile stress. Repetitive motion causing prolonged and excessive tensile stress on the ligament can stretch the ligament, resulting in ligament pathology. These structures are richly innervated and hence pain is an obvious consequence.

Nerve

The nerve, like any other mechanical structure is a mobile unit. They change in length to adapt for movement and hence have a gliding capacity. When the gliding is interrupted, the nerve is vulnerable to dysfunction. This occurs secondary to mechanosensitivity and occlusion of vascular channels within the nerve.[15]

The structure of the nerve and the milieu through which they glide have a profound influence in the maintenance of this gliding motion. The outer covering of the nerve called the paraneurium and the individual nerve fibers or fascicles are vulnerable to restriction. In addition the milieu through which the nerve glides, namely, the muscle, ligament, fibrous band and fascia can interfere with normal gliding. These structures are called nerve interfaces. Gross motion of the nerve is called 'neurodynamics' and neurodynamics tests help to assess the normalcy of nerve gliding. Examples are slump, straight-leg-rising (SLR), etc. However, due to faulty mechanics, if one of the interfaces through which the nerve glides is irritated, it can interrupt the ability of the nerve to glide through them resulting in nerve dysfunction. This specific nerve motion through a specific interface is referred to as a 'neurokinematic' restriction. This term has been coined by the author to speculate methods of assessing nerve dysfunction. A separate section is devoted to the description of this hypothesis.

In manual therapy jargon, neurodynamics would be analogous to osteokinematics (gross movement), whereas 'neurokinematics' would be analogous to arthrokinematics (specific motion). Treatment hence addresses the restricting interfaces first, before gross nerve gliding is addressed.

Hypothetical somatic concept of nerve dysfunction[16]

Osteokinematic (gross flexion, extension, etc.)	Neurodynamics (gross nerve motion SLR, slump, etc.)
Arthrokinematics (specific joint glides)	Neurokinematics (nerve gliding in specific interfaces)
Mobilizing arthrokinematic restriction restores osteokinematic motion	Mobilizing neurokinematic restriction restores neurodynamic motion/gliding

The principles of diagnosis in extremity joint dysfunction will hence follow the above philosophy which comprises the ART protocol. In this scenario the conclusive findings from an arthrokinematic standpoint will be:

Positional Fault
Radial head stuck or restricted inferiorly, or superiorly.

Movement Fault
Superior glide of radial head or dorsal glide of distal carpals producing wrist extension.

Alignment Deviation
The restricted position of the radial head should be inferiorly or superiorly.

Restricted Joint or Tissue Mobility
The radial head not moving superiorly or inferiorly (decreased superior/inferior glide) or the distal carpal bones not moving superiorly (decreased dorsal glide).

Tenderness Locally
The tenderness over the lateral epicondyle and radial head, and pain on STT of ECRB.

To summarize, the diagnosis of musculoskeletal dysfunction comprises aspects of various disciplines in healthcare. The philosophy described here is indeed unique but other components be it neurological, vascular, radiological findings, special tests, etc. should be considered. The manual therapy component of diagnosis is intricate and is often times missed out. It yields favorable results when used in conjunction with other methods of diagnosis. The astute clinician should best be eclectic in his/her methods of evaluation.

REFERENCES

1. Bourdillon JF. Spinal Manipulation.1992, 5th ed, Butterworth-Heinemann, Oxford, Sydney.
2. Greenman PE. Principles of Manual Medicine. 2nd edn, 1996, Lippincott Williams and Wilkins, Baltimore.
3. Fujii R, Sakaura H, Mukai Y, et al. Kinematics of the lumbar spine in trunk rotation: in vivo three-dimensional analysis using magnetic resonance imaging. Eur Spine J. 2007;16:1867-74.
4. Ishii T, Mukai Y, Hosono N, et al. Kinematics of the cervical spine in lateral bending: in vivo three-dimensional analysis. Spine. 2006; 31:155-60.
5. Troke M, Schuit D, Petersen CM. Reliability of lumbar spinal palpation, range of motion, and determination of position. BMC Musculoskeletal Disorders. 2007;8:103.
6. Greenman PE. Syndromes of the lumbar spine, pelvis and sacrum. Phys Med-Rehab Clin N Am. 1996;7:773-85.
7. Kaltenborn FM. Mobilization of the extremity joints. Examination and basic treatment techniques. 3rd edn, 1980, Olaf Noris Bokhandel, Oslo, Norway.
8. Patla CE, Paris SV. E1,Course Notes: Extremity evaluation and manipulation. 1996, St. Augustine Institute press.
9. Lucas N, Macaskill P, Irwig L, et al. Reliability of physical examination for diagnosis of myofascial trigger points: a systematic review of the literature. Clin J Pain. 2009;25:80-9.
10. Shah JP, Gilliams EA. Uncovering the biochemical milieu of myofascial trigger points using in vivo microdialysis: an application of muscle pain concepts to myofascial pain syndrome. J Bodyw Mov Ther. 2008;12:371-84.
11. Brezinschek HP. Mechanisms of muscle pain: Significance of trigger points and tender points. Z Rheumatol. 2008;67:653-7.
12. Cyriax J. Textbook of Orthopedic Medicine (Vols 1 and 2). 1944, Cassel and company, London.
13. Travell JG, Simons DG, Simons LS. Myofascial pain and dysfunction: The trigger point manual. 2nd edn, 1999, Williams and Wilkins, Baltimore.
14. Korr IM. The collected papers of Irvin M. Korr. American Academy of Osteopathy, 1979, Indianapolis.
15. Topp KS, Boyd BS. Structure and biomechanics of peripheral nerves: Nerve responses to physical stresses and implications to physical therapist practice. Phys Ther. 2006; 86: 92-109.
16. Sebastian D. Effects of neural interface mobilization on lower extremity radicular pain A single case design. The Journal of Manual and Manipulative Therapy. 2005;13:185.

Section 2

Spinal Manipulation

Chapter 8: Cervical Spine
Chapter 9: Thoracic Spine and Ribs
Chapter 10: Lumbar Spine
Chapter 11: The Pelvic Complex

INTRODUCTION

Every joint in the human body has a purpose worth understanding. They serve as links to the complex skeletal structures and the purpose of these intervening links is to effect movement. When we observe gross movements of the body, the careful organization and resulting grace is much owed to the neural influence of the central and peripheral nervous system. However, assuming that the neural control is intact, the normalcy of the intricate mechanics of the individual joint components is an absolute necessity for normal movement.

From a biomechanical perspective, movements in the extremity joints have been well researched and their functional basis has been well described. This advancement with regards to the extremity joints may be attributed to various reasons. For one, the gross motion produced in an extremity joint is brought about by fewer articulations which are better visualized on imaging procedures or for that matter palpable. Consider shoulder flexion and the articulations that bring about the movement. If, in your examination, you have elicited a limitation in shoulder flexion, what structures would you suspect to narrow down your diagnostic focus. Now consider a limitation in lumbar flexion. Where does your logical thinking zero in?

The more the detail in localizing the lesion, the more elaborate the examination and treatment. When we observe an experienced clinician examining an extremity joint, he/she will carefully observe alignment, test the range of motion actively, passively and stress the supporting structures. A more astute clinician may also examine joint play or arthrokinematic motion, perform special tests and look for movement deviations of the joint in question. The spine, on the contrary, may be tested for gross range of motion rarely for strength, special tests or provocative maneuvers for pain, and gross alignment with no specific detail. The serious implication here is that the articulations of the spine are synovial articulations, no different from the joints of the extremities with greater specificity in mechanics, distinctly unique with every region.

A bigger focus of this portion of the book is to enlighten clinicians to set the same standards of examination and treatment for the spine as applied to the extremities. A detail understanding of the mechanics for each region (cervical, thoracic, lumbar and pelvic) is absolutely essential to diagnose mechanical spinal dysfunction. Prior to discussing regional application of the spine, it is important for the clinician to be aware of the possible contraindications to manipulation of the spine. It should essentially be the first thing that comes to mind before any treatment procedure is initiated. The major contraindications are listed, however, as most manual therapy guru's would advise:

"when in doubt, don't"

The clinician is hence advised to exercise sound clinical judgement prior to initiating treatment. The list is as follows, but not limited to:

- Vertebral artery insufficiency
- Ligament insufficiency especially alar and transverse
- Rheumatoid arthritis and downs syndrome (especially the subcranial spine)
- Connective tissue disorders
- Recent fractures
- Acute disc pathology
- Osteoporosis
- Malignancy or tumors
- Spondylolysis/spondylolisthesis
- Instability
- Bladder bowel incontinence
- Pregnancy
- Bone and joint disease
- Surgical or anomalous joint fusion
- Congenital spinal anomalies
- Systemic disease
- Anticoagulant therapy

CHAPTER 8

Cervical Spine

The cervical spine functions to support and position the head in space for purposes of function and proprioception. This demands mobility and hence the stability in this area is relatively lesser compared to the other areas of the spine. This apparently increases their vulnerability to dysfunction. The anatomy and mechanics of the cervical area is unique and hence a clear understanding of how this area functions is an important precursor to evaluation and treatment.

RELEVANT ANATOMY

The cervical spine consists of seven vertebral segments. The first cervical vertebra or C1 is called the 'atlas' and the second cervical vertebra or C2 is called the 'axis'. The atlas articulates with the occiput above to form the atlanto-occipital joint, and the altas articulates with the axis below to form the atlantoaxial joint. The occiput, atlas and axis together with their articulations are termed the upper cervical, suboccipital or subcranial spine. The area formed by C3 through C7 is called the midcervical spine. The segments of the midcervical region differ from those of the subcranial region in structure and mechanics.[1,2]

MIDCERVICAL SPINE OSSEOUS ANATOMY

A typical midcervical vertebra consists of a body, two transverse processes and a bifid (two projections) spinous process (Fig. 8.1).

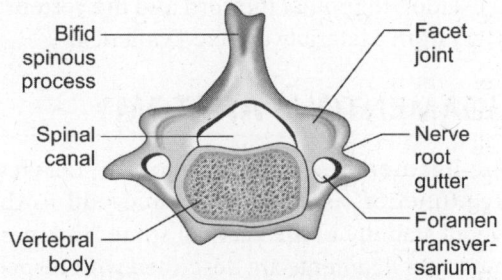

Fig. 8.1: Typical cervical vertebra.

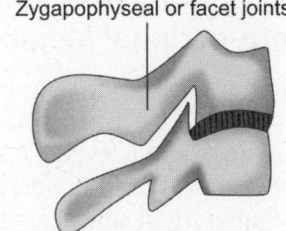

Fig. 8.2: 45° orientation of facets.

On either sides of the body are two openings called the foramen transversaria through which the vertebral artery passes. The transverse process has two projections called the anterior and posterior tubercles. A shallow depression between the two tubercles is what is known as a nerve root gutter, through which the spinal nerve passes. Between the posterior tubercle and spinous process are the articulating facets. These articulations are the zygoapophyseal or facet joints and are oriented in a 45° angle (Fig. 8.2). All manual therapy procedures, are incorporated to effect movement in these joints.

Typical Cervical Vertebra

The superior surface of the cervical vertebral bodies have bony processes that project upwards from the posterolateral rims. The inferior aspect, in conjunction is beveled so as to seat itself between the bony rims. They do so and form the lateral interbody articulations or the uncinate/unciform joints.[1] They are also known as the joints of Von Luschka who first described them. Although there is some controversy, these are not considered synovial joints. The unciform joints prevent excessive lateral bending and lateral translation to protect the cord and the vertebral artery from a laterally directed violence.

LIGAMENTOUS ANATOMY

The ligamentous apparatus of the cervical area function as check reins and add to the overall stability of the cervical spine. The more important ligaments are described with respect to their location and function.

Anterior Longitudinal Ligament and Atlanto-occipital Membrane

The anterior longitudinal ligament (ALL) is attached to the vertebral bodies and intervertebral discs at the level of C3 and all of the segments below it until the periosteum of the sacrum. Superiorly, it attaches to the body of the atlas and axis and continues upward towards the occiput and is known as the atlanto-occipital membrane. This ligament functions as a check rein for excessive extension. Pathologically, the ALL can be involved secondary to crystalline deposit disorders, and calcification.

Posterior Longitudinal Ligament and Tectorial Membrane

The posterior longitudinal ligament (PLL) runs from C2 all the way into the sacrum and on to the coccyx. It is continued upward as the tectorial membrane which bypasses the atlas and inserts into the occiput. It serves as a restraint for any posterior protrusion of the disc and is most advantageous in this area as it the widest in this location. It checks excessive flexion.

Ligamentum nuchae and supraspinous ligament: The ligamentum nuchae extends from the spinous processes of C7 and T1 and attaches into the external occipital protuberance. The anterior placement of the head to the neck causes a flexion moment on the head and this is checked by the ligamentum nuchae. The supraspinous and interspinous ligaments blend with the nuchal ligament.

Ligamentum Flavum

The ligamentum flavum is an important ligament in the cervical spine. It attaches to the inner rim of the vertebral arch and extends to the lamina of the vertebra below. By this position, it forms one of the posterior boundaries of the spinal canal. It extends from C2 to all of the caudal segments. Above C2 it is replaced by the posterior atlantoaxial membrane. This ligament checks flexion, however, on extension it shortens by way of its elastic predisposition. Extension does not cause in folding of the ligament into the spinal canal when there is normal disc height. However, in situations where there is a loss of disc height due to degenerative changes, extension of the cervical spine can cause an infolding of the ligament into the spinal canal causing spinal canal stenosis and myelopathy.

It also contributes to the formation of the anterior wall of the facet joint capsule. It has an important function of sliding the facet capsule in and out of the facet joint during movements of the spine. This mechanism is often lost during dysfunctional states of the ligamentum flavum as which occurs during a laminectomy due to a posterior denervation, resulting in a facet capsule impingement.

Hence, to summarize, ligamentum flavum by way of its attachment to the posterior wall of the spinal canal can cause spinal canal stenosis by infolding and by way of its attachment to the facet capsule can cause a foraminal stenosis due to impingement.

MUSCULAR ANATOMY

The muscles of the cervical area are categorized by side, anterior and posterior and by location, superficial and deep.

Posterior Group

Superficial

1. Trapezius
2. Levator scapulae
3. Splenius
4. Semispinalis
5. Posterior scalenes.

Deep

1. Suboccipital muscles
2. Multifidus.

Anterior Group

Superficial

1. Sternomastoid
2. Anterior and lateral scalenes.

Deep

1. Longus colli
2. Longus cervicis.

The cervical muscles effect movement but additionally it should understood that these muscles have a dense array of muscle spindles and they also function as proprioceptors. The cervical spine muscles are also required to perform unique and highly coordinated functions because of the reflex connections between the sensory organs of the head and motor neuron pools related to the cervical spine.

Their relevance to manual therapists is obvious as discussed in the principles of management that these muscles are analogous to ropes holding the pole of a tent. Their ability to stabilize alignment should be taken advantage of. In addition, the length or excursion needs to be considered as altered lengths of muscles due to tightness or injury or hyperactivity of muscle spindles may stress on vertebral alignment by virtue of their attachment to them.

The most important factor to be considered is that these muscles, on contraction not only effect movement, but also exert a compressive force on the cervical spine. Dysfunctional states of these muscles can increase these compressive forces further predisposing to mechanical dysfunction within the complex. From a manual therapy perspective two factors should be remembered with relevance to musculature. Their strength has to be maintained as they help to stabilize, maintain alignment and absorb the shock of routine activity. Secondly, their length has to be maintained so as to prevent further compressive forces on the spinal alignment and predisposition of faulty alignment due to their traction effect on the skeletal insertion.[3]

The muscles are classified by Vladmir Janda as postural and phasic muscles. It is an accepted understanding that postural muscles tighten or contract in length and phasic muscles weaken during dysfunctional states. This may not be a hard and fast rule but the case for the most part. In addition, due to their dense array of muscle spindles they can be easily involved during injury and on the other hand effectively influenced beneficially. Hence, appropriate exercise prescription following manual therapy not only produces effective outcomes but also unique to the way physical therapists manage mechanical spinal dysfunction.

The anatomy of the above muscles can be gleamed from any standard text but the major postural and phasic muscles are worth knowing for appropriate management.

Postural

- Upper trapezius
- Levator scapulae
- Sternomastoid
- All posterior cervical retractors.

Phasic

All deep anterior cervical musculature. Mid and lower trapezius.

Current literature suggests that the most important stabilizers of the cervical region are the deep neck flexors namely the longus colli and cervicis.[4]

Remember that postural muscles can weaken and phasic muscle can tighten. Their primary tendency is such as mentioned above and hence the management should be appropriate as in first lengthening a postural muscle before strengthening and vice versa for a phasic muscle.

SUBCRANIAL SPINE

The subcranial spine is unique with regard to its mechanics as it works to support the occiput or the skull. The mechanics is complicated and probably more than the other regions of the spine. The basic musculoskeletal, ligamentous and vascular anatomy are worth understanding for accuracy in evaluation.[1,2]

OSSEOUS ANATOMY

Atlas

Atlas (Fig. 8.3) is termed so from the character in greek mythology 'Atlas' who apparently supported the earth over his upper back. The atlas in the cervical spine works likewise as it supports the occiput over it. Its unique structural characteristic is that it does not have a spinous process. It, however, has two prominent transverse processes laterally. It has two superior articulating facets that articulate with the occipital condyles to form the atlanto-occipital joint. The central opening is the spinal canal that lodges the spinal cord. On the anterior aspect of the inner rim of the spinal canal lies an articulating facet for the dens of the axis.

Axis

Axis (Fig. 8.4) is termed so as it allows a significant amount of rotation occurring in the cervical area. It has a prominent spinous process and hence on palpation, inferior to the occiput, the first palpable spinous process is that of the axis (as the atlas does not have one). On the anterior aspect of the axis is a bony prominence that projects superiorly. This bony prominence is called the odontoid process, or the 'dens'. The dens articulates with the facet on the anterior inner rim of the spinal canal of the axis to form the atlantoaxial joint. The analogy hence, a large ring being spun over a finger. Axis thus provides an axis for the atlas to rotate thereby supporting the fact that a considerable amount of rotation occurs in the atlantoaxial joint.

LIGAMENTOUS ANATOMY

Although the subcranial area has several ligaments the important ones are described in more detail owing to their strong relevance to manual therapy procedures. It was mentioned earlier that the cervical spine has sacrificed a certain amount of stability owing to the mobility demands in this area. The principal structures that offer stability to this area especially subcranial area, are the ligamentous structures. Primarily, they stabilize the skeletal structures and prevent them from compromising the neural elements of the brain and spinal cord. Their anatomy, function and tests for integrity are of extreme importance to the manual therapist as the consequences of unplanned treatments may be

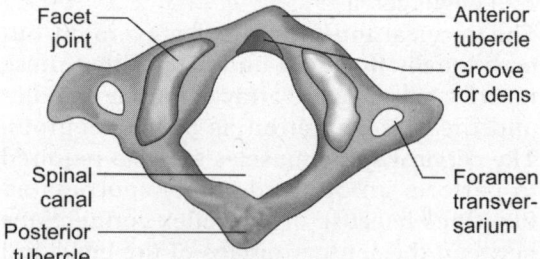

Fig. 8.3: Atlas.

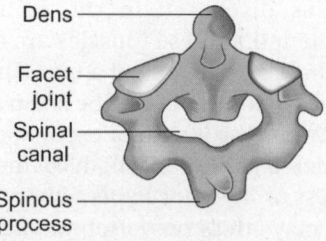

Fig. 8.4: Axis.

disastrous. The anterior and posterior atlanto-occipital membrane, tectoral ligament have been described earlier. The atlantoaxial ligament is the subcranial extension of the ligamentum flavum. The following are some of the ligaments in the subcranial region, however, only the clinically relevant ligaments are elaborated upon.

Atlanto-occipital Ligament

- Fibrous capsule
- Anterior occipitoatlantal ligament
- Posterior occipitoatlantal ligament
- Lateral occipitoatlantal ligaments are two in number

Occipitoaxial Ligament

- Occipitoaxial ligament
- Alar ligaments are two in number
- Apical ligament

Atlantoaxial Ligament

- Anterior atlantoaxial ligament
- Posterior atlantoaxial ligament
- Lateral ligaments are two in number
- Atlantal part of alar ligament

Cruciate ligament consisting of:
- Transverse ligament
- Superior longitudinal fascicles
- Inferior longitudinal fascicles.

Alar Ligaments

The alar ligaments attach laterally to each side of the dens, run upward, laterally and attach to the occiput. The atlantal part of the alar ligament runs from the dens to the facet capsule of C1 and C2 on either sides. They principally limit flexion of the occiput and also side bending and rotation. Their most important function is that they serve to make the occiput, atlas and axis to function as one unit (Fig. 8.5A). Laxity or degeneration of this ligament can severely limit this function and render this area unstable increasing the vulnerability of the neural structures.

The dens is a structure vulnerable to fractures and in such situations the alar ligaments by virtue of their attachments to the dens can cause an upward pull as they are attached to the occiput on the other end. Manual therapy procedures especially traction can cause the fractured dens to be pulled upwards into the foramen magnum and possibly compress the medulla (Fig. 8.5B). Additionally, the dens can also be involved in congenital situations as in os odontoideum.

In situations of laxity of the alar ligaments due to disease, degeneration and injury, any form of manual or manipulative treatments to the subcranial spine can be gravely dangerous and potentially life-threatening.

Transverse Ligament

The transverse ligament attaches on either sides of the inner rim of the spinal canal of the atlas and encircles and reinforces the dens (Fig. 8.6A). By this position it offers a great deal of stability to the dens. It serves as a fence to the spinal cord immediately posterior to it within the spinal canal and prevents the dens from compromising the spinal cord. When the integrity of this ligament is lost due to disease or injury, the fence between the dens and spinal cord does not exist (Figs. 8.6B and C). The alar ligament may be the

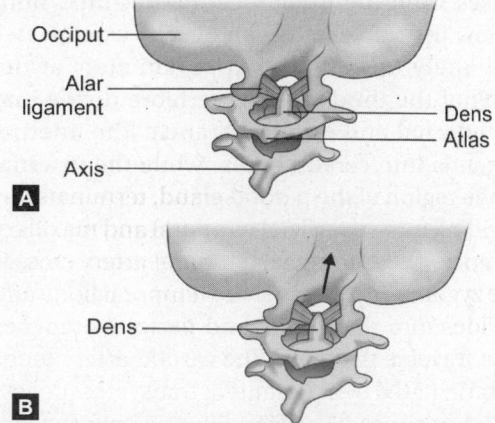

Figs 8.5A and B: (A) Alar ligament and consequence of injury (B) Fractured dens pulled up by alar ligament into foramen secondary to traction.

next line of defense, however, not reliable. Any form of flexion, forward translation or rotation of the subcranial spine can bring the dens closer to the spinal cord resulting in a compromise. Hence in unstable situations of the transverse ligament, manual therapy procedures of the subcranial spine especially those involving flexion, forward translation or rotation can cause a serious spinal cord compromise.

VASCULAR ANATOMY

Vertebral Artery

The vertebral artery originates from the subclavian and ascends upwards into the sixth cervical vertebra. It passes into the openings on the transverse processes known as the foramen transversaria. When it exits out of the altas, it turns inwards and horizontally owing to the wide nature of the transverse processes of the atlas. It then runs upwards into the foramen magnum joins the vertebral artery on the other side to form the basilar artery (Fig. 8.7).

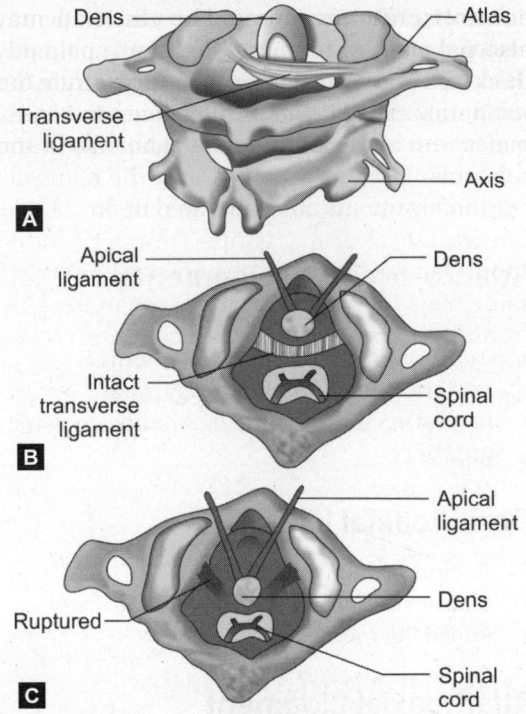

Figs. 8.6A to C: Transverse ligament compromise and consequence.

Carotid and Temporal Artery

The left common carotid artery arises from the aortic arch and the right common carotid artery arises from the brachiocephalic trunk. Both follow the same course and each vessel passes obliquely upward and approximately at the level of the third cervical vertebra divide into an internal and external branch. The internal ascends into cerebral area, while the external at the region of the parotid gland, terminates by dividing into superficial temporal and maxillary arteries. The superficial temporal artery crosses the zygomatic process of the temporal bone and divides into the frontal and parietal branches that traverse the scalp. The carotid artery tends to be irritated by a prominent transverse process of C1 at times. Occasionally one can develop a condition called atherosclerotic carotidynia that can be serious if undetected. Typically the patient has a vascular history, tenderness on palpation of the carotid artery and pain on

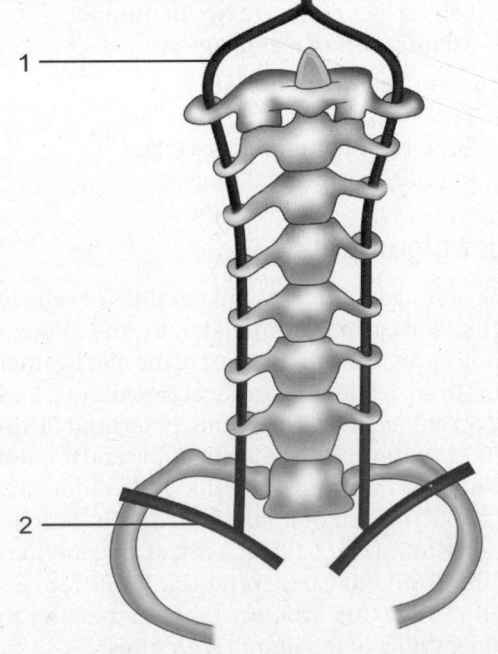

Fig. 8.7: Basilar artery: (1) Vertebral artery; (2) Subclavian.

contralateral movement. The clinician may also palpate the temporal area for a palpably thick and pounding temporal artery to rule out temporal arteritis. This is often seen in elderly males with a coexisting occipital headache and a vascular history.

The brain requires blood supply to survive. The vertebral artery is one source of blood supply, and owing to its position in the cervical spine, may be kinked. It can occur in the subcranial area if the occiput is extended and rotated to the same side. The individual may not have an adequate back up from the carotids and proceed to have signs and symptoms of cerebrovascular ischemia.[5]

Manual therapy procedures to the subcranial spine involving excessive or violent extension or rotation can cause a compromise of the vertebral artery and there lies the risk of a hemiparesis and possible death.

MUSCULAR ANATOMY

Suboccipital Triangle

The suboccipital triangle is formed by the arrangement of the small muscles related to the occiput, atlas and axis. In the mid-line are the rectus muscles:
1. The rectus capitis posterior minor
2. The rectus capitis posterior major

The rectus capitis posterior minor arises from the posterior arch of the atlas and inserts into the occiput. The rectus capitis posterior major arises from the spine of the axis and ascends to the occiput. Lateral to the recti are the obliquus muscles:
1. The obliquus capitis superior
2. The obliquus capitis inferior

The large inferior oblique muscle arises from the spinous process of the axis and adjacent lamina and attaches to the transverse process of the atlas. The superior oblique muscle arises from the transverse process of the atlas and runs superiorly to attach to the occiput (Fig. 8.8).

The two recti draw the head backwards and so does the obliquus capitis superior. The rectus capitis posterior and the obliquus capitis inferior rotate the head to the same side and the obliquus capitis superior to the opposite side.

The posterior division of the second cervical nerve emerges from the spinal canal between the posterior arch of the atlas and the lamina of the axis below the inferior obliquus. It supplies a twig to this muscle and receives a communicating filament from the first cervical nerve. It then divides into an internal and external branch. The internal branch, called the greater occipital nerve ascends obliquely inwards between the obliquus inferior and the complexus. It pierces the latter muscle and the trapezius near their attachment to the cranium. It is now joined by a filament from the posterior division of the third cervical nerve, and ascending on the posterior part of the head with the occipital artery, divides into two branches. This supplies the integument of the scalp as far as the vertex, communicating with the lesser occipital nerve. It gives off an auricular branch to the posterior part of the ear and a muscular branch to the complexus (Fig. 8.9).

The occipital nerve is of clinical significance as it is the irritation of the occipital nerve that results in muscular headaches by virtue of their supply to the integument of the scalp. The pain

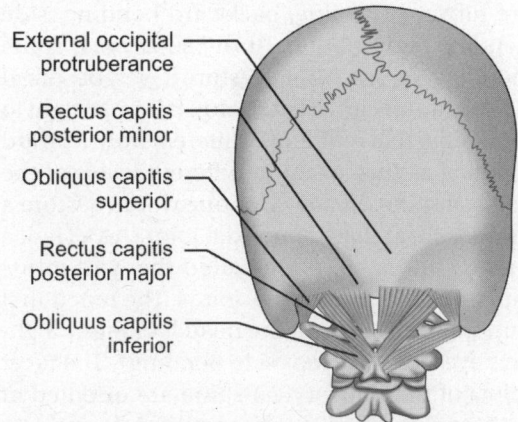

Fig. 8.8: Suboccipital musculature: (1) External occipital protuberance; (2) Rectus capitis posterior minor; (3) Obliquus capitis superior; (4) Rectus capitis posterior major; (5) Obliquus capitis inferior.

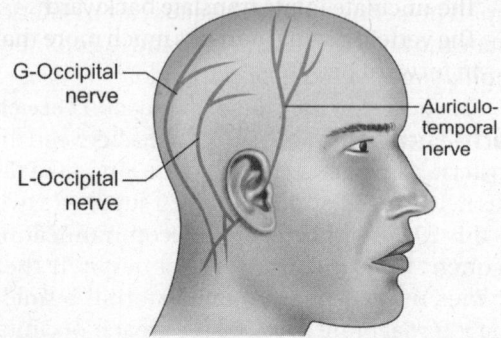

Fig. 8.9: Innervation relevant to headaches.

typically occurs behind the head, vertex and temporal areas. The irritation of this nerve occurs secondary to a dysfunction of the suboccipital muscles, occipitoatlantoaxial joint or both.[6] Additionally, irritability of the rectus capitis posterior minor may aggravate symptoms of a headache as it is in direct communication with the duramater.[7]

COMBINED MECHANICS OF THE UPPER AND MIDCERVICAL SPINE

The combined mechanics are as follows.[2] The movements possible at the midcervical spine are forward bending, backward bending, side bending and rotation. At the subcranial spine 'nodding', as one would gesture a 'yes', occurs at the atlanto-occipital (AO) joint. It is important to remember that nodding is different from forward bending as they occur at different levels of the cervical spine. Rotation, as one would gesture a 'no' occurs at the atlantoaxial joint (AA). Hence the AO joints are often called the 'yes' joints and the AA joints, the 'no' joints. The functional importance is to have the head looking straight and eyes level (except side bending). The facet joints of the midcervical spine are oriented at a 45° angle and hence the movements occur as follows.

Forward bending causes all of the facet joints to slide upward and forward relative to the facet joint below them.

Backward bending causes all of the facet joints to slide backward and downward relative to the facet joint below them.

Rotation, say right rotation, will cause the right facet joints to slide downward and backward and the left facets to slide upward and forward.

The same occurs with side bending as well, due to the 45° orientation and right side bending will cause the right facets to slide down and back and the left facets to slide up and forward.

During forward bending, the head and face look down and the reverse occurs during backward bending where the face looks up.

If the joints were flat, during rotation and side bending, the face and head would look straight over the shoulder as a perfect turn would occur. When the joints are oriented at a 45° angle, side bending and rotation will technically cause the face to look down on the shoulder, but the head continues to look straight for purposeful function. This occurs due the the following reasons.

Neurophysiologically all movements occur in diagonals and for that matter all function. If walking is considered a function then on one would argue that the fact holds true for walking being a diagonal activity. If that be the case then we would be walking at an angle sideways and not purposefully straight. When we march on forward it is right arm, left leg, left arm, right leg. Hence there exists the reciprocal activity. PNF principles describe this as reciprocal diagonals. Hence all movement are compensated reciprocally at some level. Now recalling the first rule of Fryette, neutral mechanics is side-bending and rotation coupled in opposite directions. If this be neutral then the structures in the motion segment are not unduly stressed. However, since the midcervical spinal joints, being oriented at a 45° angle have side bending and rotation coupled to the same side an opposite movement will need to occur elsewhere in the cervical complex. Hence as side bending occurs in the midcervical spine, an opposite rotation of the axis occurs to the opposite side. The same is true for rotation which is compensated by a side bending of the occiput to the opposite side.[8] The two factors that influence this are the neurophysiological basis and ligamentous tension.

The second important point to know is that the atlas always follows the occiput except during rotation. Hence forward bending will cause the atlas to slide forward, backward bending will cause the atlas to slide backwards. Side bending will cause the atlas to slide to the SAME direction as the side bend, however, rotation will cause the atlas to slide in the OPPOSITE side of the rotation because the occiput side bends to the opposite direction. This is very important to understand as it is an essential to diagnose a subcranial dysfunction. The clinical significance here is that, if one has to improve rotation, mobilizing the midcervical joints and AA articulation alone may not suffice. Side bending of the OA joints should also occur in the opposite direction, hence this should be restored. The same case with side bending as in to fully improve side bending mobilizing the midcervical joints and AA articulation alone may not suffice. Rotation of the AA joints should also occur in the opposite direction, hence this should be restored. Hence to summarize the combined mechanics of the midcervical and subcranial spine, the following is the sequence that every manual therapist should absolutely understand.

Forward Bending

- The occiput rolls forward on the atlas
- The atlas slides forward over the axis following the occiput
- The midcervical facet joints slide forward and upward
- The uncinate joints translate forward
- The vertebral canal narrows slightly.

Backward Bending

- The occiput rolls backward on the atlas
- The atlas slides backwards following the occiput
- The midcervical facet joints slide backward and downward
- The uncinate joints translate backward
- The vertebral canal narrows much more than in forward bending.

Side Bending (e.g. Right Side Bending)

- The occiput rolls down and in on the right over the atlas
- The atlas first slides right following the occiput
- The atlas then rotates left on the axis below to keep the face looking straight
- The midcervical facets on the right slide down and back
- The midcervical facets on the left slide up and forward
- The uncinate joints on the right translate backward
- The uncinate joints on the left translate forward.

Rotation (e.g. Right Rotation)

- The occipital condyle on the right rolls back and forward on the left
- The atlas rotates right and slides left, opposite to the occiput
- The occiput then side bends left over the atlas to keep the face looking straight, hence the atlas is still following the occiput
- The midcervical facets on the right slide down and back
- The midcervical facets on the left slide up and forward
- The uncinate joints on the right translate backward
- The uncinate joints on the left translate forward
- The reverse occurs with left side bending and rotation.

MECHANISM OF DYSFUNCTION

The first thing to consider in the management of mechanical cervical dysfunction is posture. The cervical spine with its soft tissue stabilizers work to support the head and position/move the head for function. A neutral and erect posture of the head and neck provide optimal balance, muscular coordination and adaptation with minimal expenditure of energy and minimal stress on the supporting structures. If the posture is not neutral and balanced, the weight is either anterior or posterior to the joint. The head and neck is then counter balanced by passive tension in the soft tissues or increased muscular activity. The most common postural deviation of the cervical area is the forward head posture (Fig. 8.10).

Components of the Forward Head Posture

The forward head posture is seen either as a habit, natural tendency, slouching or wearing bifocals. It is also seen in individuals who function looking down as in a desk job. The dynamics are as follows:

To maintain the head in neutral a subcranial backward bending occurs. This can cause a shortening of the soft tissue structures including the suboccipital muscles. Restriction can occur in the OA and AA joints. The greater occipital nerve can be irritated causing occipital and temporal headaches.

In the midcervical area, the facets are in forward bending to compensate resulting in a loss of the normal cervical lordosis. The restriction in the subcranial area can be compensated by increased mobility in the midcervical area, resulting in increased wear and tear and conventional 'cervical spondylosis'. The cervical musculature, especially the guide wires namely upper trapezius, levator scapulae and sternomastoid can contract and be altered in their length tension relationships. Their attachment to the cervical vertebra can alter alignment resulting in extension, rotation, sidebending (ERS) and flexion, rotation, sidebending (FRS) (opening and closing) dysfunctions. This can in turn affect the facet joints and the capsule compromising the foramen and spinal nerve resulting in radiculopathies.[9] The disc can be sheared predisposing to disk herniations, wear and tear. The muscle shortening can also cause a compressive effect on the joints and discs further leading to wear and tear. Contraction of the scalenes can compromise the thoracic outlet and elevation of the first rib due to its distal attachment on the first rib. This can compromise the costoclavicular space leading to the symptoms of a thoracic outlet syndrome.

Due to the forward head position, the jaw is forced to open. To keep the mouth closed the masseter and temporalis become hyperactive, causing increased compressive forces on the temporomandibular joint (TMJ) leading to dysfunction.

The shoulder girdle protracts including the scapula which can cause an impingement of the supraspinatus tendon at the shoulder. The internal rotators including the pectoralis minor can tighten leading to symptoms of the thoracic outlet.

The abdominal wall can constrict due to a chronic forward head decreasing diaphragmatic breathing and increases upper respiratory breathing. This increases activity of the scalenes which is an accessory muscle of breathing leading to symptoms of a thoracic outlet syndrome.

The vicious cycle is obvious and the clinician should remember that these dysfunctions not only occur due to faulty posture, but also due to weakness of cervical muscles and overuse. Weakness and overuse can fatigue muscle which respond by contracting or tightening and on persistence can cause dysfunctions described above. The function of the cervical musculature

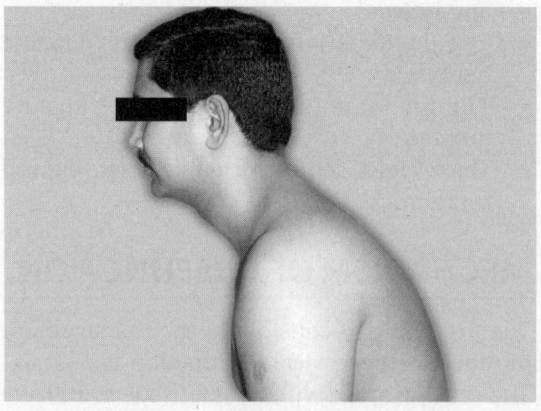

Fig. 8.10: Forward head posture.

to draw the head backwards also increases their vulnerability to dysfunction. Prolonged flexion of the head for extended periods of time, as a surgeon or a writer would do for example (looking down on the operating table or the desk), can fatigue these muscles.[10] The immediate response to excessive fatigue is a contraction which can be continual in occupational situations. This results in dysfunctional states.

Trauma

The most common cause for trauma and subsequent irritation of the cervical area are whiplash injuries. Often occurs secondary to being hit from behind by a moving vehicle or being violently pushed from behind. The resultant momentum causes the head to violently snap back into extension and subsequently flexion. This results in trauma of the suboccipital and cervical muscles and the facet joints of the subcranial more than the midcervical complex.

The previous causes described were secondary to faulty posture, fatigue and overuse, however, whiplash injuries cause actual trauma to the cervical musculature especially the sternomastoid, longus colli and cervicis as they are anteriorly placed and contract heavily to prevent the head from snapping back.[11] The facet joints of the subcranial spine more than the midcervical spine are most involved. They hence result in a wider array of symptoms including intense headaches making their management relatively difficult.

Owing to the strain of the facet capsule and subsequent muscle guarding, the joints of the subcranial complex can exhibit a greater deal of restriction and pain with more intense headaches. (The suboccipital muscles are intimately related physiologically to the extrinsic and intrinsic ocular muscles other neck and trunk musculature.) Hence, pain in the region of the eye is a common feature. Proprioceptive impulses from them are conveyed (over the first and second spinal nerves) to the upper cord and thence re-distributed to appropriate stations at the segmental and suprasegmental levels.

The direction of gaze, visual axes and accompanying head, neck and trunk posturing are produced and maintained by movement and fixations, among which these small suboccipital muscles play a major role. The principal interconnecting pathways between ocular and neck musculature include the medial longitudinal fasciculi and the reticular substance of the brainstem, both of which receive proprioceptive, exteroceptive and interoceptive modalities essential for the integration and regulation of external orientation and internal homeostasis. These brainstem and cord functions guide and are governed by higher stations of neural integration including the neuropsychic levels. It is not surprising, therefore, that disturbances of equilibrium and autonomic functions, both subjective and objective occur in a traumatic situation since deep pain in the neck and head, together with evidence of cervical muscle spasm, head and neck alignment changes are prominent features in whiplash injuries.[12]

It may be of value to add that these symptoms are not only seen in whiplash situations, but also in prolonged and chronic overuse/fatigue syndromes of the subcranial spine. Their occurrence in whiplash injuries, however, are relatively more common.[3]

EXAMINATION

Midcervical Spine

Midcervical examination is relatively straight forward as the facets slide only in two directions, forward and backward. The possibility of a muscular restriction should first be ruled out to conclude that the restriction is at the facet joint.

Active Movement

Forward Bending

The patient is asked to nod the head and gently drop the neck down towards the chest. Note for any restriction and possible signs of transverse ligament involvement (Fig. 8.11).

Backward Bending

The patient is instructed to look upward toward the ceiling without leaning the trunk backwards (Fig. 8.12). Note for restriction. This movement is not often tested and should be avoided in the elderly to avoid a possible vertebral artery compromise.

Side Bending

The patient is instructed to drop the ear towards the shoulder with the face looking straight. Note for restriction. Now the shoulder on the opposite side is raised as in a shrug and the elbow is supported by the examiner. This will slacken the muscles on that side. Now if the range of motion in side bending increases then the restriction was probably more muscular. If the range appears restricted despite slacking the musculature by shrugging, then the restriction is probably more in the facet joints (Figs. 8.13 and 8.14).

Rotation

The patient is instructed to turn the head towards the side and vice versa. The opposite shoulder is shrugged upwards and a change in range, if any, is noted to rule out a muscular restriction (Figs. 8.15 and 8.16).

Passive Movement

As mentioned earlier the facets in the midcervical area slide only in two directions. Up and forward and down and back. In other words there is either an up slide or a down slide. The clinician should hence be able to examine this movement occurring in every segment of the midcervical spine. The up and forward is called an 'open' position and the down and back is called a 'closed' position of the facet joint. The reason for segmental testing versus gross motion is absolutely important.

The reason being that even if one joint is restricted the other joints may move excessively and compensate to complete the gross motion. This may give the clinician a wrong impression that the motion is normal. In reality, however, there may be a segment that is restricted and being compensated by the segment above or below it

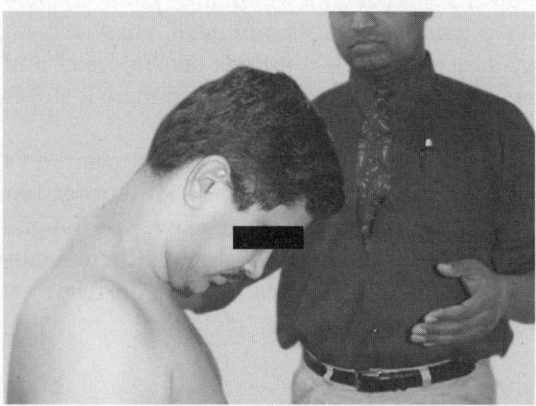

Fig. 8.11: Forward bending.

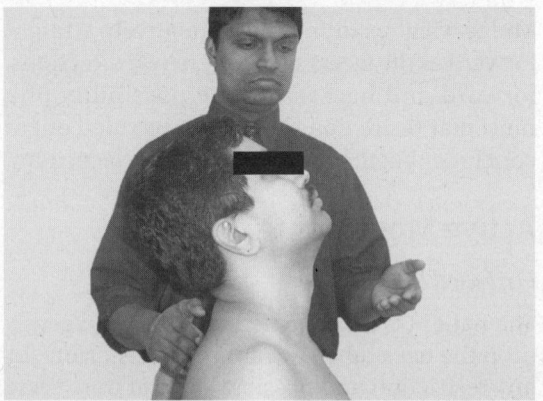

Fig. 8.12: Backward bending.

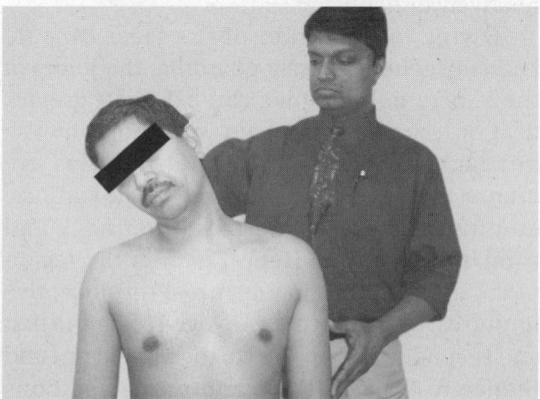

Fig. 8.13: Side bending.

Cervical Spine

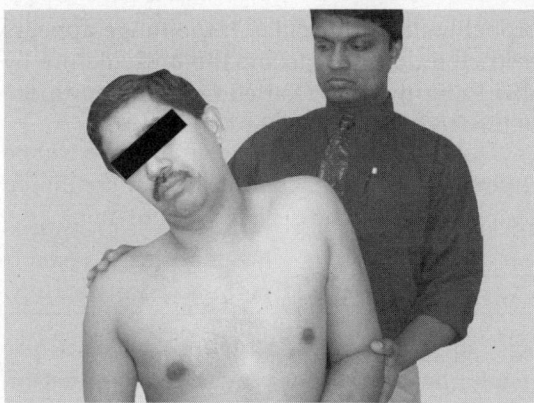

Fig. 8.14: Side bending with shoulder shrug to slacken musculature.

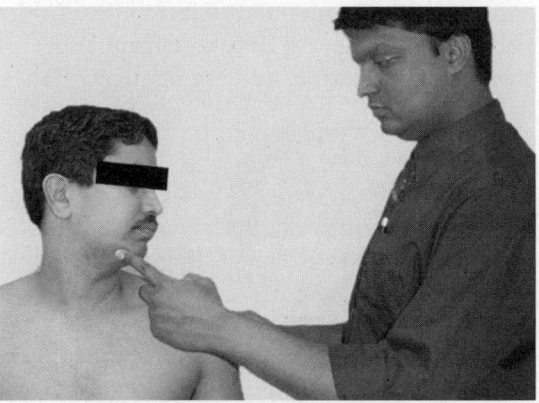

Fig. 8.15: Rotation with overpressure at end range.

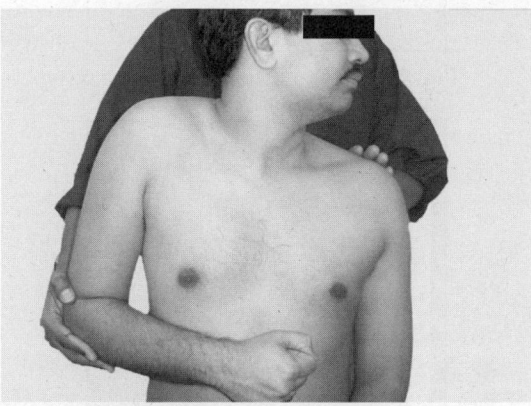

Fig. 8.16: Rotation with shoulder shrug to slacken musculature.

which invariably is rendered hypermobile and predisposed to further dysfunction.

The movement is tested both with the neck in flexion and extension. Caution should be exercised when the movement is tested in extension for possible vertebral artery compromise and should be done with extreme caution in the elderly.

MIDCERVICAL SPINE SOMATIC DIAGNOSIS

Basic Hold (Fig. 8.17)

Normal movements occur in patterns or diagonals. It is usually a combination of movements in all three cardinal planes (flexion/extension, side bending, and rotation). The movements of the vertebral column occur in diagonal patterns and two possibilities can exist and are as follows:

- Extension, rotation side bending (ERS) opening restriction (not opening)/ERS flexion restriction (not flexing)
- Flexion, rotation, side bending (FRS). Closing restriction (not closing)/FRS extension restriction (not extending).

Opening Restriction (Not Opening)/ERS Flexion Restriction (Not Flexing)

On reviewing spinal joint motion we inferred that during flexion the facets slide equally forward and the exact opposite during extension. Let us consider two segments, C4 and C5. Assume the left facet of C4 is restricted, or stuck in extension (closed). On blocking the level of the thyroid with the second MP on the left and side bending to that level, right rotation is attempted and chin deviation is observed. This is done with the neck flexed. Assume the chin deviates half as much to the right in comparison with chin deviation to the left. Then one can assume that the left C4 is stuck in extension, rotation, side bending left (ERS left C4) or an opening restriction of C4 on the left since it does not flex or open (Fig. 8.18).

Closing Restriction (Not Closing)/FRS Extension Restriction (Not Extending)

Assume the right facet of C4 is restricted, or stuck in flexion (open). On blocking the level of the thyroid with the second MP on the left and side bending to that level, right rotation is attempted and chin deviation is observed. This is done with the neck extended. (Fig. 8.19). Assume the chin deviates half as much to the right in comparison with chin deviation to the left. Then one can assume that the right C4 is stuck in flexion, rotation, side bending (FRS left not right of C4 as you go by the posteriority) or a closing restriction of C4 on the right since it does not extend or close (Fig. 8.20).

It is obvious that both sides be tested for both ERS and FRS dysfunctions. The principles thus described are with regards to the midcervical spine in isolation. However, the midcervical and subcranial spine work so closely to each other that dysfunctions occur as a combination due to the combined mechanics.

Examination of the subcranial spine will be described next and identification of combined dysfunctions will be described thereafter.

SUBCRANIAL SPINE

The subcranial spine owing to its unique mechanics has a more intricate examination protocol with specific attention to localize findings. The reason being that movement and symptoms may also arise from the midcervical spine. The orientation of the facet joints in the subcranial spine are different from those of the midcervical area, and are relatively flatter.

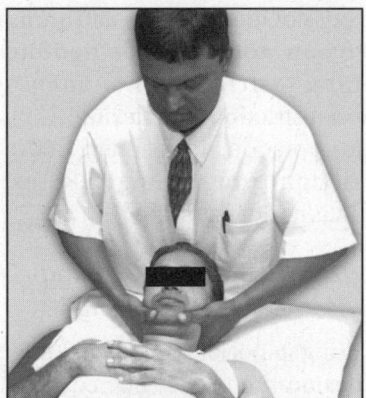

Fig. 8.17: Basic hold.

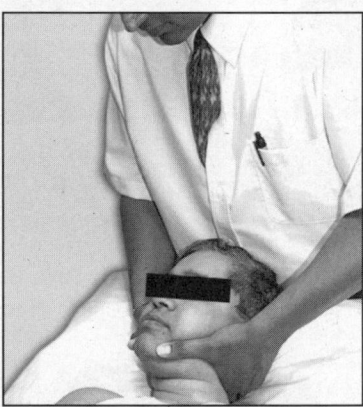

Fig. 8.19: Left-mid cervical opening.

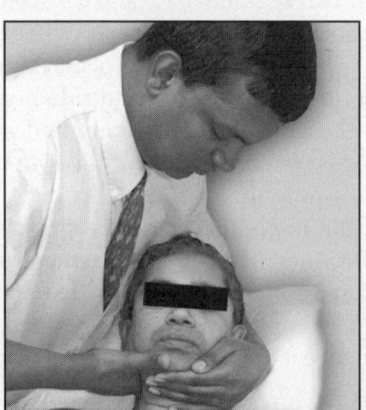

Fig. 8.18: Testing opening restriction on the left

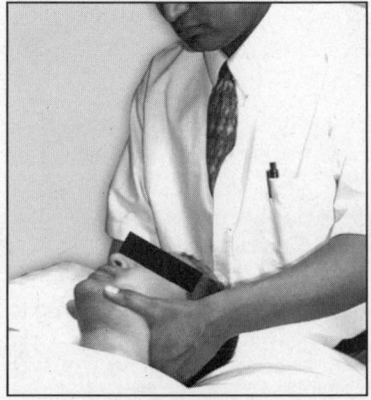

Fig. 8.20: Right-mid cervical closing.

Hence examination is more straightforward. The key is to lock the midcervical spine to localize movement. They will be dealt specifically.

The only exception is that the FRS and ERS concepts do not apply in the subcranial joints (OA/AA). Their examination is more unique. The other area where they do not apply as well is the pelvic complex (sacrum and ilium).

Active Movement

Forward Bending

From what we inferred from the previous chapters, forward bending and backward bending occurs in the atlanto-occipital joint (AO). The movement is technically not forward bending, but rather forward 'nodding', the 'yes' joints, as was described. Hence the patient is asked to nod forward as in saying 'no'. The landmark to be observed is the chin in relation to the midline. If there is a deviation of the chin from midline, an OA dysfunction should be suspected. The side of the deviation is the side of the dysfunction. For example, if the chin deviates to the right then the restriction is probably at the right OA joint (Fig. 8.21).

Backward Bending

Similarly, the patient is asked to backward 'nod' (not bend and look up to the ceiling). In a backward nod the chin deviation is observed and the deviation is opposite to the side of the dysfunction. Hence, if the right OA joint is restricted in backward bending, the chin deviates to the left. Backward bending dysfunction in the subcranial spine is not a common dysfunction (Fig. 8.22).

Rotation

Rotation predominantly occurs in the atlantoaxial joint. Remember, however, that rotation also occurs in the midcervical spine. The key is to localize this movement to the AA joints so that the rotation being tested is pure AA rotation. This is not accurately possible as an active movement, hence the clinician must rely on the passive

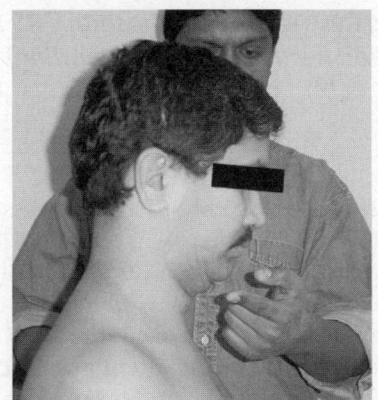

Fig. 8.21: Atlanto-occipital forward nod.

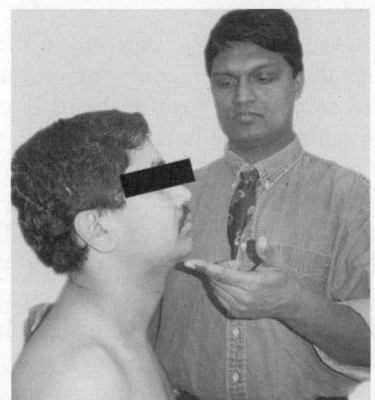

Fig. 8.22: Atlanto-occipital backward nod.

motion test to obtain information. It is described in the section on somatic diagnosis.

Passive Movement Tests and Musculoskeletal Red Flag Assessment

Passive motion testing in the subcranial spine involves a greater risk of stressing the vulnerable structures as described earlier. Hence these structures should be tested first for integrity before any other testing procedures, or for that matter, treatment procedures are done. The three structure to be tested first are alar and transverse ligaments, and vertebral artery.

Alar Ligament

The patient is seated and the clinician places one hand over the vertex of the head and the thumb of the other hand is placed over the spinous process of C2 (which is the first palpable spinous process at the base of the occiput). The patient is instructed to relax fully and informed that the head is going to be side bent gently on either sides for just a few degrees (Fig. 8.23).

On side bending, the spinous process will be felt to deviate immediately to the opposite side. So for example, if the head is side bent to the right the spinous process will be felt to deviate to the left. If this does not occur then one should suspect a laxity of the ligament or a fracture of the odontoid process, or both. Any subcranial treatment procedure, mainly traction is strictly contraindicated if a laxity of the alar ligament is suspected.

The same test can be performed in supine lying with the clinician facing the patient from the head side. The patients head is cradled with the palms of the hand while both middle fingers are placed on either sides of the C2 spinous process. The patient is instructed on the procedure and asked to side bend for no more than 10 to 15 degrees. On side bending, the spinous process will be felt to deviate immediately to the opposite side and felt by the opposite finger. So for example, if the head is side bent to the right the spinous process will be felt to deviate to the left and can be felt by the left middle finger. If this does not occur then one should suspect a laxity of the ligament or a fracture of the odontoid process, or both.

The alar ligament is commonly stretched or injured during whiplash injuries and injuries to the cervical spine. Owing to its attachment to the odontoid process, a fracture of the odontoid can allow the ligament to cause a stretch on it leading to instability. Any excessive motion, especially side bending can add to the instability and can be life-threatening. A traction maneuver can possibly dislodge the odontoid and cause it to compress the neural structures in the foramen magnum. A compromise on alar ligament integrity is seen in disease states especially rheumatoid arthritis. It is also seen in an individual with Down syndrome. Other conditions that can affect alar ligament stability are advanced stages of pregnancy and collagen disorders like os odontoideum, Marfans syndrome, systemic lupus erythematosis, etc. These situations are strict contraindications for manual therapy of the subcranial spine.

Transverse Ligament

The patient is sitting and is asked to perform a subcranial forward bending by retracting the chin backwards and inwards. A careful overpressure is added at the chin counter-pressure over the spinous process of C2 (Fig. 8.24).

A positive test can produce sharp pain that is shock-like-sensation with tingling numbness in the extremities. Sometimes a 'clunk' can be heard in situations of instability.

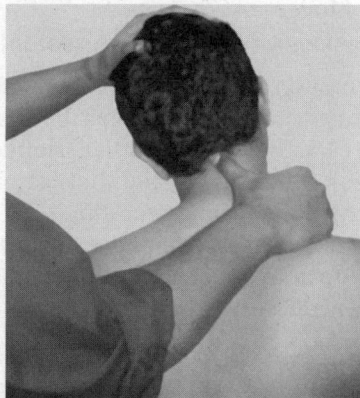

Fig. 8.23: Assessing alar ligament integrity in sitting.

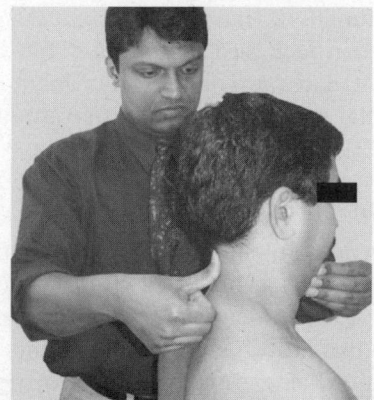

Fig. 8.24: Assessing transverse ligament integrity in sitting.

The transverse ligament prevents the atlas from sliding forward during forward bending. Hence, this ligament can be injured during forced forward bending. A laxity of this ligament can allow the atlas to slide forward bringing the odontoid process close to the cord (Figs. 8.6 A to C). Hence on testing it is not just pain that is produced but cord signs as well such as tingling and numbness in the extremities.

Cervical Flexion

Owing to the aggressive nature of the test an alternate simple test may be performed. The patient is sitting and the clinician faces the patient from the side and places the palm of the hand in front of the forehead of the patient as a potential support. The patient is asked to gently flex the neck forward (Fig. 8.25). On reviewing subcranial mechanics, the atlas follows the occiput and hence would translate forward. This brings the odontoid closer into the spinal canal and to the cord. If the transverse ligament is intact, no consequence is noted. However, if the ligament is lax the possibility a cord compromise exists. A positive test can produce sharp pain that is shock-like-sensation with tingling numbness in the extremities.

Manual therapy procedures especially sub-cranial forward bending can seriously compromise the cord if the transverse ligament is lax and hence is strictly contraindicated. A patient with a compromise of the alar and transverse ligaments present with severe muscle guarding and hence sometimes these tests cannot be performed and may also be dangerous to do so. They present with a heavy head and difficulty in holding their head up. They may also present with severe headaches. All of the above warrant immediate medical attention.

Vertebral Artery

The patient is lying supine and the clinician faces the patient from the head side. The clinician explains to the patient that he/she is about to extend and rotate the neck to one side and hold it there for 15 to 20 seconds. Ideally it is best not to suggest to the patient as to what he/she may experience. The procedure is begun and ideally the head is not brought over the edge of the table. Either the head end of the treatment table can be tilted down or a pillow can be arranged in the scapular area. The reason being that in case the patient tests positive, the head rest can be immediately brought to neutral or the pillow can be removed. The clinician supports the head with both hands and first extends the head fully backward. The patient is asked to keep the eyes widely open and the clinician monitors for signs. The head is then rotated to one side and held in that position for 15 to 20 seconds (Fig. 8.26). The patient is asked to count backwards from 15 to 1 as this requires alert cognition. In the 15 to 20 seconds period the clinician observes with full attention and caution for:
- Dizziness
- Diplopia

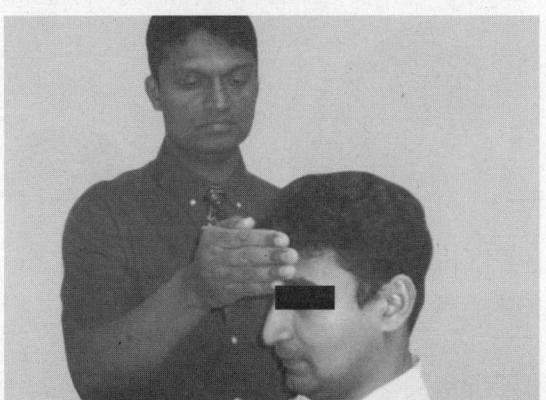

Fig. 8.25: Assessing transverse ligament integrity in sitting.

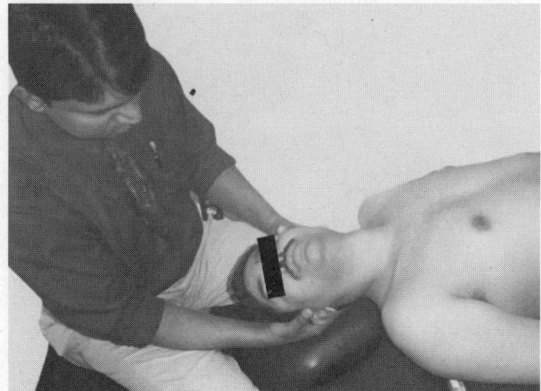

Fig. 8.26: Vertebral artery testing in supine.

- Dysarthria
- Dysphagia
- Drop attacks

If any of the above are suspected the clinician should immediately bring the head back to neutral and elevate the leg with pillows to facilitate circulation to the head. Manual therapy, especially to the subcranial spine is strictly contraindicated if the patient tests are positive for vertebral artey insufficiency.

Contemporary research questions the validity of the standard vertebral artery test. Hence it is suggested the clinician should probably follow this as a rule. All cervical procedures should be tested at the end range of that particular procedure by holding for 15 seconds at least, and observing for positive vertebral artery signs. This should be done routinely and a negative finding may encourage proceeding with the technique.

Other important tests to be performed to rule out the presence of red flags are as follows:

Vertex Compression

The patient is seated and the clinician faces the patient from the side. A mild compression is applied over the vertex (Fig. 8.27). Moderate-to-severe pain seen with an associated history of trauma and severe muscle guarding can indicate serious pathology as in a Jefferson fracture. A Jefferson fracture is a fracture of the ring of the atlas. The causes are due to a hit on top of the head as in standing up from a stooped position where the ceiling is very low. The vertical compression can crack the atlas line, a glass bangle (atlas) placed under a hard ball (occiput) and compressed. A positive test with a pertinent history may require immediate medical attention.

Pupil Light Reflex

The patient is seated with the clinician facing the patient. The patient is asked to focus his gaze on the index finger of the clinician which is held at eye level. Using a pen torch, light is flashed into the patient eye and the clinician observed for the pupil to contract (Fig. 8.28). Contraction of the pupil on the same side indicates an intact optic nerve. Contraction of the opposite side when light is flashed on the same side indicates an intact oculomotor nerve. The reason for doing this test is two fold that are:

- Sometimes a whiplash injury can cause a concussion. This helps to determine if there is a brainstem involvement.
- Whiplash causes soft tissue lesions, especially of the small intervertebral muscles and joints which are rich in proprioceptors. These proprioceptors fire chaotically and may establish a proprio-autonomic reflex which might impair the function of the brainstem. (This reflex causes a disturbance in the pupillary motor activity after whiplash. Pupillary motor activity improved after injection of local anesthetics into the cervical muscles). The clinician should note that other

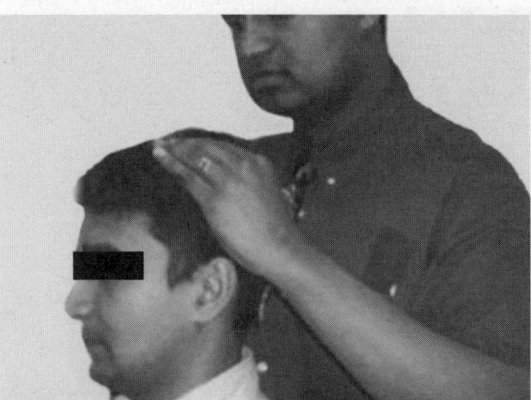

Fig. 8.27: Vertex compression.

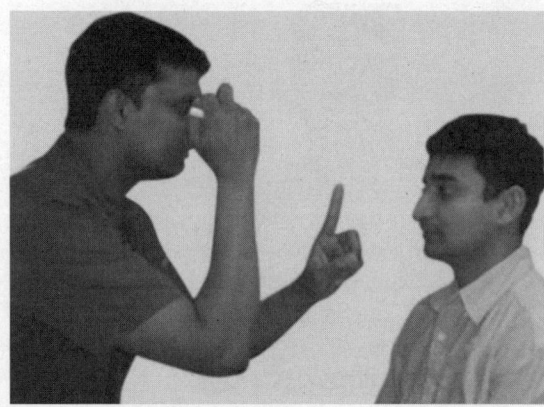

Fig. 8.28: Pupillary reflex testing.

conditions can cause diminished pupil reflex including medications (barbituates).[13]

Battle Sign and Raccoon Sign

Patient's presenting with a hit on the head, fall on the head and other forms of concussion should be inspected behind the ear for hyperemic areas. A presence is called a 'battle sign'. Additionally puffiness with redness around the eyes is looked for as they resemble the eyes of a raccoon. A presence of the two may indicate a basal skull fracture and warrants immediate medical attention.

Clay-Shoveler's Fracture

A clay-shoveler's fracture is the fracture of the spinous process of C7. It is seen in laborers who perform activities involving lifting weights rapidly with the arms extended. Examples of these activities include shoveling and pulling. The severe contraction force of the muscles (trapezius and rhomboid muscles) pulling on the spine at the base of the neck actually avulse the spinous process of the vertebral body. Symptoms include burning, "knife-like" pain at the level of the fractured spine between the scapulae. The pain can sharply increase with repeated activity that strains the muscles of the upper back. The C7 spinous process and nearby muscles are exquisitely tender.

With the patient sitting the clinician supports the head and gently runs the fingers down the spinous processes (Fig. 8.29). Acute tenderness over the lower cervical area especially over C7 may indicate a clay-shoveler's fracture with an appropriate history.

SUBCRANIAL SPINE SOMATIC DIAGNOSIS

Dysfunction

The occiput for purpose of reference is termed C0, as the atlas and axis being C1 and C2, respectively. The dysfunctions in the subcranial spine are grouped as C0, C1 (OA) and C1, C2 (AA) dysfunctions, respectively. The dysfunctions are termed according to the direction of the restriction.

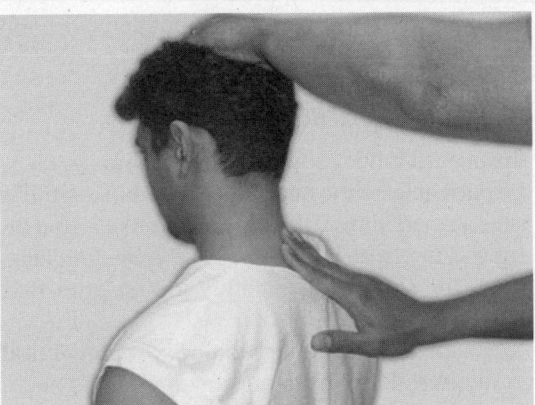

Fig. 8.29: Assessing Clay-shoveler's fracture.

C0, C1 (OA Dysfunctions)

The movements possible at C0 and C1 are forward and backward nodding and side bending. The principles of diagnosis then would be to detect restriction of these movements specific to the direction of restriction.

C0, C1 Forward Bending Restriction

The patient is lying supine and the clinician faces the patient from the head side. The occiput is cradled in both palms with the fingers directed towards the occipital protruberance and mastoid. The thumbs grip the temporal areas. The examiner gently glides the occipital condyles backward by applying a downward pressure on the occiput (Fig. 8.30).

When this is done the occipital condyles roll backward and the atlas slides forward. When either of these are restricted a restriction will be felt on performing this maneuver.

With the face looking straight, both condyles are being tested. However, to localize and detect restriction on one side, the head is rotated slightly and the same maneuver is applied. For example, if the head is rotated right and if a downward pressure is applied, then the right OA joint is being tested.

If a restriction is present the patient typically feels pain and discomfort when the maneuver is applied. Also, when the maneuver is localized to one side as in rotating the head to the right or left, the discomfort is usually felt locally on one side more than the other.

C0, C1 Backward Bending Restriction

The patient is lying supine and the clinician faces the patient from the head side. The hold is similar as described above. The only difference is that an upward pressure is directed on the occiput (Fig. 8.31). The side being tested is similar to testing forward bending.

When this maneuver is done, the occipital condyles roll forward and the atlas slides backward. A restriction will be felt if this does not occur.

Testing backward bending should be done with caution for the risk of possible vertebral artery compromise. The most common restriction seen, however, is forward bending. If one recollects that in a forward head posture the subcranial spine is stuck in backward bending and hence forward bending is often felt to be restricted on testing.

One should always remember that when the term forward bending restriction is used, it denotes that the forward bending 'movement' is restricted and that the segment is stuck in backward bending.

C0, C1 Side Bending Restriction

Upon recollection it was inferred that the atlas follows the occiput with all movements except rotation. Hence on side bending, if not restricted the atlas should be felt to slide to the same side as the side bending. It also rotates to the opposite side and hence the transverse process is felt slightly anterior.

Hence the patient is sitting with the clinician facing the patient from behind. Both transverse processes of C1 are palpated with the tips of the fingers slightly anterior to the transverse process (Fig. 8.32). The patient is asked to side bend to either side and the clinician palpates for an increase in prominence. For example, if the head is side bent left, the transverse process on the left is felt as an increased prominence. If this is not felt then it denotes a side bending restriction of the atlanto-occipital joint on the left. The same theory applies on the right.

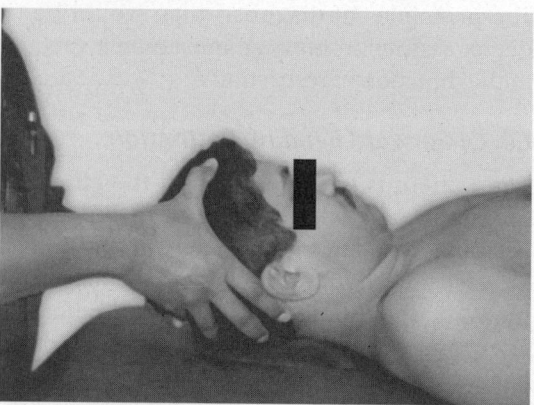

Fig. 8.30: OA passive forward nod.

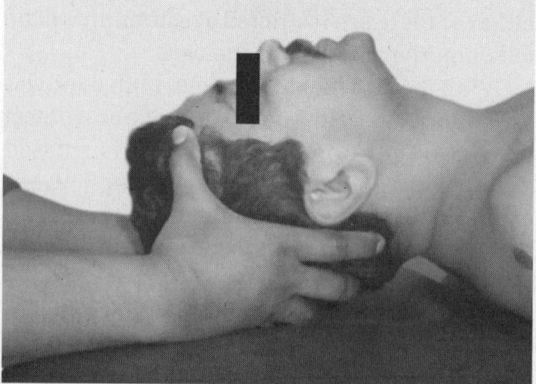

Fig. 8.31: OA passive backward nod.

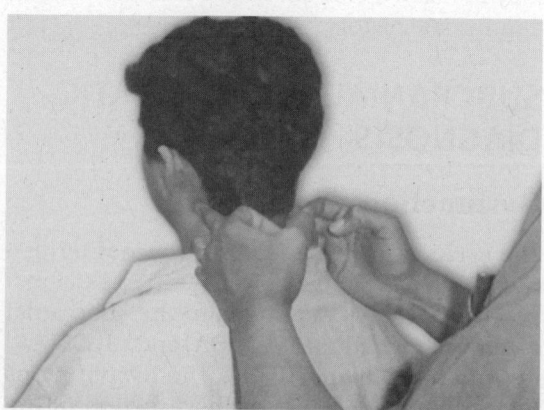

Fig. 8.32: Assessing OA side bending.

C1, C2 (AA Dysfunctions)

The movements occurring at the atlantoaxial joint is exclusively rotation hence that will be the only movement to be examined. Rotation in the AA joint is, however, accompanied by midcervical spine rotation and this has to be avoided during testing. So to localize rotation at the AA joint the midcervical spine should be locked. This is achieved by either side bending or forward bending the midcervical spine and then rotating the occiput. Side bending is preferred as it is a more aggressive locking of the midcervical spine. Forward bending is used if there is excessive restriction or guarding that does not allow adequate side bending.

Rotation Restriction

The patient is lying supine and the clinician faces the patient from the head side. The clinician holds the occiput in flexion and gently side bends the neck to the side, as allowed by available range. The neck is then rotated to the opposite side. This exclusively tests the AA joint (Fig. 8.33). The test is done ideally with the shoulder in a shrug position bilaterally as this helps to ease the soft tissue that may interfere with the test (sternomastoid).

Determining the side being tested is of importance when performing this test. As the neck is in flexion, the side being tested will be the side opposite to the side of the rotation. For example, if the neck which is in flexion is side bent left and rotated right, it is the left AA joint that is being tested.

Tissue Tenderness

Tissue texture abnormality in the subcranial and midcervical spine is usually felt as a palpable thickening which is often times tender. It can be felt on suboccipital muscles, on lamina and the transverse process. It is of a greater significance when the tenderness is felt exclusively on the site of dysfunction.

Treatment

The progression for treatment is based on the findings. If the dysfunction is identified exclusively at the subcranial or midcervical spine then it should be addressed as appropriate. This is, however, relatively rare as dysfunctions are seen as a combination of both subcranial and midcervical. The progression should then be cephalocaudal, in that the subcranial dysfunction be addressed first before the midcervical dysfunction is addressed.

Treatment of the subcranial spine will incorporate techniques to free:

C0, C1 (OA Dysfunctions)

1. Forward nodding restriction
2. Backward nodding restriction
3. Side bending restriction.

Soft Tissue Inhibition

The soft tissues especially the muscle and myofascia are strong supportive barriers for the skeletal alignment. Hence intervention of techniques to free joint restriction should always be preceded by soft tissue inhibition. Traditional soft tissue mobilization and massage may most definitely be effective, but for specificity and time constraints inhibition techniques may be adopted.

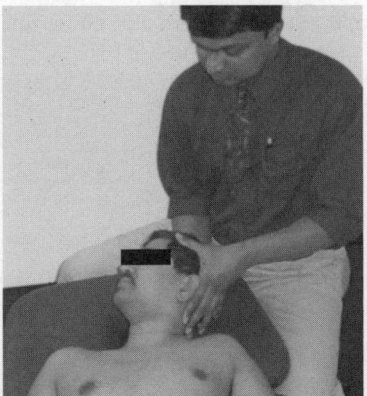

Fig. 8.33: Assessing atlantroaxiel rotation.

Inhibitive Distraction of the Subcranial Spine (Suboccipital Release)

The patient is lying supine and the clinician faces the head side of the patient. The clinician places the index, middle, and ring fingers of each hand on either sides of the occipital rim, just distal to it.

The fingers first direct a gentle upward compression, and is then followed by a long axis traction which is held for several seconds and released (Fig. 8.34).

This is a powerful technique and is strictly contraindicated in situations of ligament insufficiency especially in alar-and transverse ligaments.

Forward Nodding

The patient is lying supine and the clinician faces the patient from the head side. Assume forward nodding is restricted on the right. The head is gently rotated to the right. The forehead of the patient is grasped with the palm of the right hand. Subcranial nodding is induced with the right hand while the left index, middle and ring finger blocks the atlas from sliding back due to the restriction (because ideally the atlas should slide forward during forward nodding, but since it is restricted on the right it may slide backward as the occipital condyles roll backward). This will help free the atlas to slide forward freeing the restriction (Fig. 8.35).

Alternately, the patient is lying supine with the clinician facing the patient from the head side. The cervical area is cradled with one hand and the index, middle and ring fingers of the other hand are placed on the suboccipital aperture. Maintaining slight flexion, the clinician brings the anterior aspect of the shoulder to the forehead of the patient (Fig. 8.36). A gentle downward and forward compression is applied through the shoulder. Subcranial nodding is induced with the right shoulder, while the index, middle and ring finger blocks the atlas from sliding back due to the restriction (because ideally the atlas should slide forward during forward nodding, but since it is restricted on the right it may slide backward as the occipital condyles roll backward). This will help free the atlas to slide forward freeing the restriction.

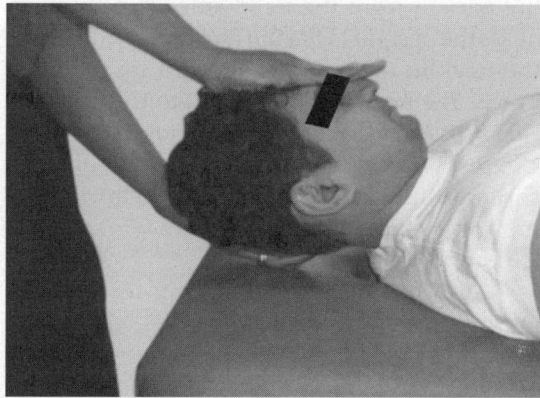

Fig. 8.35: OA forward nod mobilization.

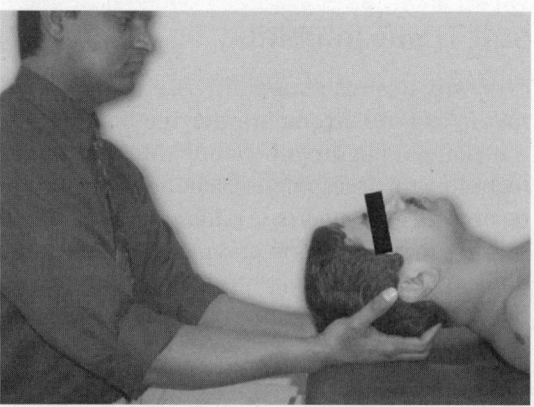

Fig. 8.34: Suboccipital release.

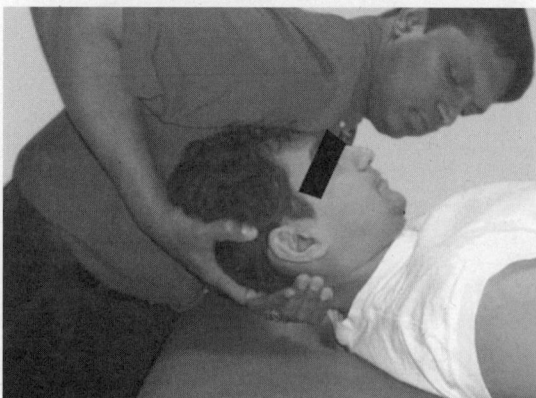

Fig. 8.36: OA forward nod with shoulder reinforcement.

Cervical Spine

Backward Nodding

The patient and clinician position are as above. The fingers of the clinicians' hand are placed on the external occipital protuberance on both sides. The patient is asked to push backwards with the head, against the fingers of the clinicians' hand (Fig. 8.37). This contracts the rectus capitis posterior minor and the obliqus capitis superior. These muscles attach to the occiput and atlas and on contraction they pull the atlas backward, which is stuck forward. This aids to free the restriction.

Side Bending

The patient is lying supine and the clinician faces the patient from the head side. Assume side bending is restricted on the right. The head is gently rotated and side bent to the right. The forehead of the patient is grasped with the palm of the right hand. Subcranial nodding with side bending is induced with the right hand in a downward and diagonal direction, while the left hand supports the occipital area (Fig. 8.38).

C1, C2 (AA Dysfunctions)

Rotation restriction: Assume right rotation is restricted and the restriction is at the left AA joint. Hence, for a restriction in right rotation, the head is side bent fully to the left and slightly rotated right. The opposite hand holds the chin and cradles the head in the forearm. The abdomen of the clinician supports the head in position. The right metacarpophalangeal joint (MCP) contacts the right transverse process of C1 (Fig. 8.39). The right MCP now exerts a lateral and downward pressure on the right transverse process of C1 to rotate it towards the right. This will restore rotation of the atlas to the right, restoring rotation of the AA joint to the right. Remember to always assess and monitor for signs of vascular compromise or instability.

In the illustration, ideally, the head is rotated slightly to the right.

MIDCERVICAL SPINE

Treatment of the midcervical spine will incorporate techniques to free:

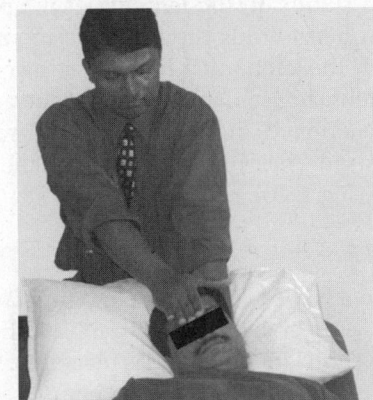

Fig. 8.38: OA side bending mobilization.

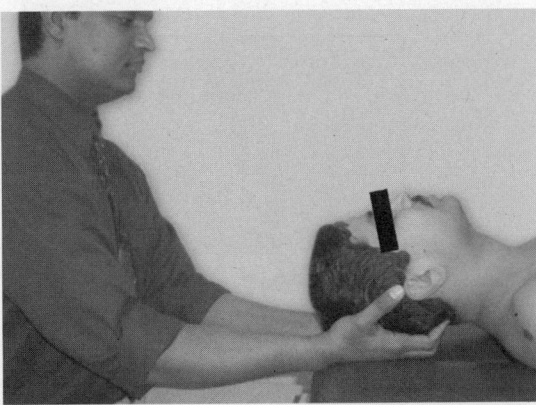

Fig. 8.37: OA backward nod mobilization using rectus capitis posterior major and obliquus capitis superior.

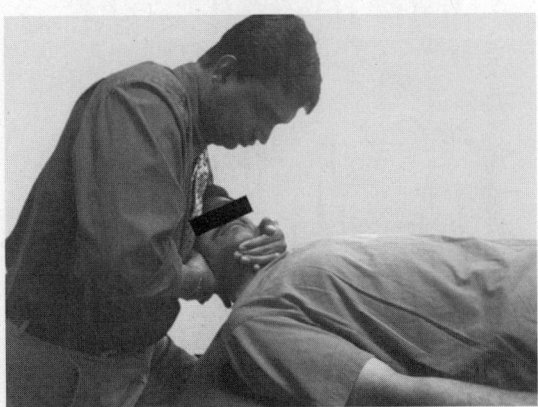

Fig. 8.39: Atlantoaxial rotation mobilization.

C3 to C7 (Midcervical Dysfunctions)

1. Extended, rotated, side-bent (ERS) restriction not opening
2. Flexion, rotation, side bending (FRS) restriction not closing.

Soft Tissue Inhibition

Soft tissue inhibition for the midcervical spine can be initiated using inhibitive distraction as described for the subcranial spine, followed by:

Lateral Stretch

Method 1

The patient is lying supine and the clinician stands on the side of the patients head. If the clinician stands on the left side of the patient, the right hand holds the forehead to stabilize the head. The left hand is placed on the cervical paravertebral musculature. A lateral and anterior stretch is applied and held for several seconds and released. The same is repeated on the opposite side (Fig. 8.40).

Method 2

The patient is lying supine and the clinician faces the head side of the patient. To inhibit the right side, the clinicians' left hand is placed under the occiput of the patient. The right hand is cupped over the clavicle, first rib and scapula of the right shoulder. The occiput is laterally bent to the left while a downward counter-pressure is applied over the right acromion. The head is then rotated slightly left to inhibit the right levator scapula and posterior scalenes, and rotated slightly right to inhibit the right trapezius. The procedure is repeated in neutral for the middle scalenes and in extension for the anterior scalenes. Vertebral artery sign are monitored, especially in extension. Both sides are alternated, one muscle at a time.

Levator Scapula

Side bend and rotation away (Fig. 8.41).

Trapezius

Side bend away and rotation to the same side (Fig. 8.42).

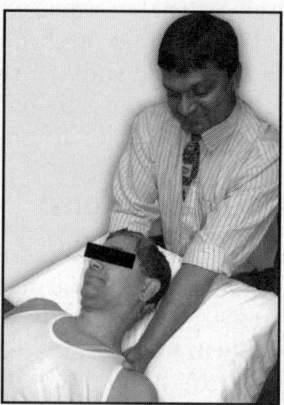

Fig. 8.41: Levator scapula stretch.

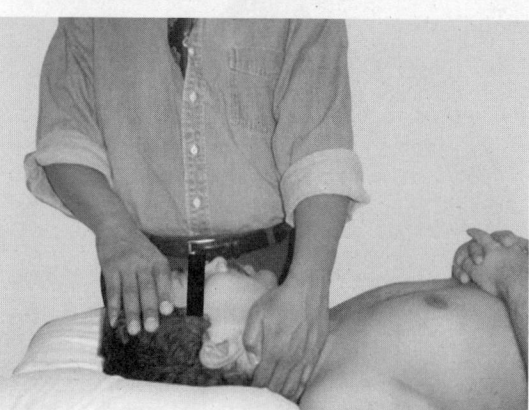

Fig. 8.40: Lateral stretch.

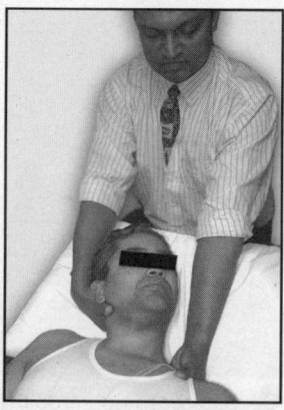

Fig. 8.42: Trapezius stretch.

Scalenes

Side bending away with slight extension (Fig. 8.43).

Technique to Free an ERS Restriction on the Right (Right not Opening)

Basic Hold

The basic hold is to cradle the occiput with the forearm of one hand and the fingers are placed under the chin. The head MUST be in a neutral position. The second MP of the other hand is placed on the articular pillars of the opposite side with the thumb resting on the chin (Fig. 8.44).

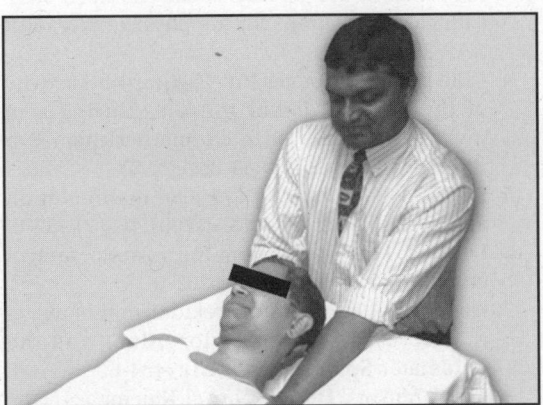

Fig. 8.43: Scalene stretch with neck in slight extension.

Note: These techniques are precedents to thrust techniques and are done by experienced clinicians. The practitioner is advised to exercise caution at all times for instability and vascular signs.

Assume the left facet of C4 is restricted, or stuck in extension (closed). On blocking the level of the thyroid with the second MP on the left and side bending to that level, right rotation is attempted and chin deviation is observed. This is done with the neck **flexed**. Assume the chin deviates half as much to the right compared to chin deviation to the left. Then one can assume that the left C4 is stuck in extension, rotation, side bending right (ERS left C4) or an opening restriction of C4 on the left since it does not flex or open (Fig. 8.45). Now the clinician maintains this position at the barrier or end range and gently oscillates the joint to free it into an open position.

Technique to Free an FRS Restriction on the Left (Right not Closing)

Assume the right facet of C4 is restricted, or stuck in flexion (open). On blocking the level of the thyroid with the second MP on the left and side bending to that level, right rotation is attempted and chin deviation is observed. This is done with the neck **extended**. Assume the chin deviates half as much as the chin deviation to the left. Then one can assume that the right C4 is stuck in flexion, rotation, side bending (FRS left not right

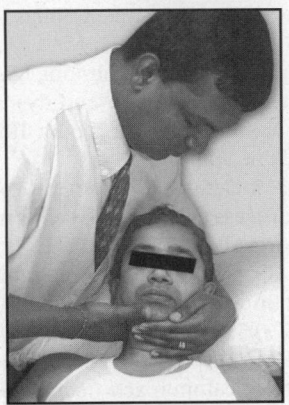

Fig. 8.44: Basic hold.

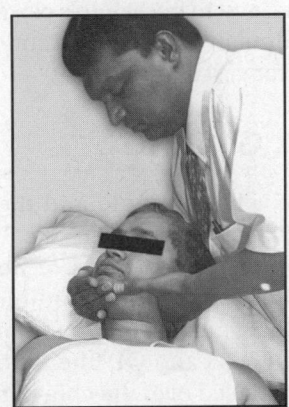

Fig. 8.45: Left midcervical opening.

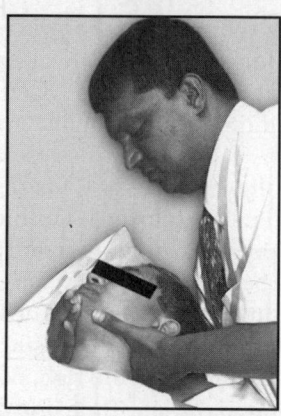

Fig. 8.46: Right midcervical closing.

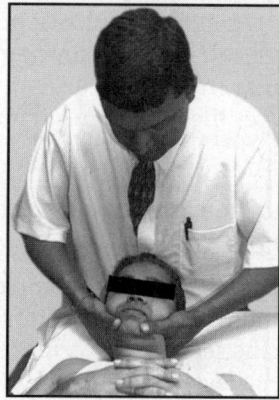

Fig. 8.47: Midcervical side gliding.

of C4 as you go by the posteriority) or a closing restriction of C4 on the right since it does not extend or close. Now the clinician maintains this position at the barrier or end range and gently oscillates the joint to free it into a closed position (Fig. 8.46). Monitor and exercise caution for both techniques for vascular signs.

LATERAL GLIDING

The patient is lying supine and the clinician faces the patient from the head side. The second metacarpophalangeal joints of both hands are placed just below the mandible over the lateral articular pillars. The mandibular angle corresponds to C3 and C4. The thumbs of the clinician are placed over the chin of the patient on either sides (Figs. 8.17 and 18). A gentle lateral motion is induced on either sides to induce a lateral translation in the cervical facet joints. Note that when a lateral glide is introduced from right to left, there is a downslide of the right facet which technically is a closing and an upslide of the opposite side of the same facet which is an opening (Fig. 8.47). Research suggests that this is an effective and safe method to open and close the facet joints, hence effective for radicular pain and cervical range of motion.

REFERENCES

1. Porterfield JA, DeRosa C. Mechanical Neck Pain, 6th edn. WB Saunders. Philadelphia, 1995.
2. Paris SV. S3 course notes, Institute press, St. Augustine, 1988.
3. Sebastian D. Extracranial causes for head pain: Clinical implications for the physical therapist. JIAP. 2002;1:9-16.
4. Falla D, Jull G, Hodges PW. Feedforward activity of the cervical flexor muscles during arm movements is delayed in chronic neck pain. Exp Brain Res. 2004;157(1):43-8.
5. Kapral MK, Bondy SJ. Cervical manipulation and the risk of stroke. CMAJ. 2001;165(7):907-8.
6. Lewitt K. Pain arising from the posterior arch of atlas. Euro Neurol. 1977;16:263-9.
7. Hack GD, et al. Anatomic relationship between the rectus capitis posterior minor and the duramater. Spine. 1995;20(23):2484-6.
8. Ishii T, Mukai Y, Hosono N, et al. Kinematics of the cervical spine in lateral bending: in vivo three-dimensional analysis. Spine. 2006;31(2):155-60.
9. Rosomoff HL, Fishbain D, Rosomoff RS. Chronic cervical pain; Radiculopathy or brachialgia. Noninterventional treatment. Spine. 1992;17:S362-6.
10. Travell JG, Simons DG, Simons LS. Travell and Simon's Myofascial pain and dysfunction: The trigger point manual. 2nd edn. 1999, Williams and Wilkins, Baltimore.
11. Van Der Muelen JCH. Present state of knowledge on the process of healing in collagen structures. Int J Sports Med. 1982;3:4-8.
12. Kunkel RS. Diagnosis and treatment of muscle contraction headaches. Med Clin North Am. 1991;75(3):595-603.
13. Hinoki M. Vertigo due to whiplash injury: aneurotological approach. Acta Otolaryngologica. 1985;419:9-29.

CHAPTER 9

Thoracic Spine and Ribs

Mechanical dysfunctions of the thoracic spine occur in isolation but often associated with dysfunctions of the cervical spine. Vice versa, dysfunctions of the thoracic spine predispose to a cervical spine dysfunction. This is more with regards to the upper thoracic spine. The same principle applies to the lower thoracic spine and dysfunctions of the lumbar spine. The upper thoracic spine behaves more like the cervical spine in structure and mechanical characteristics as does the lower thoracic spine in relation to the lumbar vertebrae.

The thoracic vertebrae are intimately attached to the ribs and hence predispose to chest pain in dysfunctional states. It may be of interest to know that in the United States, almost 40% of patients going to cardiac emergencies have chest pain of a skeletal origin. Accurate identification and treatment of thoracic dysfunction can alleviate pain that is often thought to arise from a visceral origin.[1]

OSSEOUS ANATOMY

A typical thoracic vertebra consists of a body, two transverse processes and a spinous process (Fig. 9.1). Superiorly and inferiorly, it has two articulating facets that articulate with the segment above and below it to form the facet joints. Posteriorly, between the body and articulating facets are two demi facets on either sides, above and below. These facets articulate with the head of the rib. Laterally, on the transverse processes, are two facets on either sides that articulate with the tubercle of the rib. Hence, a typical thoracic vertebra has 12 articulations namely 4 facets, 4 for the head of the rib, 2 for the tubercle of the rib and 2 intervertebral (disc).

Typical Thoracic Vertebra

The uniqueness of the osseous anatomy in the thoracic spine is the relationship of the levels of the transverse processes to the spinous process. They vary at different levels of the thoracic vertebral column.

This is important to know for the fact that to make a somatic diagnosis, the spinous process is located first to determine the level and the corresponding transverse process is located. However, the transverse processes in the thoracic spine do not correlate to the same level as the spinous processes. The reason being that the transverse processes are placed at a higher level as compared to the spinous processes. The corresponding levels are described by different

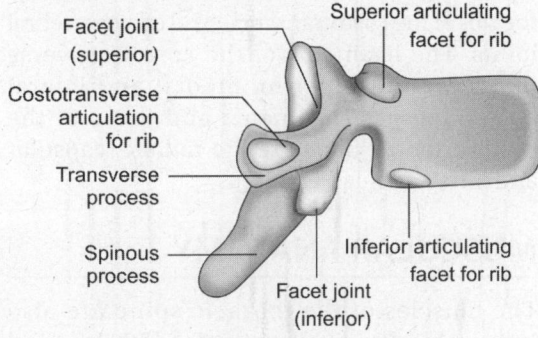

Fig. 9.1: Typical thoracic vertebra.

authors, however, do not correlate well. The most common description is called the rule of 3s, and is as follows.[1]

1,2,3	same level
4,5,6	½ level
7,8,9	1 level
10,11,12	same level

Hence, from a palpation/diagnosis perspective, to make it practically easier, when the palpable area of the spinous process is palpated, the corresponding transverse process will be at the level of the spinous process one level above.

The reason for this is that the palpable area of the spinous process (especially for the segments that extend further down) is not the tip but the body of the spinous process. It is the tip that extends one to one and a half segments below (more so T5,6,7) and is not always the prominent palpable area.

So, from a practical perspective, if the clinician is palpating the spinous process of T8, then to locate its corresponding transverse process the clinician palpates one level up, which is hence corresponding to the spinous process of T7.

LIGAMENTOUS ANATOMY

There are no specific ligaments that arise from the thoracic spine but rather the ligaments that run through the thoracic area. The principal ligaments are the anterior longitudinal ligament (ALL), posterior longitudinal ligament (PLL), supraspinous ligament, ligamentum flavum and intertransverse ligaments. However, there are ligaments that attach the thoracic vertebrae to the ribs at the costotransverse and costovertebral joints. The ligaments of the costotransverse joints are the superior, medial and lateral costotransverse ligaments and those of the costovertebral joints are the radiate, capsular and intra-articular ligaments.

MUSCULAR ANATOMY

The muscles of the thoracic spine are also intimately related to the muscles of the cervical area. The bigger function of the muscles of the thoracic spine are to support the segments from being exaggerated further in their kyphotic predisposition. As this may lead to a forward head and protracted scapulae predisposing to cervical and shoulder dysfunctions. Lower down, an increased thoracic kyphosis may lead to an increase in the lumbar lordosis, predisposing to lumbopelvic dysfunctions.

The musculature, for convenience may be categorized as musculature that attach the thoracic spine to the cervical area and those that attach the scapulae to the thoracic area.

Muscles Attaching Thoracic Spine to the Cervical Area

- Trapezius (upper)
- Splenius capitis
- Splenius cervicis
- Semispinalis.

Muscles Attaching Thoracic Spine to the Scapula

- Rhomboid major
- Rhomboid minor
- Trapezius (middle and lower).

Thus, essentially the thoracic muscles attaching to the cervical spine, especially the occiput, function to retract and support the head in a neutral position. The thoracic muscles that attach to the scapula retract the scapula backwards to maintain an erect posture with normal thoracic kyphosis. They also help to maintain the patency of the space between the acromion and head of humerus.

Other muscles that are clinically relevant to thoracic pain are:
- Serratus posterior superior
- Erector spinae
- Serratus anterior
- Pectoralis minor
- Subclavius
- Levator scapula.

Dysfunctional states of these muscles can cause pain in the thoracic region.

NEURAL ANATOMY

- **Dorsal scapular nerve**
  5th cervical—supplies rhomboids
  3,4th cervical—supplies levator scapula.
- **Thoracodorsal**—supplies latissimus dorsi.
- **Long thoracic**—supplies serratus anterior.

When the corresponding nerves are involved, since the muscles supplied are in the thoracic region, there is a predisposition to pain and dysfunction.

Posterior and Anterior Rami of the Thoracic Spinal Nerves

- Posterior rami medial supplies. 1-6 semispinalis, multifidus, 7-12 transversospinalis, longissimus. Posterior rami lateral supplies longissimus, iliocostalis, costotransverse joints.
- Anterior rami consists of the intercostals, muscular branches and subcostal nerves.

Intercostal Nerve Supplies

- Internal and external intercostals, serratus posterior superior
- Second intercostal brachial nerve joins the medial brachial cutaneous nerve to supply the medial arm.

Muscular Branches Supply

- About 7-11 innervate abdominals.
- Subcostal nerve supplies the skin of iliac crest, lateral hip and lower abdominals. The intercostal nerve is clinically significant as an irritation of this nerve close to the costovertebral joint can cause pain in the rib region resulting in a condition called 'intercostal neuralgia'.

MECHANICS

The mechanics of the thoracic spine is complex owing to the thoracic kyphosis. Hence, the following is a simplified version of the mechanics to avoid confusion. The facet orientation in the upper and midthoracic spine are almost in the same plane as the midcervical spine and hence side bending and rotation occur in the same direction. However, the facet orientation in the lower thoracic spine are almost in the sagittal plane and hence behave more like the lumbar spine. In this case, side bending and rotation will occur in the opposite direction.

MECHANISM OF DYSFUNCTION

When the function of the thoracic musculature is disturbed secondary to overuse, fatigue, weakness or injury, it predisposes to mechanical dysfunction. The most common causes for dysfunctions in the thoracic area is due to faulty posture, overuse/fatigue and weakness.[2] Faulty head posture or constant flexion stresses the insertion sites of the muscles that work to retract the head which is in the thoracic spine. If prolonged, they can contract in length due to fatigue and affect the mechanics of the thoracic facet joints, predisposing to a restriction and dysfunction. Pain in the upper back and the shoulder blades are a common symptom. Traumatic contraction of these muscles are seen due to jerky movements of the head (whiplash) and also the arm as in trying to pull, push or lift a weight. This can predispose to thoracic dysfunctions giving rise to symptoms and pain.

Muscular headaches also have a origin from the thoracic spine, especially the upper thoracic spine. The semispinalis capitis muscle arises from the transverse processes of C7 and T1-6 or 7 and inserts into nuchal line of the occiput. The greater occipital nerve pierces this muscle near its insertion into the occiput. Dysfunctional states of this muscle for the reasons described above can irritate the greater occipital nerve giving rise to headache. The semispinalis is also called the complexus.

Also, forward bending of the upper thoracic spine as seen in faulty forward head postures can increase backward bending at the subcranial spine contracting the suboccipital muscles and giving rise to headache.

The first rib has an attachment to T1 and is commonly a source for dysfunction and pain. The first rib usually tends to be elevated due to faulty postures or due to excessive activity of the accessory muscles of respiration. An elevated position of the first rib can compromise the thoracic outlet and cause symptoms of a thoracic outlet syndrome.

The special tests for a thoracic outlet syndrome have a high incidence of false positives, like Adson's maneuver, Allen maneuver, etc. Manual therapy tests incorporating examination of the first rib, tightness of the scalenes, and the pectoralis minor and weakness of the upper back retractors will help confirm the diagnosis as dysfunctions of these structures contribute to compromise of the thoracic outlet.

Tissue texture abnormality is an obvious finding in the thoracic spine. Dysfunctional segments will exhibit tenderness over their corresponding transverse processes and also over the corresponding musculature. Greenman describes this as a fourth layer hypertrophy where the deepest layer of the four layer of muscles of the back tend to be hypertrophied and tender secondary to dysfunctional states of the thoracic facet joints.

Rib dysfunctions are yet another area that predispose to thoracic pain. The costovertebral, costotransverse and costochondral joints are mediators. Hypomobility of the glenohumeral joint or scapulohumeral dysfunction are also mediators of thoracic pain.

EXAMINATION

Examination of the upper thoracic spine is done preferably in sitting. Examination of the upper thoracic spine involves detection of an elevated first rib and ERS or FRS dysfunctions.

THORACIC SPINE SOMATIC DIAGNOSIS

Elevated First Rib

The patient is sitting and the clinician stands behind the patient. The first rib is palpated by placing the hands on the upper trapezius and retracting the upper fibers of the trapezius backwards. The bony structure palpable between the retracted upper fibers of the trapezius and the clavicle is the angle of the first rib.

The clinician palpates the first rib on either sides and asks the patient to inhale deeply (Fig. 9.2). The first rib on both sides are felt to rise up. Now, as the patient exhales in continuation with the breathing process, ideally both first ribs should descend downwards. In the event of the first rib not descending downwards and is palpated as being elevated, then that rib is stuck in an elevated position. This is usually tender on palpation and is felt as a palpable bony prominence.

Assessment of Closing and Opening Restriction

ERS/Opening Restriction (Upper Thoracic Spine) T1-T5

The patient is in the sitting position and the clinician stands behind the patient. The clinician first palpates, e.g. the spinous process of T1 which is the prominent bony projection in the center of the spine at the base of the neck just below C7. The corresponding transverse process is palpated at the same level of the spinous process. The patient is then asked to drop the head and shoulders forward without rotating the trunk. The transverse processes are palpated on either sides to see if there is a posteriority

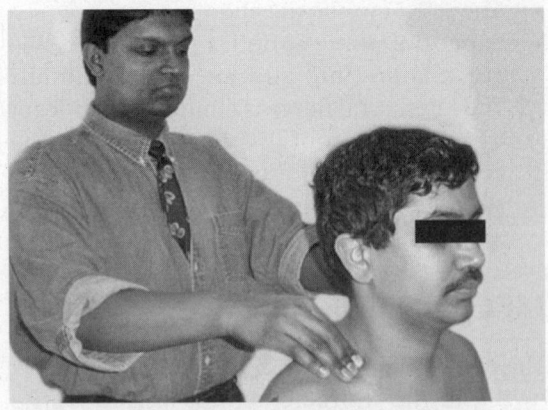

Fig. 9.2: Palpation of the first rib.

(Fig. 9.3). Assume as the head and shoulders are flexed forward and the transverse process of T1 appears posterior on the right. Then one can assume that the left facet is sliding forward into flexion and the right is not as it is stuck in extension and appears posterior (not opening).

To confirm, the transverse process is palpated in a neutral straight position and backward bent position. If the transverse processes appear even then it can be assumed that the facets are able to slide back into extension. Hence, the only positive finding was a posteriority on the right transverse process in flexion as it is stuck in extension (not opening). Hence, the diagnosis is an ERS right of T1 (not opening).

A similar principle is applied for segments T1 to T5 in sitting.

FRS/Closing Restriction (Upper Thoracic Spine) T1 To T5

The patient is in the sitting position and the clinician faces the patient from the back. The transverse processes of T1 are palpated as above and the patient is asked to arch backward and look up to the ceiling. The transverse processes are palpated on either sides to see if there is a posteriority (Fig. 9.4). Assume that the transverse process on the right appears posterior when the upper back and head is arched backwards. Then one can assume that the right facet is sliding backwards and appears posterior but the left facet is not as it is stuck in flexion (not closing).

To confirm, the transverse processes are palpated in a neutral straight position and in a forward bent position. If they appear neutral, then one can assume that the facets are able to slide forward into flexion. Hence, the only positive finding was a posteriority of the right transverse process in extension (arching back) as the left facet is stuck in flexion. Hence, although it is the left facet that is stuck in flexion, the diagnosis is always by the side of the posteriority and will hence be an FRS right of T1 (not closing on the left).

A similar principle is applied for segments T1-T5 in sitting. This is a common dysfunction seen in the upper thoracic spine.

ERS (Mid and Lower Thoracic Spine) T6-T12

The position and testing is as described for the upper thoracic spine except that for the mid and lower thoracic spine, the patient is asked to bend forward to a point where both arms drop between the knees (Fig. 9.5).

FRS (Mid and Lower Thoracic Spine) T6-T12

The patient is positioned prone and is asked to prop up on the elbows with the chin resting on the palms. Now the patient is in an extended position. The clinician is on the side facing

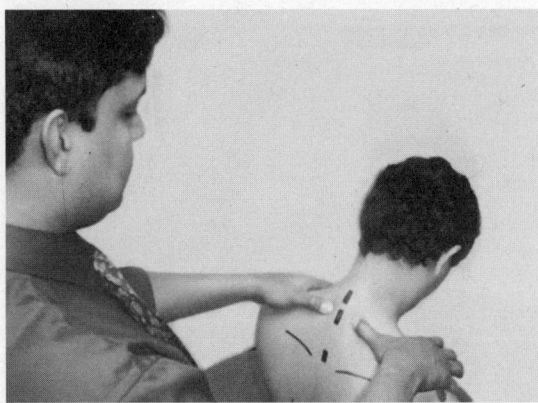

Fig. 9.3: Assessment of ERS/opening restriction.

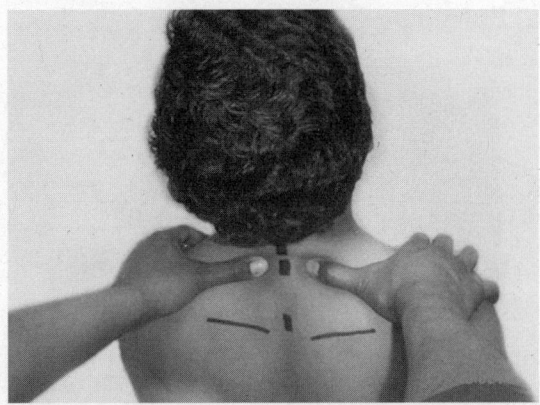

Fig. 9.4: Assessment of FRS/closing restriction.

the patients head diagonally. The transverse processes of the mid to lower thoracic spine are palpated to observe for a posteriority (Fig. 9.6).

Assume the right transverse process of T7 appears posterior. Then it can be assumed that the right facet can slide backward into extension but the left does not as it is stuck in flexion.

To confirm, the patient is asked to assume an erect sitting posture and then asked to bend forward. If the transverse process appears neutral then it can be assumed that the facets are able to slide forward into flexion and the posteriority is observed only on extension because the left facet is stuck in flexion. Since the side of the diagnosis is by the side of the posteriority the diagnosis will be an FRS right of T7 (not closing on the left).

TREATMENT

Soft Tissue Mobilization

The patient is in prone lying and the clinician faces the patient from the side. The thenar eminence and palmar surface of the thumb is used for this technique. The thumb is placed on the long axis of the muscle just adjacent and lateral to the spinous process on the opposite side of the clinician. Now the thumb is reinforced by the palmar surface of the other hand and a gentle laterally directed pressure is applied over the erector spinae which is gradually increased based on patient tolerance. The pressure is held for about 10 to 20 seconds and repeated along the length of the thoracic spine. Care should be taken to direct the pressure away from the spinous process and not toward (Fig. 9.7).

The patient is in prone lying and using an index knobbler, trigger-point compression is applied to the right and left paraspinals of the upper thoracic region primarily focusing on the levator scapula, upper and middle trapezius and rhomboids (Fig. 9.8).

Prone Unilateral and Cross-Hand Stretch for the Levator Scapulae and Upper/Middle Trapezius

Patient is lying prone with clinician facing the patient from the head side. The clinician places

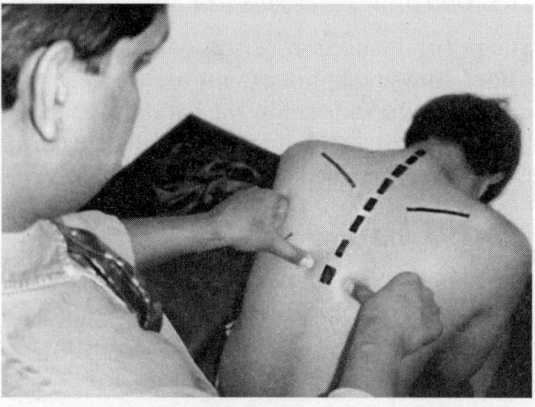

Fig. 9.5: Assessment of ERS/opening restriction.

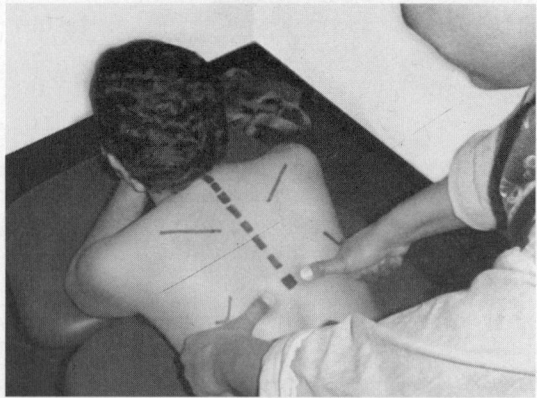

Fig. 9.6: Assessment of FRS/closing restriction.

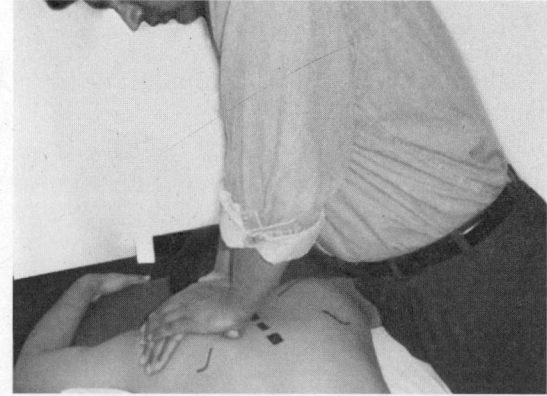

Fig. 9.7: Soft tissue mobilization mid-thoracic paraspinals.

Thoracic Spine and Ribs

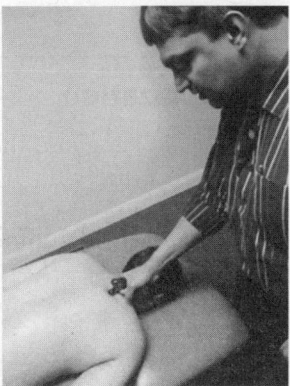

Fig. 9.8: Soft tissue mobilization of the upper thoracic region using an index knobbler.

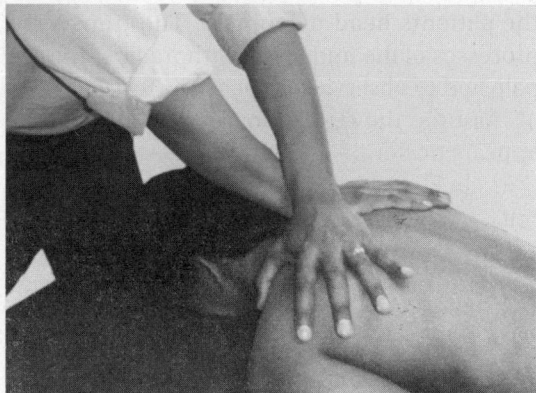

Fig. 9.10: Soft tissue mobilization of the upper thoracic region.

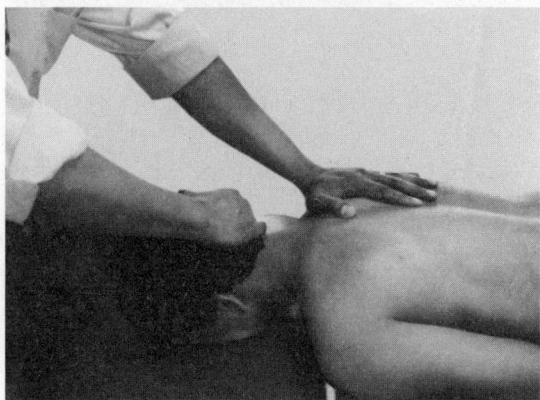

Fig. 9.9: Soft tissue mobilization of the upper thoracic region.

one hand at the base of the occiput. The other hand is placed on the shoulder girdle. A gentle stretch is applied by pulling the hands in opposite directions (Fig. 9.9).

The technique is now repeated with both hands being placed on the shoulder girdle and mid scapular area and applying a longitudinal stretch (Fig. 9.10).

Correction Technique

General Mobilization of the Upper Thoracic Region

With the patient sitting and arms folded above the neck with the elbows forward the clinician faces the patient from the head side. The hands of the clinician are slide under the forearm and placed under the spinous processes of T1, T2, and T3. Gentle oscillations are performed in an upward direction into extension. This maneuver assists in mobilizing the thoracic vertebral segment into a closing position (Fig. 9.11).

With the patient lying prone the clinician faces the patient from the head side. A pincer grip is used over the spinous processes of T1, T2, and T3. With reinforcement from the palm of the other hand, gentle oscillations are performed in a caudal direction. This maneuver assists in mobilizing the thoracic vertebral segment into a closing position (Fig. 9.13).

Elevated First Rib on the Right

Patient is sitting with clinician standing behind. The arm opposite to the involved side is placed on the thigh of the clinician. One arm of the clinician cups the head with elbows resting on the patients shoulder girdle. The web space of the other hand is placed on the elevated 1st rib. The patients head is rotated and side bent to the same side to relax the upper trapezius. The patient is asked to breathe deeply and on exhalation the web space of the hand applies a downward pressure on the rib so as to depress it (Fig. 9.12). The depression is continued through the inhalation process for one or two cycles.

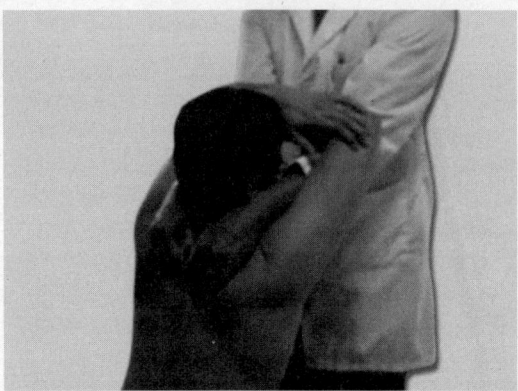

Fig. 9.11: General mobilization of the upper thoracic region into closing.

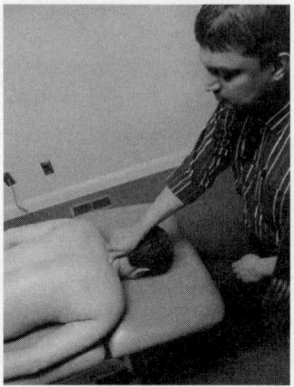

Fig. 9.13: Closing mobilization by using a pincer grip.

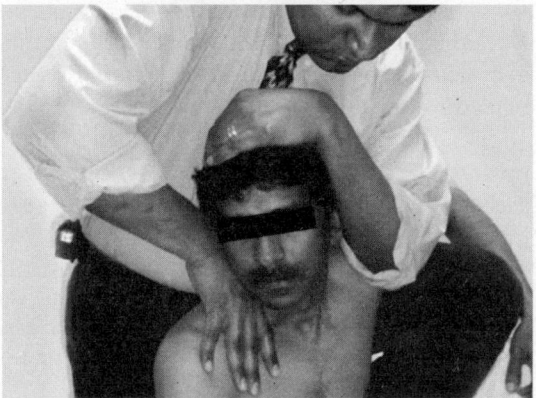

Fig. 9.12: First rib depression manipulation.

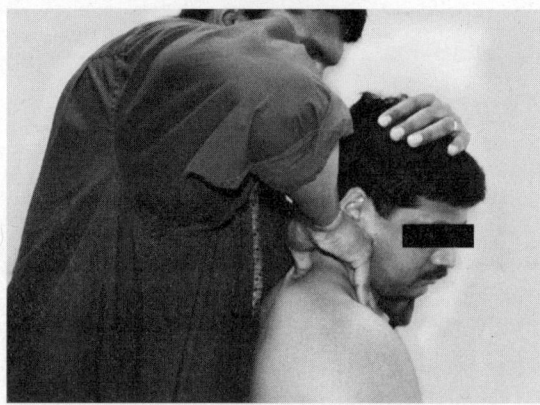

Fig. 9.14: Manipulation for opening restriction of the upper thoracic spine.

ERS (Upper Thoracic Spine) T1-T5 (Not Opening)

The patient is sitting and the clinician faces the patient from behind. Assume the dysfunction is an ERS left of T1. The clinician places the left upper arm on the patients shoulder girdle and the palm supports the top of the head. The right thumb is placed on the right lateral aspect of the spinous process of T1. The clinician flexes the neck until T1 is felt to move, then side bends the head to the right and rotates to the head to the right until T1. This locks the spinal segments until T1. In this position, the left hand of the clinician support the vertex of the patient's head while the right thumb exerts a lateral force from right to left (Fig. 9.14). This frees the left facet of T1 into flexion which was originally stuck in extension (not opening).

FRS (Upper Thoracic Spine) T1-T5 (Not Closing)

The patient is sitting and the clinician faces the patient from behind. Assume the dysfunction is an FRS left of T1. The clinician places the left upper arm on the patients shoulder girdle and the palm supports the side of the head preferably at the mastoid or vertex (Fig. 9.15). The right thumb is placed on the right lateral aspect of the spinous process of T1. The clinician extends the neck until T1 is felt to move, then side bends the head to the left and rotates the head to the right until T1. This locks the spinal segments until T1.

Thoracic Spine and Ribs

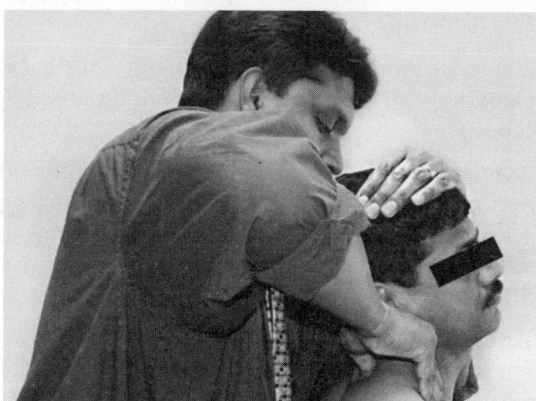

Fig. 9.15: Manipulation for closing restriction of the upper thoracic spine.

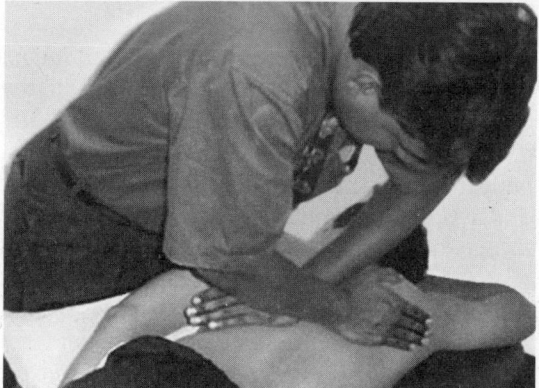

Fig. 9.17: Manipulation for opening restriction of the mid-thoracic spine.

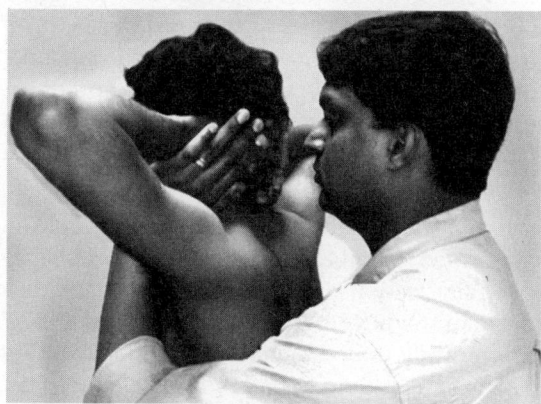

Fig. 9.16: Distraction manipulation of cervicothoracic junction and upper thoracic spine.

In this position, the left hand of the clinician support the occiput of the patient and exerts an upward stretch, while the right thumb exerts a lateral force from right to left. This frees the right facet of T1 into extension which was originally stuck in flexion (not closing).

Technique to Close Upper Thoracic Spine

Patient is sitting with the hands behind the head and the clinician faces the patient from the back. The arms of the clinician pass through the arms of the patient and the hands are placed behind the patients head. Care is taken not to flex the patients head. The forearms of the clinician are placed over the lateral pectoral areas of the patient (Fig. 9.16). The patient is asked to inhale and upon exhalation a thrust is applied in the posterosuperior direction.

Caution: This is a thrust technique and should be performed by trained clinicians, strictly exercising contraindications.

ERS (Mid and Lower Thoracic Spine) T6-T12

The patient is lying prone and the clinician faces the patient from the left side. Assume the dysfunction is an ERS right of T8. The upper trunk is flexed by bending the table or with pillows, until T8. The upper trunk is then side bent to the left and rotated to the left until T8 by arranging pillows under the left shoulder.

The pisiform bone of the right hypothenar eminence of the clinician contacts the right transverse process of T8. The left palm of the clinician is placed on the left transverse process below as in T9 to block the movement. This is now a 'cross hand position'. As the left hand provides a counter pressure, the right hypothenar/pisiform contact exerts an inferiorly directed force on the right transverse process of T8 (Fig. 9.17). This frees the right facet of T8 into flexion which was originally stuck in extension.

FRS (Mid and Lower Thoracic Spine) T6-T12

The exact same technique is adopted as above for an FRS right of T8. The only difference being that the upper trunk is extended instead of being flexed (Fig. 9.18).

ERS Mid-thoracic Spine

Patient is lying supine with the clinician facing the patient from the side. The patient lies with the arm crossed over his chest and knees flexed. The clinician holds the head and neck of the patient with one hand and the space between the thenar and hypothenar eminence is placed on the mid-thoracic segments. Assuming the hand is placed at the level of the inferior angle of scapula at the level of T7, the trunk of the patient is flexed, rotated and side bent right to open the left facet of T7. The mobilization impulse is applied over the patient's arms with the clinicians chest (Fig. 9.19). The same technique is executed in extension to close right facet of T7.

FRS Mid-thoracic Spine

The technique is the same as above but the leg is extended and the thoracic spine is maintained in relative extension.

Caution: This is a thrust technique and should be performed by trained clinicians, strictly exercising contraindications.

Sitting (Opening and Closing)

Patient is sitting with arms folded across the chest, and the clinician faces the patient from the back. The clinician folds a towel and places it on the segment to be mobilized at T7. The clinician brings both arms around the patient and cups on both elbows of the patient (Fig. 9.20). The trunk of the patient is flexed to the level of the towel rotated and side bent right to open the left facet of T7. A mobilization with impulse is applied in the upward and posterior direction to open left facet of T7. A similar procedure is attempted with the trunk extended to close right facet of T7.

Caution: This is a thrust technique and should be performed by trained clinicians, strictly exercising contraindications. The incidence of thoracic disk herniations have been reported in literature.[3] Remember that the thoracic spinal canal is much smaller than the other levels of the spine. Additionally, there has been reports in literature of calcified disks injuring the spinal cord during manipulation.[4,5] It is advisable for the clinician

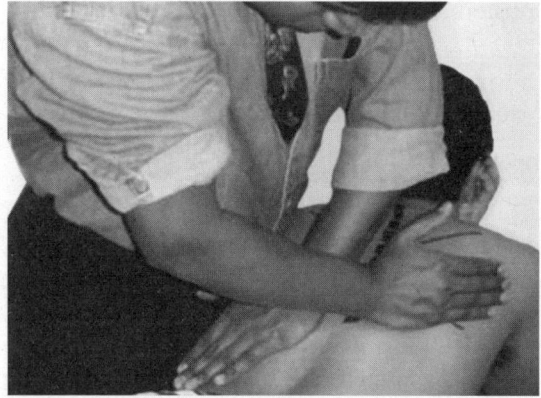

Fig. 9.18: Manipulation for closing restriction of the mid-thoracic spine.

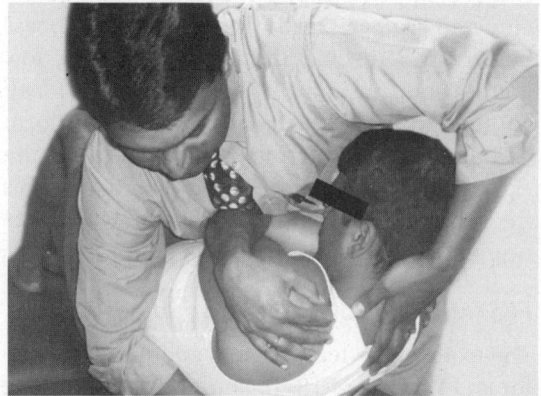

Fig. 9.19: Manipulation for opening restriction of the mid-thoracic spine.

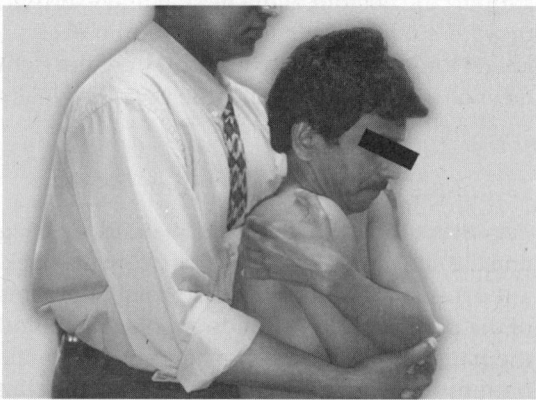

Fig. 9.20: Manipulation for opening/closing restriction of the mid-thoracic spine.

to routinely test for the Babinski sign as a positive finding warrants an immediate medical referral and is a strict contraindication for manipulation.

Remember, the key in the mid and lower thoracic spine is to side bend and rotate the upper trunk to the opposite side of the posteriority.
- The upper trunk is flexed for an ERS.
- The upper trunk is extended for an FRS.

PROPHYLAXIS

Cervicothoracic Complex

Exercise Prescription

The prophylaxis of mechanical dysfunctions of the cervicothoracic complex will most definitely involve stabilization of the musculature. As discussed in the principles of management, the musculature function as ropes to hold the alignment and minimize shock of functional activities. Appropriate exercise prescription will help to address this. The one important thing that the clinician should remember is to never make a home exercise program too elaborate. This will decrease motivation, considering the routine day-to-day schedule of work and family responsibilities of the average individual. Exercises addressing the target structures and most appropriate to the dysfunction is recommended. Since exercises are dysfunction specific inappropriate exercise prescription can deter outcomes hence the appropriateness is of importance.

The musculature of the upper quarter sometimes span the entire length of the three regions. They may originate at the subcranial spine and run across the midcervical spine to insert into the mid-thoracic spine. Hence, stabilization will involve the entire complex. Dysfunctions may occur in a similar manner. Functionally it is the effect of the combined mechanics of the three regions. The three regions will need to share the work of supporting and effecting function in the upper quarter. Hence a restriction in one region is usually compensated by increased work or the activity of the other. This is so often seen in the cervical spine. We often see a diagnosis of cervical spondylosis or cervical radiculopathy of the midcervical spine commonly C5, C6, up to C8, T1. But how often have we seen a diagnosis involving C1, C2 or T4, T5. This is often missed and in many instances, in patients with a midcervical diagnosis an associated upper cervical or an upper/mid-thoracic dysfunction can be identified. Hence, as a matter of fact, altered mechanics of the upper cervical and upper thoracic can stress the midcervical area as it compensates for the altered mechanics and function. This may be picked up as the conventional cervical diagnosis we see in our day-to-day practice. An astute manual therapy diagnosis of an upper cervical or an upper/midcervical dysfunction may help to address the cause for the midcervical diagnosis rather than treating the symptom only, (e.g. traction) which is the nerve root pain arising from the midcervical dysfunction.

Hence, as much as manual treatment should ideally address dysfunctions of the entire complex, exercise prescription should also address mobility and strength of the supporting musculature of the entire cervico-thoracic complex. The common soft tissue restriction patterns are:
- Backward bending of the subcranial spine with shortening of the suboccipital muscles and Spleneus/semispinalis and weakness of cervical flexors.
- Side bending and rotation of the midcervical spine with shortening of the upper fibers of trapezius, scalenes and levator scapulae.
- Protraction of the scapulae with shortening of the upper pectoralis major and pectoralis minor, and increased thoracic kyphosis.

All of the above muscles are postural muscles and as discussed earlier postural muscles tighten and hence lead to shortening leading to the above alignment dysfunctions. Hence, it is obvious that postural muscles will need to be lengthened and most appropriately done with active stretching exercises to prevent recurrence of an alignment dysfunction.

The muscles that attach the thoracic spine to the scapulae are phasic muscles and they weaken

to cause the above alignment dysfunction. The common weakness patterns are:
- Subcranial backward bending secondary to weakness of the anterior cervical musculature.
- Midcervical forward bending secondary to weakness of the upper trapezius.
- Scapular protraction with rounded shoulders and increased thoracic kyphosis secondary to weakness of the mid and lower trapezius and rhomboids.
- Intervertebral instability and weakness secondary to weakness of the multifidi.

This weakness pattern is most appropriately addressed by active strengthening exercises to prevent recurrence of an alignment dysfunction. Current literature suggests that the deep cervical flexors are the key muscles contributing to stability in the cervical region.[6]

MYOFASCIAL TENDER POINTS

The concept of addressing myofascial tender points is to decrease actin and myosin cross-bridging and myofibrillar restriction. Their continual presence may encourage chemical accumulation, early fatigue and decreased muscle performance with accompanying pain and dysfunction. Their attachment to the spine can further cause alignment issues. They may be best treated with frictions and electrotherapy. Tender points secondary to aberrant gamma efferents may require an alternate positional release approach and the reader is encouraged further reading in the area of 'strain counterstrain' methods. The following are some common dysfunctional points of the cervicothoracic region (Figs. 9.21 and 9.22).

RIBS

Ribs are thin, flat, curved bones that form a protective cage around the organs in the upper thorax. They are comprised of 24 bones arranged in 12 pairs. The ribs are divided into three categories. The first seven ribs are called the

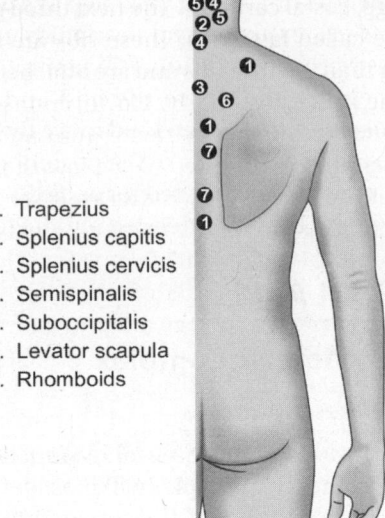

1. Trapezius
2. Splenius capitis
3. Splenius cervicis
4. Semispinalis
5. Suboccipitalis
6. Levator scapula
7. Rhomboids

Fig. 9.21: Myofascial tender points: Cervicothoracic (posterior).

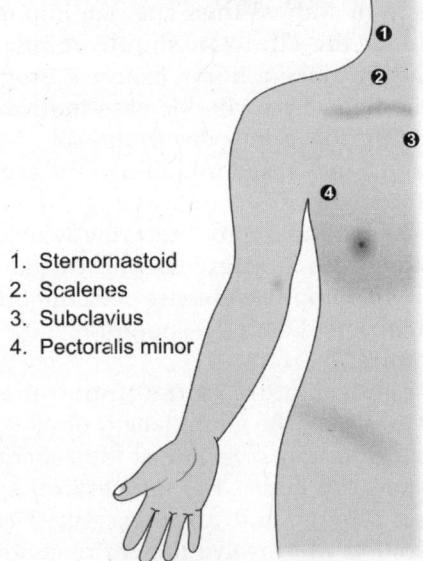

1. Sternomastoid
2. Scalenes
3. Subclavius
4. Pectoralis minor

Fig. 9.22: Myofascial tender points: Cervicothoracic (anterior).

true ribs. These ribs are attached to the thoracic spine posteriorly. In the front, the true ribs are connected directly to the sternum by strips of cartilage, costal cartilage. The next three pairs of ribs are called false ribs. These ribs are slightly shorter than the true ribs and are attached to the thoracic spine posteriorly. However, instead of being attached directly to the sternum, anteriorly, the false ribs are attached to the lowest true rib which is the seventh rib. The last two sets of ribs are called floating ribs. Floating ribs are smaller than both true ribs and false ribs. They are attached to the spine posteriorly at the level of T11 and T12, but do not have an anterior attachment, hence floating.

The typical rib is attached to the thoracic spine by the costovertebral and costotransverse joints. The rib attaches to the costotransverse joint of a thoracic vertebra and the head attaches to the superior costovertebral joint of the same vertebra and inferior costovertebral joint of the vertebra above (Fig. 9.23).

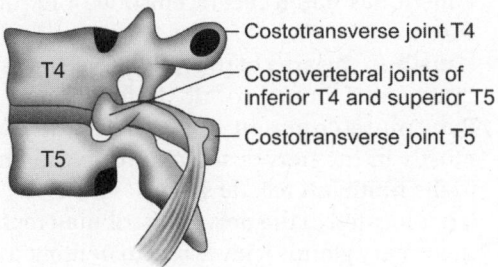

Fig. 9.23: Depicted rib belongs to T5.

Since the articulations in the upper levels are concave over convex, the ribs move in a pump handle fashion. The relatively flatter articulating surfaces in the lower levels help with lateral expansion and hence move in a bucket handle fashion (Figs. 9.24A and B).

Mobility in the costovertebral and costotransverse joints can be rendered in excess resulting in hypermobility. The causes are varied and could be secondary to repeated activity related stress or frequent cracking or popping of the thoracic articulations as in repeated manipulations. When the ribs move into an inspiratory position there is a relative anterior movement of the rib owing to its movement in a pump handle fashion. The instability of the posterior rib joints are taken advantage of by the anteriorly placed tight pectoralis minor and posterolaterally placed weak serratus anterior. This relative 'anterior slipping' of the ribs can result in a sudden instability like feature resulting in a spasm or catching sensation of the supporting musculature namely serratus posterior superior, serratus anterior and intercostals. While this occurs, there is potential for the head of the rib to irritate the exiting intercostal nerve resulting in a winding, sharp pain in the intercostal spaces. This feature is called intercostal neuralgia. Thus, rib dysfunctions can cause the following clinical syndromes:

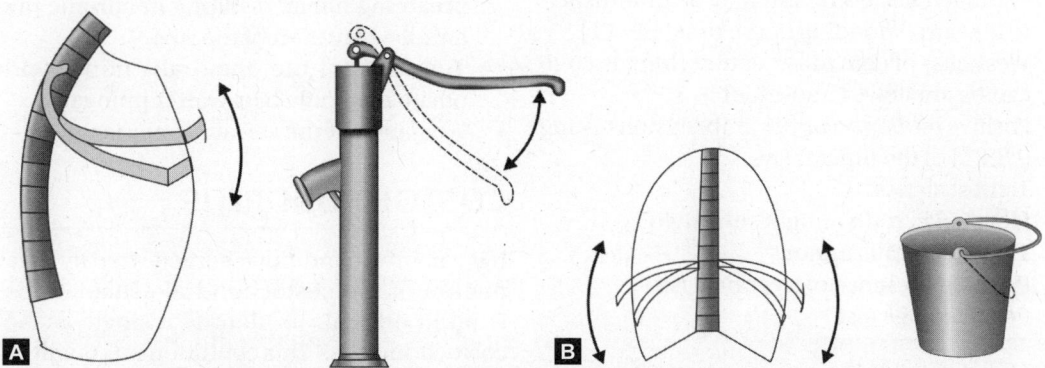

Figs. 9.24A and B: Depiction of pump handle and bucket handle motion.

COSTOCLAVICULAR SYNDROME/THORACIC OUTLET SYNDROME

The first two ribs receive the insertions of the anterior and middle scalene, respectively. As they are accessory muscle of inspiration they assist in elevating the first and second ribs. Anteriorly the first rib lies just below the clavicle. This space is called the costoclavicular space. A tight set of scalenes can elevate the first rib compromising the costoclavicular space and compressing the lower trunk of the brachial plexus, or the circulatory vessels, namely subclavian. This condition is the costoclavicular contribution to a thoracic outlet syndrome.

Examination Findings

- Forward head posture
- Restricted range of motion with painful muscle trigger points (commonly levator scapula, upper and middle trapezius and scalenes)
- Muscle tightness may be evident especially the superficial groups (mainly the scalenes, pectoralis minor)
- Closing or opening restrictions of the mid cervical spine
- Restricted OA/AA mobility
- Sensation may be diminished to the corresponding nerve root (C8, T1)
- Manual muscle strength may be diminished to the corresponding nerve root (C8, T1)
- Weakness of core musculature (longus colli, capitis and lower trapezius)
- Positive finding on upper limb tension testing (ULTT) of the ulnar nerve
- Tight scalenes
- Elevated first rib or tight subcalvius
- Tight pectoralis minor
- Possible presence of a cervical rib
- Positive Roos test.

INTERCOSTAL NEURALGIA

It is a neuralgia of one or more of the intercostal nerves.[7] The intercostal nerves are 12 in number and consist of an anterior and posterior ramus. These nerves run in a groove in the lower edge of the ribs called the intercostal groove. Common causes are anemia, cold exposure, pressure from tumors, or an aortic aneurysm. Clinical relevance to the physical therapist is that it can arise from dysfunctions of the thoracic vertebrae. In mechanical dysfunctions of the thoracic vertebrae (degeneration with foraminal narrowing or disc herniation) and associated rib dysfunctions (anterior or rib instability), faulty postures and muscle imbalances secondary to weakness of the serratus anterior and tightness of the pectoralis minor can cause rib dysfunctions[8] and associated intercostal neuralgic pain.

Examination Findings

- The pain is sharp shooting and can wind around the rib cage
- Patient has had a recent episode of herpes zoster
- Usually in the area of the fifth nerve
- Presence of thoracic or rib dysfunction
- Pain more common on the left side and mostly in the nerves situated from the fifth to the ninth intercostal space
- If it is located in the nerves distributed to the mammary glands it gives rise to neuralgia of the mammary gland
- History of repeated cracking, popping or manipulations
- Prolonged slouched postures and sort, shallow breathing habits resulting in chronic pump handle, elevation of the ribs
- Tightness of the pectoralis minor with a positive scapula backward tipping test
- Weakness of the serratus anterior.

COSTOCHONDRITIS

It is a painful condition characterized by inflammation of the costochondral articulations. It is often difficult to identify a single cause of costochondritis.[8] This condition is thought to be commonly secondary to repetitive microtrauma, or overuse. The most frequently affected age group is young adults between 20 and 40 years old. Costochondritis can also occur as an overuse injury in athletes. In particular this condition has been identified in competitive rowers or activities that involve frequent repetitive horizontal adduction. It can also be found after a traumatic injury. Commonly secondary to a car accident where the driver's chest strikes the steering wheel and injuring the ribs and cartilage in the costochondral area. Viral infections, usually upper respiratory infections have also been identified as a cause of costochondritis. Individuals with rheumatological pathology are also susceptible.

Examination Findings

- Local tenderness in the costochondral area
- History of heavy or repetitive physical activity as in lifting, rowing, bench pressing, etc.
- History of rheumatological pathology as in rheumatoid arthritis
- History of blunt trauma
- Muscle imbalance as in strong powerful anterior groups (pectorals) and weak posterior groups (lower trapezius, rhomboids)
- Rib dysfunction, anterior and posterior
- Repeated manipulation of the thoracic spine.

INTERCOSTALS MUSCLE STRAIN

The intercostal muscles are located between the ribs, in the intercostal space. There are two divisions internal and external. The internal intercostal muscles originate on ribs 2-12 and have their insertions on ribs 1-11. The internal intercostals are responsible for the depression of the ribs decreasing the transverse dimensions of the thoracic cavity which aid in forced expiration. This is called a pump handle movement. The external intercostal muscles originate on ribs 1-11 and have their insertion on ribs 2-12. The external intercostals are responsible for the elevation of the ribs, and expanding the transverse dimensions of the thoracic cavity which aid in quiet and forced inhalation. This is called a bucket handle movement. Both external and internal muscles are innervated by the intercostal nerves (the ventral rami of thoracic spinal nerves). A pathology of these nerves has been discussed in the section on instability of the costovertebral and costotransverse joints/intercostal neuralgia. The intercostal muscles are also reported to be stressed on repeated vigorous activity as in rowing. It is also described to be associated with stress fractures of the rib.

Examination Findings

- Local rib tenderness with possible bruising
- Pain on position changes especially supine to sit
- Pain on valsalva
- History of repeated cracking, popping or manipulations
- Prolonged slouched postures and sort, shallow breathing habits resulting in chronic pump handle and elevation of the ribs.
- Tightness of the pectoralis minor with a positive scapula backward tipping test
- Weakness of the serratus anterior.

ANTERIOR INTERCOSTAL COMPRESSION SYNDROME

Anterior intercostal compression syndrome (AICS) is a differential screen for anterior chest and thoracic pain.[11] It is a condition where the intercostal space is compromised resulting in anterior chest and thoracic pain. While intercostal neuralgia exists as a clinical entity, several other structures within the intercostal space are speculated to be potential pain mediators. In the presence of AICS the exact structures however are difficult to specify. When visceral mediation has been ruled out and in the absence of neuralgic radiating pain, AICS may be considered.

Forward head posture with protracted scapulae can cause cervical, thoracic and shoulder dysfunction. The consequence of a forward head posture on the ribs is worth mentioning. The upper ribs assist respiration by moving in a pump handle fashion assisted by the pectoralis minor which narrows the intercostal space. Rib widening or the bucket handle movement is assisted by the serratus anterior which helps widen the intercostal space.[9] This is accomplished with a fixed scapula whilst stabilizing the ribs from an excessively anterior displacement.[10] Dysfunctional states as in a prolonged forward head and scapula protraction, can render the pectoralis minor tight and the serratus anterior weak in addition to other factors (subcranial, cervical and thoracic dysfunction). This can cause a relative approximation of the intercostal space resulting in pain. In the absence of intercostal neuralgia, the structures within the intercostal space that are speculated to cause pain are the periosteum of the ribs, intercostal muscles, and intercostal artery and vein.

Management should hence address all components of a forward head but more specifically pectoralis minor stretching, mobilizing the intercostal space into opening and serratus anterior strengthening. Differentials include intercostal muscle cramp or tear, rib fractures, costochondritis, Tietze syndrome, rib infection or metastasis in rare cases, and post-operative thoracic surgery particularly coronary artery bypass.

Examination Findings

- History of a dull achy pain in the anterior and lateral rib area.
- Prolonged slouched forward head postures and short, shallow breathing habits resulting in chronic pump handle and elevation of the ribs.
- Tightness of the pectoralis minor with a positive scapula backward tipping test
- Weakness of the serratus anterior
- History of repeated cracking, popping or manipulations.

SLIPPING RIB SYNDROME

This condition occurs mainly in the floating ribs and a feature of instability of the eleventh and twelfth ribs at the costovertebral and costotransverse articulations. Occasionally the lower ribs may be involved with an instability of the costal cartilage anteriorly. The slipping rib syndrome is also called 'Cyriax' syndrome. This condition may mimic many visceral types of discomfort. The syndrome is diagnosed by a clinical test called the hooking maneuver where the clinicians fingers are hooked to the lower ribs and pulled up or anteriorly reproducing the pain.[12]

Examination Findings

- Intense pain in the lower chest or upper abdomen above the costal margin mostly lower and floating ribs
- A tender spot on the costal margin
- Reproduction of the pain by pressing the tender spot or by external pressure
- Signs and symptoms are usually unilateral, however there are also cases where patients reported bilateral pain
- Positive 'hooking maneuver'.

ASSESSMENT AND TREATMENT

Assessment of rib dysfunction is qualitative and the location of symptoms is usually the first clue to the clinician. The following are common collective signs and symptoms. A history of a dull achy pain in the anterior and lateral rib area. Prolonged slouched forward head postures and short, shallow breathing habits resulting in chronic pump handle and elevation of the ribs. Tightness of the pectoralis minor with a positive scapula backward tipping test. Weakness of the serratus anterior. History of repeated cracking, popping or manipulations.

The ribs can be dysfunctional in the following directions:

1. Superior (mostly 1st and 2nd ribs)
2. Posterior (expiratory)
3. Anterior (inspiratory)

Superior (Elevated) Rib Dysfunction

Elevated First Rib on the Right

The clinician faces the seated patient from behind and the hands palpate the first rib between the clavicle anteriorly and the bulk of the upper trapezius posteriorly. This is done on both sides. The patient is asked to take a deep inhalation

Thoracic Spine and Ribs

breath and the first rib is felt to rise on both sides. Upon exhalation, the clinician palpates and feels the descent of the rib. Assuming the right rib does not descend on exhalation and the rib on the left is felt to descend, one can assume it is an elevated first rib on the right.

The treatment for an elevated first rib on the right is as follows. The patient is sitting with the clinician standing behind. The arm opposite to the involved side is placed on the thigh of the clinician. One arm of the clinician cups the head with elbows resting on the patients shoulder girdle. The web space of the other hand is placed on the elevated 1st rib on the right (Fig. 9.25). The patients head is rotated and side bent to the same side to relax the upper trapezius. The patient is asked to breathe deeply and on exhalation the web space of the hand applies a downward pressure on the rib so as to depress it. The depression is continued through the inhalation process for one or two cycles.

Posterior Rib Dysfunction

Posterior Rib Dysfunction on the Right (If Symptomatic)

Posterior rib dysfunction is similar to palpating for a posterior transverse process except that the palpating fingers are move more laterally to palpate the rib angle for posteriority and tenderness. Remember the costotransverse joint is the extension of the rib from the thoracic spine. Posterior rib dysfunction is seen in a direct hit on the chest as in a steering wheel or hypertrophy and spasm of the serratus anterior and serratus posterior superior. (Figs. 9.26A and B)

Treatment technique for a posterior rib dysfunction is similar to performing an opening or a closing mobilization of the mid thoracic spine, however, the supporting hand is now moved slightly laterally to the angle of the ribs and not the spinous process.

Anterior Rib Dysfunction

Assessment of an anterior rib dysfunction is similar to assessing a posterior rib dysfunction, except that the patient is in supine lying and the angles of the anterior ribs are palpated for a more anterior position. Dysfunction is considered only when symptoms are present.

Anterior rib dysfunction can occur at the level of the first five ribs. This is commonly seen in patients with slouched postures, a direct hit

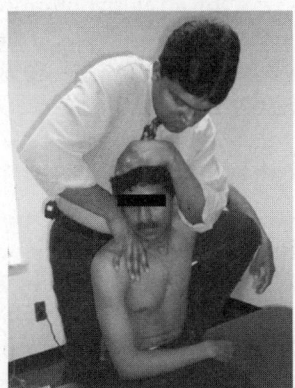

Fig. 9.25: First rib depression.

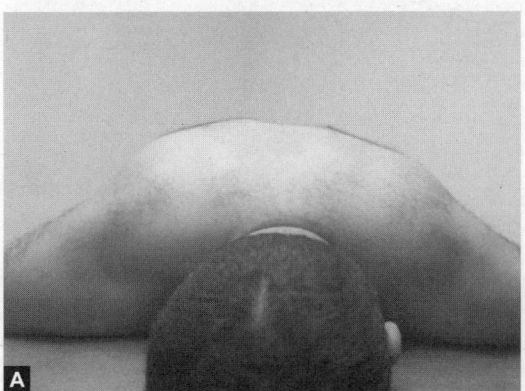
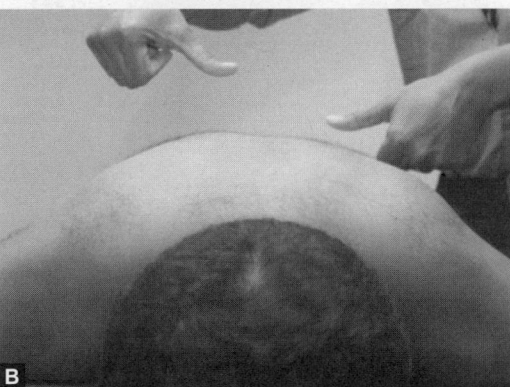

Figs. 9.26A and B: Posteriority observed over the right posterior ribs.

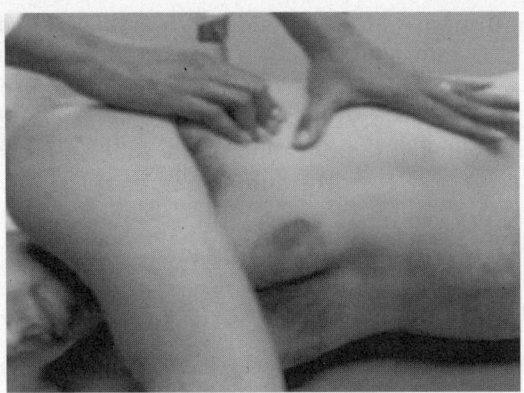

Fig. 9.27: Intercostal stretch.

on the back, hypertrophy of the pectoralis minor and most important weakness of the serratus anterior. The patient is lying supine and the clinician palpates the clavicle and the rib space below it. The next rib that is palpable is the second rib. Both sides are palpated at the same time to observe for a relatively more elevated position of the rib in question. Tenderness can also be elicited in the rib that appears more elevated or anterior.

Intercostal Space Stretching

With the patient in a side lying position the clinician uses the thumb of one hand to fix the rib lower to the intercostal space. The tips of the fingers of the other hand are placed in the intercostal space above the thumb. A gentle stretch is imparted in an upward direction so as to stretch the intercostal spaces (Fig. 9.27).

Serratus Anterior Strengthening

The serratus anterior has an attachment to the medial and anterior inner portion of the scapula to the lateral five ribs. When activated they hold the medial border of the scapula down on the rib cage preventing winging and draw the ribs backward and downward so as to stretch the intercostal spaces.

The patient is either standing or supine lying. The arms are in the 90° shoulder flexion position with the elbows fully extended. A resistance band is used as shown in the figure and is wrapped around the scapular area and held by the hands. In the lying position, a pair of dumbbells are used. In this position the patient protracts both scapula as if to reach forward in standing, or reach for the ceiling in supine lying. The elbow, as a mandate, does not flex throughout the procedure and the clinician ensures the protraction is not too excessive (Figs. 9.28A and B).

REFERENCES

1. Greenman TW, Flynn PE. Thoracic spine and rib cage: Musculoskeletal evaluation and treatment. 1996, Butterworth - Heineman, Boston.
2. Flynn TW. Thoracic spine and rib cage disorders. Orthop Phys Ther Clin North Am. 1999;8:1-20.

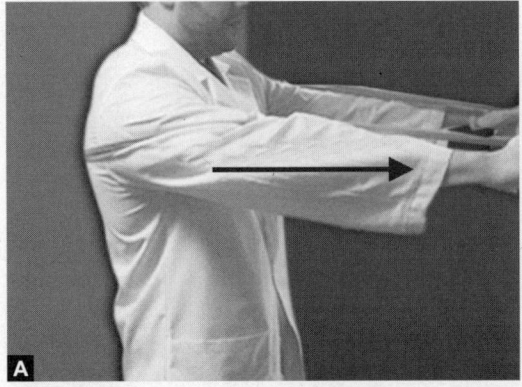
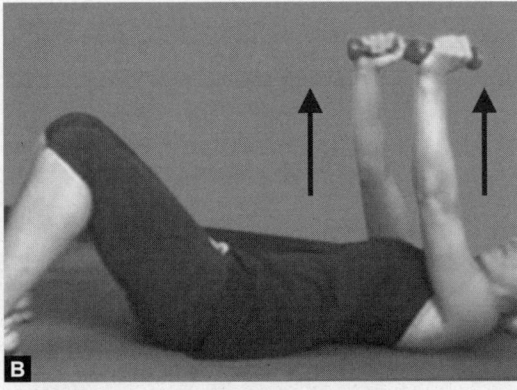

Figs. 9.28A and B: Serratus anterior strengthening.

3. Deitch K, Chudnofsky C, Young M. T2-3 Thoracic disc herniation with myelopathy. J Emerg Med. 2009;36(2):138-40.
4. Lopez-Gonzalez A, Peris-Celda M. Acute paraplegia after chiropraxis. Eur Spine J. 2011;20 (Suppl 2):S143-6.
5. Wang CC, Kuo JR, Chio CC, et al. Acute paraplegia following chiropractic therapy. J Clin Neurosci. 2006;13(5):578-81.
6. Falla D, Jull G, Hodges PW. Feedforward activity of the cervical flexor muscles during voluntary arm movements is delayed in chronic pain. Exp Brain Res. 2004;157(1):43-8.
7. Gonzalez-Darder JM. Thoracic dorsal ramus entrapment. Case report. J Neurosurg. 1989;70(1):124-5.
8. Ayloo A, Cvengros T, Marella S. Evaluation and treatment of musculoskeletal chest pain. Prim Care. 2013;40(4):863-87.
9. Brand RA. Origin and comparative anatomy of the pectoral limb. Clinical Orthopaedics and Related Research. 2008;466(3):531-42.
10. Flynn TW. The Thoracic Spine and Chest Wall. Butterworth-Heinemann Boston, 1996.
11. Sebastian D. Anterior intercostal compression syndrome. Sebastian D (ed) In differential screening of regional pain in musculoskeletal practice). 2015; Jaypee Brothers Medical Publisher, New Delhi.
12. Kumar R, et al. The painful rib syndrome. Indian Journal of Anaesthesia. 2013;57(3):311-13.

CHAPTER
10

Lumbar Spine

INTRODUCTION

The lumbar spine continues to be a clinical dilemma from a diagnosis perspective. The structures involved as a source for pain are often difficult to identify as most symptomatology are invariably identical. They predominantly tend to be pain in the back with pain radiating down to the leg. Clinician's often narrow down their conclusions to the disk and a few to a foraminal compromise.[1] But the root of the problem is not always the structures mentioned above. As a matter of fact a discogenic pathology or a foraminal compromise may be an end result of a source elsewhere.[2] The lumbar spine is a region subjected to significant functional demands. They are also placed between the two transitional zones namely thoraco lumbar junction and lumbosacral junction. In addition, bony anomalies are common in this region. This collectively increases its vulnerability to dysfunction.

Back pain is an universal entity. Treatments may either address symptoms or the cause, may be palliative or functional, may be relief oriented or management oriented. In any case the clinician should understand first that it is a complex that is being dealt with. The lumbar, pelvic and hip area essentially work as a combination to function and may do the same in situations of a dysfunction. Not to forget that the supporting pillars of the lumbo-pelvic-hip complex are the lower extremities and dysfunctional states of the lower extremities especially the foot and ankle may predispose to the entity 'back pain'.[3]

The strategies described in this piece of literature, or for that matter any other chapter in this book is based on an assumption that the source of dysfunction is mechanical and not one originating from a malignant, vascular or visceral entity. However, some of the mechanical causes are intricate and may be missed and be continuously treated with multiple approaches including surgery. The reasoning for back pain may be debated endlessly and often times an enlightenment to reality which includes our limitations. Indeed we are humbled every single day in our respective practice environments. The point that is to be made is that no back pain is identical in a collective population, neither is the cause for back pain with pain radiating down the leg from a single cause even if it is purely mechanical. The management be it palliative, functional, etc. is decided and based on the individual characteristics[4] of the solution seeking subject on your treatment table. Hence, very subjective but one reason for sure that they are resting their hopes on your ability to treat and manage.

OSSEOUS ANATOMY

The lumbar spine consists of five vertebra numbered L1 to L5. The lumbar vertebral bodies are different from the rest of the segments in that they have a larger and thicker body. Like any other typical vertebral body they have two transverse processes on either sides and one spinous process in the midline (Fig. 10.1). The facet joints of the lumbar segments are almost in the saggital plane and the movement patterns are accordingly determined. The spinous process of L5 is flatter compared to the rest of the lumbar segments and is sometimes missing as a congenital anomaly. The curvature of the lumbar spine is lordotic and has a wider range of motion as it has no ribs attached to it.

The lumbar vertebrae support the upper part of the body and transmit their weight to the pelvis and lower extremities. It is often debated that the vertebral body is the shock absorbing agent and not the disk.[5] It is of worth to discuss the structure and role of the disk and the facet joints in this section, and essentially this discussion speaks for the entire spine.

Intervertebral Disk

The intervertebral disk as it is called is found between all the bodies of the vertebrae except the sacral and atlantoaxial segments. They make up for approximately 25% of the whole length of the spine and almost 50% at birth. The shape of the disk contours to the shape of the vertebral body and curvature. Hence in a lordotic situation as in the cervical and lumbar spine they are thicker anteriorly than posteriorly. The disk has principally three functions according to Dr Paris which are as follows:[5]

1. They bind and hold the vertebral bodies together.
2. They form a smooth surface to allow movement within the vertebral segments.
3. They equalize and distribute loads and do not absorb them.

The disk has three parts namely the vertebral end plate, annulus fibrosis and nucleus pulposis. Between the vertebral body and the disk is a thin layer of hyaline cartilage known as cartilaginous end plate. This is the structure from which the annular rings arise. The outer annulus consists of about 6 to 10 concentrically arranged tough fibrous rings. These function contain the nucleus, stabilize the vertebral bodies, provide movement and offer minimal shock absorption.

The inner aspect of the disk which is encased by the annulus fibrosis is a gel-like structure called nucleus pulposis. The nucleus pulposis is in the center most part of the disk. Its functions are as follows:

- The morphology of the nucleus pulposis is such that it has a property of imbibition and it is able to absorb nutrients by virtue of its osmotic properties. This occurs through the cartilaginous end plates and the nutrient fluids are derived from the vertebral bodies. The imbibition occurs at rest and results in an expansion of the nucleus. Once weight bearing commences the fluids are forced out. This is the reason why one tends to be relatively taller in the morning on waking up and gradually lose some height by the end of the day. The clinical implication is that the annulus is most stretched in the mornings and offers a greater risk for injury.
- The nucleus functions to transmit force, equalize stress and offer movement. It not only provides movement but also provides a rocking action to it. Its hydrodynamic properties enhance its stress equalization ability.

Facet Joint

These are formed by the superior and inferior articulating processes of the vertebra above and

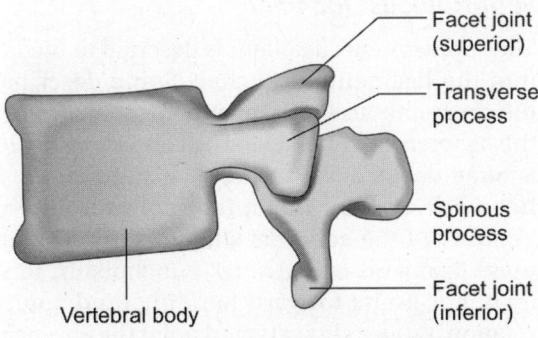

Fig. 10.1: Typical lumbar vertebra.

below. The facet orientation is such that it is between the frontal and horizontal planes in the cervical region, between the frontal and sagittal plane in the thoracic region and in the sagittal plane in the lumbar region.

The facet joint[6,7] consists of an articular cartilage. It is somewhat compressible in younger individuals. It also has a tendency to swell with brief periods of exercise and subsides with rest. The facet joints, like any other synovial joint possess an articular capsule which is partly elastic and blend with the ligamentum flavum. The multifidi and the ligamentum flavum prevent the articular capsule from being nipped between the bony facets. The elastic elements of the capsule also help to maintain the facets in close contact to each other.

The principal functions of the facet joints are to allow movement within the segments. All movements in the vertebral segments involve the intervertebral disk and this is controlled by the movements of the facet joints. The intervertebral disk is described as an unique structure that permits movement and transfers loads received by it. The disk, however, has no potential for independent movement and depends on the facet joint for mobility. Hence minor alterations of the mechanics of the facet joint as we see in extended rotated side-bent (ERS) and flexed rotated side-bent (FRS) dysfunctions can have a profound effect on the mechanics of the disk predisposing to injury.[8] Furthermore, altered movement of the disk secondary to altered facet mechanics can lead to a decreased ability of the disk to derive nutrition by imbibition and predispose to disk degeneration.

LIGAMENTOUS ANATOMY

The ligaments of the lumbar spine as in the other areas of the spine function to limit and modify movement, in addition to their proprioceptive potential. All of the major ligaments in the lumbar area are multisegmental in that they span the entire length of the spinal column. In addition, there are what are known as segmental ligaments which are specific to each segment in the spinal column.[5]

Multisegmental Ligaments

Anterior Longitudinal Ligament

The anterior longitudinal ligament (ALL) as was previously described in the cervical spine section has an attachment to the anterior and lateral surface including the disks of all the segments and finally terminates into the periosteum of the sacrum. The ALL functions to resist distraction of the vertebrae, and backward bending. It also supports the weight of the lumbar spine especially at the lumbosacral junction. The most important function that it clinically relevant is that it prevents the lumbar segments from slipping into the pelvic cavity and is probably the principal restraining structure in spondylolisthesis.

Posterior Longitudinal Ligament

This ligament is attached to all of the vertebral segments including the disks on their posterior surface except atlas. They span over the lumbar area and extend into the sacrum and coccyx. This ligament has a central portion and lateral expansions. The lateral expansions are thinner than the central portion and hence the reason as to why the disk moves posterolaterally following a protrusion. Apparently the ligament is narrow at the lowest two segments of the lumbar spine and hence the restraining effect to a disk prolapse is decreased. The intervertebral space narrows during degeneration of this ligament and maybe of significance in spinal cord disease in the upper levels.

Supraspinous Ligament

The supraspinous ligament is descried to blend into the ligamentum nuchae. Some describe the supraspinous ligament as being replaced by the ligamentum nuchae in the cervical spine. It is often debated as to where the supraspinous ligament ends in the spinal column and a majority of the cadavers studied showed that these ligaments ended at L4. Functionally, this ligament limits forward bending, and some rotation. From a clinical stand point the absence of these ligaments in the lower two levels of the lumbar spine is indeed unfortunate as these levels also have the lesser efficient posterior longitudinal ligament. This further adds to a lack of restraining forces for a disk prolapse.

Segmental Ligaments

Ligamentum Flavum

A description of this ligament is provided in the section on the cervical spine. The only significance is that in the lumbar region, this ligament reaches a thickness of about 8 mm. Due to this, more than in any other level, this ligament a constant pull on the capsule of the facet joint. Hence, it constantly works to prevent the facet capsule from being pinched between the articular surfaces of the facet joints. This function is impaired during dysfunctional states of this ligament leading to facet capsule impingement. In chronic degeneration, there is a tendency for infolding of this ligament into the spinal canal during backward bending predisposing to myelopathy.

Interspinous and Intertransverse Ligament

The interspinous ligaments run backwards and upwards from the superior aspect of the spinous process below to the inferior aspect of the spinous process above. It is seen that following the age of 20 there appears to be degeneration of these ligaments especially at L4, L5 and L5, S1 levels. Since they run backwards, they allow for a greater range while they resist forward bending.

The intertransverse ligament is described as being interposed between adjacent transverse processes and well developed in the lumbar area only. A clinical significance of importance has not been described except that they help to limit side bending and rotation.

Iliolumbar Ligament

The iliolumbar ligament extends from the transverse process of L5 to the superior aspect of the adjacent sacroiliac joint and ilium. In the female, it is further reinforced by another cord from the tip of L4. Paris described this difference and speculates it as an additional reinforcement for the female pelvis on grounds of stability.

The iliolumbar ligament is initially a muscle in the early years of life and later develops into a ligament in the twenties and matures fully in the forties. The clinical significance of this ligament is that it forms the roof of the iliolumbar canal as it runs from the transverse process of L5 to the superior aspect of the sacroiliac joint and adjacent ilium. Inflammatory conditions of this ligament is described to cause a compression of the L5 nerve root causing radicular pain in the corresponding leg.

MUSCULAR ANATOMY

Refer to section on muscular anatomy in Chapter 11, titled 'pelvic complex'.

MECHANICS

The facet joint orientation in the lumbar spine is in the sagittal plane, hence side bending and rotation always occurs in the opposite directions. Hence, if one rotates to the left the lumbar spine also rotates to the left but side bends to the right.[9] This minimizes the stress and shearing effect on the intervertebral disk and the facet/ligamentous structures. However, in situations of a dysfunction, side bending and rotation can occur to the same side and this significantly increases the stress on the corresponding soft tissue structures. The vulnerability increases further if this occurs in flexion. Consider an individual bending forward to pick up an object and rotating to one side in a flexed position to place it to the side. If this is also accompanied by side bending of the lumbar segments to the same side, then the stress on the disk increases significantly. This is also the most common mechanism for back strains. In the presence of ERS and FRS dysfunctions in the lumbar spine, this type of faulty mechanics tends to occur at an arthrokinematic level and needs to be corrected to minimize stress on the supporting structures. Chapter 7 titled 'Principles of Diagnosis'.

The next aspect that is important to note that in the lumbar spine, the thoracolumbar junction and lumbosacral junction are the areas capable of rotation. If you observe the facet orientation of the mid lumbar region, the plane is saggital and no capability of rotation. At T12/LI, L4/L5 and L5/S1, the plane is closer to frontal and is capable of rotation. The mid lumbar is well suited for side bending. Recalling neutral mechanics, rotation is coupled by opposite side bending. Hence, in the lumbar while rotation occurs in the junction, side bending is occurring in the mid lumbar spine.

MECHANISM OF DYSFUNCTION

Chapter 7 titled 'Principles of Diagnosis'. The example of an alteration in the alignment of L4, L5 has been described earlier and hence is just reiterated. Abnormal alignment/mechanics, be it on ERS or on FRS can produce clinical scenarios we see in our day-to-day practice. If movement continues to occur in this abnormal position it can significantly shear the disk (which is part of the motion segment) and may result in a disk pathology. The size or the patency of the foramen is altered and as the nerve exits through the foramen it can be pinched resulting in a radiculopathy. The facet due to abnormal weight bearing stresses of faulty alignment can be susceptible to cartilage and facet capsule shearing. The effusion that occurs due to this can be poured into the foramen increasing nerve root symptoms. Hence, by freeing the facet restriction and correcting the alignment, the patency of the foramen is restored, the shearing of the disk is reduced and the facet joints are rendered less susceptible to loading stresses. This can significantly minimize symptoms.

The large muscle groups that effect movement in this motion segment can be stressed due to faulty mechanics. Hence, correcting vertebral alignment can reduce workloads of these large spinal and pelvic muscles which can later be effectively stabilized to maintain alignment.

Mechanical traction may temporarily open the foramen. Facet injections may temporarily relieve facet and nerve root [2, 10] pain so do other aspects of management including medication. They most definitely have their place as acute pain has to be addressed by these means, but in combination, if the mechanics and alignment are addressed, it may continue to address the 'cause' of the dysfunction.

EXAMINATION

Examination of the lumbar spine is done in sitting and in the 'sphinx' position. The sphinx position is where the patient lies prone and props up on the elbows with the chin resting on the hand. Hence, sitting is the position feasible for forward bending and assessing ERS dysfunctions and the sphinx would be the position feasible for backward bending to assess FRS dysfunctions. This method of examination has shown good reliability.[11]

LUMBAR SPINE SOMATIC DIAGNOSIS

Extended Rotated Side-bent (L1-L5) (Not Opening)

The patient is sitting on a stool and the clinician faces the patient from behind. The clinician then palpates the posterior superior iliac spine (PSIS) on both sides and then moves slightly upwards and medial towards the midline. The first bony landmark is the spinous process of L5. The clinician then moves about an inch lateral and slightly upwards to palpate the corresponding transverse process (Fig. 10.2). The patient is then

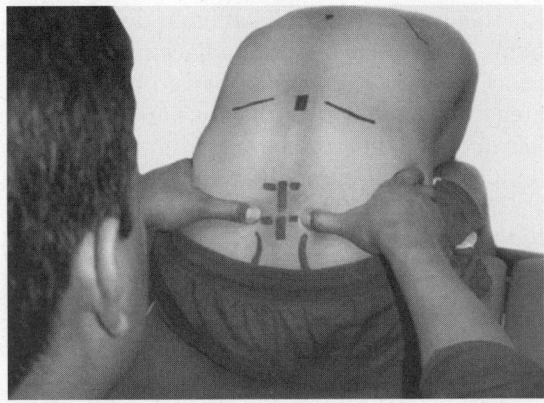

Fig. 10.2: Forward bending to assess ERS or opening restrictions.

asked to bend forwards by taking both arms towards the floor and between the legs.

Assume that the clinician is palpating the transverse processes of L4. When the patient is asked to bend forward and if the transverse process on the right appears more posterior in this position then it can be assumed that the facet on the right is not sliding forward and is stuck in extension. To confirm, the same segment is checked in neutral (sitting, or prone lying with a pillow under the abdomen) and backward bending (sphinx) positions to see if the transverse process returns to neutral. If they appear neutral then the diagnosis will be an ERS right of L4 (not opening on the right).

Flexed Rotated Side-bent (L1-5) (Not Closing)

The patient is lying prone in the prop up position (sphinx). The clinician faces the patient diagonally from the side in the direction of the patient's head. Assume the clinician is palpating the transverse processes of L5 (Fig. 10.3). In the prone prop up position the lumbar spine is technically in backward bending. In this position, if the transverse process of L5 appears more posterior on the right then it can be assumed that the facet on the right is sliding backward and the facet on the left is not as it is stuck in flexion. To confirm, the same segment is checked in neutral (prone lying) and forward bending (as above in sitting) to see if the transverse processes return to neutral. If it does then the diagnosis will be an FRS right of L5 (remember it is the left that is not closing) as the diagnosis is always by the side of the posteriority.

TREATMENT

Soft Tissue Inhibition

Soft tissue inhibition of the lumbar spine is similar to the thumb reinforcement technique described in the thoracic spine section and a similar technique is used over the lumbar area (Fig. 10.4).

Long Axis Tissue Stretch

This is yet another technique that is effective for soft tissue inhibition in the lumbar area prior to manipulative treatment.

Techniques

The patient is in prone lying and the clinician faces the patient from the side. The clinician uses the palmar surfaces of both hands in a crisscross fashion and one hand is placed on the base of the sacrum and the other over the thoracolumbar junction, or the lower thoracic area. A long axis stretch is imparted by the clinician moving both palmar surfaces away from each other with a gentle compression (Fig. 10.5).

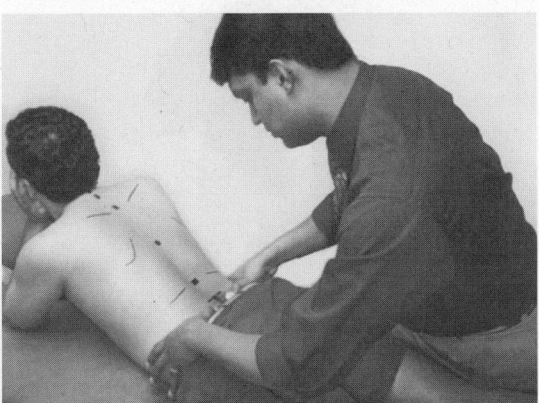

Fig. 10.3: Backward bending (sphinx) to assess frs or closing restrictions.

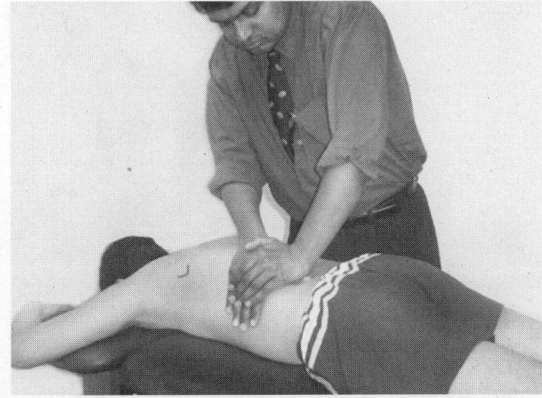

Fig. 10.4: Soft tissue mobilization with thumb reinforcement.

A similar stretch can be applied in side lying with a pillow under the waist and between the knees to support the spine in neutral (Fig. 10.6).

Extended Rotated Side-bent Dysfunction (L4-L5): The patient is in side lying and the clinician faces the patient from the side. Remember the rule that the patient always lies in the side of the posteriority for an ERS in the lumbar spine.

Hence, If it is an ERS left, then the patient lies on the left. Assume the dysfunction is an ERS left of L5. Then the patient lies on the left side and the clinician faces the patient from the side.

Since it is an ERS left the segment is technically in left rotation and extended. Hence the treatment is to free the left facet of L5 into flexion and right rotation.

Patient in Left Side Lying: The upper torso of the patient is rotated to the right by gently pulling the upper arm until L5 is felt to move.

The right leg is flexed at the hip and knee with the foot resting on the left knee.

The left leg is gently moved forward to induce flexion until L5 is felt to move.

The right hand of the clinician is taken under the right arm of the patient and the forearm of the clinician rests on the patient's right arm pit.

Now the right thumb of the clinician is used to block the spinous process of L5 on the superior aspect.

The left forearm of the clinician is placed on the right hip of the patient (Fig. 10.7).

The clinician then takes up the slack and asks the patient to breathe in and as the patient breathes out the slack is taken further. Now the clinician imparts a stretch by exerting a downward pressure using the left forearm with the right thumb blocking the superior aspect of the spinous process of L5, to rotate L5 towards the right, in flexion. This will free the left facet of L5 into flexion (opening) and rotation to the right as it is stuck in extension on the left.

Flexed Rotated Side-bent Dysfunction (L4-L5): The patient is in prone lying and the clinician faces the patient from the side. Assume the patient has an FRS right of L5.

Then technically the L5 segment is in right rotation and stuck in flexion on the left.

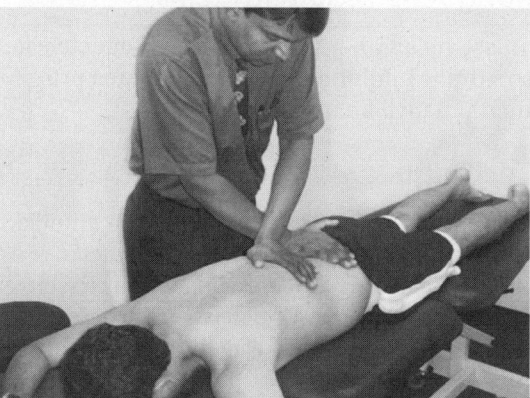

Fig. 10.5: Long axis tissue stretch in prone position.

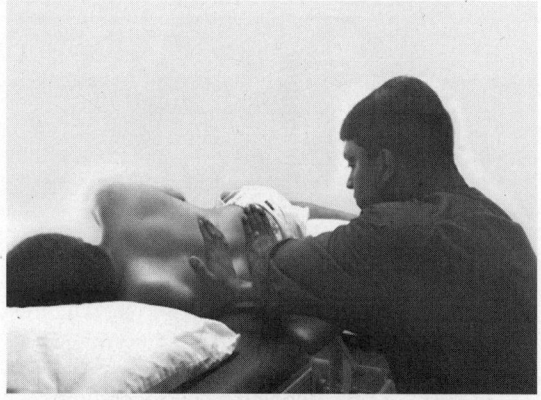

Fig. 10.6: Long axis tissue stretch side lying.

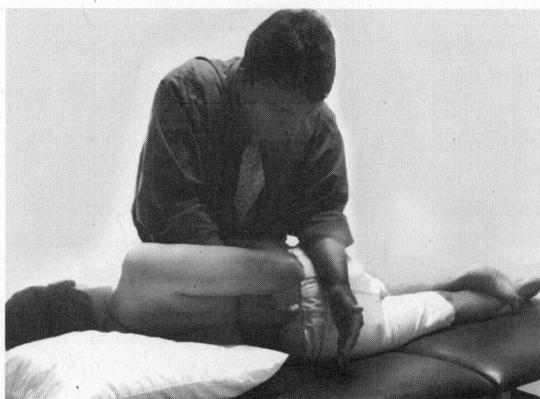

Fig. 10.7: Side lying technique for ERS dysfunction.

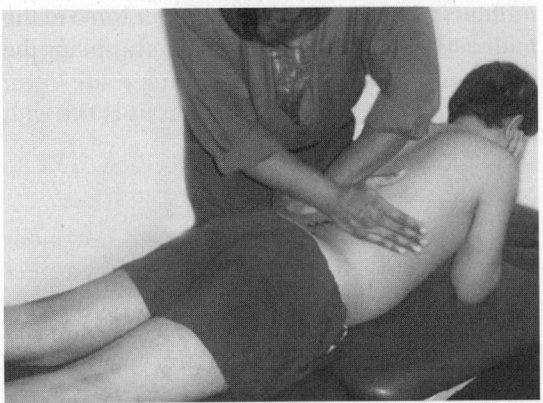

Fig. 10.8: Prone lying technique for FRS dysfunction (Depicts a higher level for visual ease).

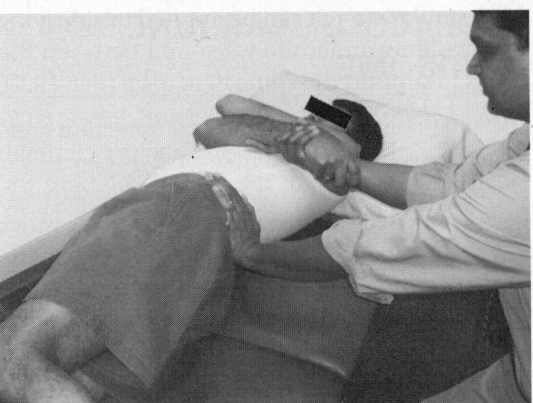

Fig. 10.9: Side lying technique for FRS dysfunction.

Treatment should hence free the left facet into extension and left rotation.

Prone Lying Technique: Clinician faces the patient from the left.

The right pisiform of the clinician is placed on the right transverse process of L5.

The left hypothenar eminence/pisiform of the clinician is placed on the left transverse process of S1 or the base of the sacrum.

The patient is asked to take a deep breath and as he exhales, the clinician takes up the slack and imparts a spring on the right transverse process of L5, while maintaining a counter pressure on the left transverse process of S1 or the base of the sacrum (Fig. 10.8).

This will free the left facet of L5 into extension and left rotation (closing on the left).

Side Lying Technique: Assume patient has an FRS right of L5. Patient is in right side lying and is rotated until L5 begins to move. The trunk is then extended and the clinician faces patient from the back. The right hand of the clinician grasps the right wrist of the patient and the patient does the same to the right wrist of the patient. The left hand is placed on the left sacral base (Fig. 10.9). The patient is asked to inhale deep and the clinican takes the slack and at the end of the exhalation phase, imparts a mobilization with impulse.

Caution: This is a thrust technique and should be performed by trained clinicians, strictly exercising contraindications.

Technique to Free Side Bending: Assume left side bending is to be restored. The patient is in left side lying and the clinician faces the patient. The right arm of the clinician is slide under the right arm of the patient and the fingers hook under the inferior surface of the midlumbar region (Fig. 10.10). The left forearm of the clinician is placed over the right pelvic area of the patient and the fingers hook under the inferior surface of the midlumbar region. Now the patient is asked to inhale and on exhalation the clinician imparts a stretch in an upward direction to restore left side bending.

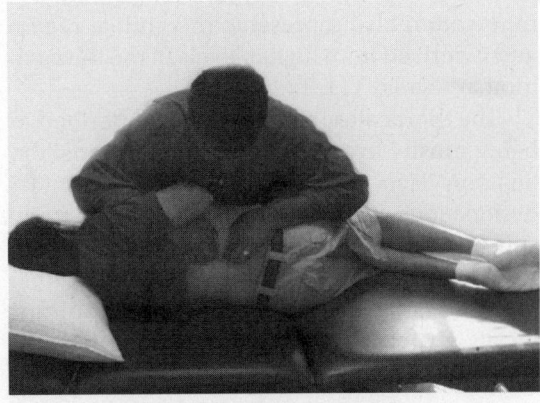

Fig. 10.10: Side bending mobilization (left).

THORACOLUMBAR JUNCTION SYNDROME

The thoracolumbar junction is a transition zone between two regions, lumbar and thoracic T12/L1. In the T12 vertebra, the superior facet is inclined as in the thoracic spine in a more frontal plane and the inferior vertebra, as in the lumbar spine in a more sagittal plane. Since most of the thoracic rotation is restricted by the presence of the ribs, and the midlumbar area by the saggital orientation of the facet joints, the thoraco lumbar junction is described as being one that possesses a significant amount of rotation.[12] In the lumbosacral junction, the orientation of the facet joints are in the frontal plane as opposed to the midlumbar articulations, which are more in the saggital plane.[13] Hence, a considerable amount of rotation also occurs in the lumbosacral junction. Pain from a thoracolumbar dysfunction is seldom felt in the thoracolumbar region. The primary site of referral is the iliac crest and gluteal region with the trochanteric and groin areas being other sites. The reason being the nerve representation. The posterior primary rami of the thoracolumbar spinal nerves innervate the skin of the back and the intrinsic muscles of the apophyseal joints and the supra-and interspinous ligaments. The cutaneous branches penetrate the lumbar fascia, descend in the subcutaneous tissue and end in the skin of the lower lumbar area. Cutaneous innervation also represents the gluteal region and is derived from higher levels of the thoracolumbar region, T11, T12, L1.

The thoracolumbar junction is described as being mostly hypomobile due to its transitory anatomy. Hence, the presence of an ERS or FRS dysfunction with local tenderness is possible and should be examined. The reason for mandatory assessment and treatment of the thoracolumbar junction is more than addressing symptoms locally. Hypomobility of the thoracolumbar articulation may cause a compensatory increase in mobility and stress in the lumbosacral junction and subsequent dysfunction.[14] Assessment and treatment are similar to that done in the lower thoracic spine except that the focus is the T12, L1 segment.

REFERENCES

1. Garfin SR, Rydevik B, Lind B, et al. Spinal nerve root compression. Spine. 1995;20:1810-20.
2. Paris SV. Anatomy as related to function and pain. Orthopedic Clinics of North America. 1983;14:475-89.
3. Porterfield JA, DeRosa C. Mechanical Neck Pain. Perspectives in functional anatomy. 1995. WB Saunders, Philadelphia
4. Waddell G. 1987 volvo award in clinical sciences. A new clinical model for the treatment of low-back pain. Spine. 1987;12:632-44.
5. Paris SV, Loubert PV. Foundations of clinical orthopaedics, course notes. 1990. Institute Press. St. Augustine, FL.
6. Lippitt AB. The facet joint and its role in spine pain.Management with facet joint infections. Spine. 1984;9:746-50.
7. Mooney V, Robertson J. The facet syndrome. Clin Orthop Relat Res.1976;115:149-56.
8. Greenman PE. Principles of manual medicine. 1996, Williams and Wilkins, Baltimore.
9. Fujii R, Sakaura H, Mukai Y, et al. Kinematics of the lumbar spine in trunk rotation: in vivo three-dimensional analysis using magnetic resonance imaging. Eur Spine J. 2007;16:1867-74.
10. Bogduk NLT. Clinical anatomy of the lumbar spine and sacrum. 1997,3rd edn. Churchill Livingstone: New York.
11. Sebastian D, Chovvath R. Reliability of palpation assessment in non-neutral dysfunctions of the lumbar spine. Orthopaedic Physical Therapy Practice. 2003;16:23-6.
12. Maigne R. Low back pain of a thoracolumbar origin. Arch Phys Med Rehabii. 1980;61:389-95.
13. Van Schaik Jan PJ. Lumbar facet joint morphology. J Spinal Disord. 2000;13:88-9.
14. Sebastian D. Thoraco lumbar junction syndrome: A case report. Physiother Theory Pract. 2009;22:53-60.

CHAPTER 11

The Pelvic Complex

The pelvis is the link between the upper torso and the lower extremities. In addition, it is the area of location of the center of gravity as well. The greater functional significance of the pelvic girdle is its role in maintaining the mechanics of the walking cycle. It is one structure that is often underestimated in its capacity and if appropriately addressed, can help diminish back pain and radicular pain. Its close relationship to the lumbar spine is the essential gist of this chapter in addition to the role of the sacrum.

OSSEOUS ANATOMY

The pelvic complex consists of three bones and nine joints (2 inferior articulating facets of L5, S1, 1 intervertebral disk, 2 sacroiliac, 2 coxa femoral (hip), 1 sacrococcygeal and 1 symphysis pubis) and hence highly mobile. The sacrum which is placed in the center is formed by the fused elements of S1 to S5. It articulates superiorly with the lumbar spine and inferiorly with the coccyx. They are termed as lumbosacral and sacrococcygeal joints, respectively. Laterally, the sacrum articulates with ilia or innominate bones to form the sacroiliac joints. The two innominates are joined anteriorly by the symphysis pubis joint.

The sacrum is a triangular structure which has a broad upper surface and a tapering, narrow inferior surface (Fig. 11.1). The upper surface of the sacrum is called the sacral base. Inferiorly, the lateral edge of the sacrum that appears prominent to palpation is due to the curved ends are inferior lateral angles (ILA). The sacral base and inferior lateral angles of the sacrum are the two main bony landmarks that the clinician incorporates to diagnose a sacral dysfunction. On the superior surface, just lateral to the midline are two articulating facets which articulate with the inferior articulating facets of the fifth lumbar vertebra to form the lumbosacral joints. Laterally on the upper surface are two facets which articulate with ilia or innominates bilaterally to form the sacroiliac joints.

The ilia or innominates are two in number and placed laterally on either sides of the sacrum. The superior and anterior aspect of the innominates have a curved projection which are anterior superior iliac spines (ASIS). Anteriorly and inferiorly is a palpable bony landmark just lateral to the groin area which is slightly higher in the male. These are known as pubic tubercles. The superior aspect of the innominate is a curved structure and this area is called the crest of the ilia. These crests taper posteriorly and medially and curve inwards forming a palpable depression inferiorly. These are known as posterior superior iliac spines (PSIS).

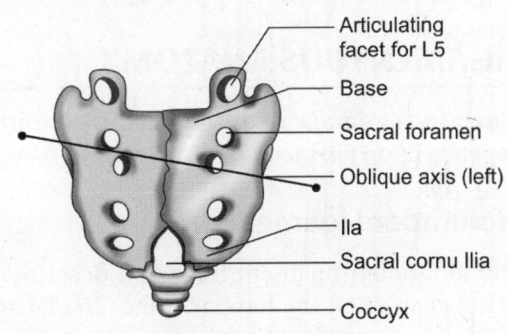

Fig. 11.1: Sacrum.

The greater clinical significance of the pelvic complex originates at the lumbosacral junction. Most dysfunctions of the pelvic complex are viewed as dysfunctions at the sacroiliac joints and may be erroneous. As most times dysfunctions of the sacroiliac joint are caused by a dysfunction that occurs at the lumbosacral junction. The reason being that the lumbar spine is one that determines the mechanics of the sacrum at the lumbosacral joint which in turn determines the mechanics of the ilium or innominate at the sacroiliac joint. Hence, the clinician should always remember that when addressing dysfunctions of the pelvic complex, first consider mechanics at the lumbosacral joint prior to addressing the sacroiliac joint which are mechanically two different areas but complimentary in causing a dysfunction. A more logical explanation to this can be gleamed when the walking cycle is described.

The next area that warrants attention in the pelvic complex is the symphysis pubis. This is an articulation that possesses movement and technically is an anterior attachment of the innominate with relevance to its posterior attachment which is the sacroiliac joint. Hence, a dysfunction in this area can contribute to dysfunctions in the sacroiliac joint posteriorly. Overall, one should understand that the sacroiliac joint that receives attention in a pelvic complex dysfunction could essentially be a secondary effect or be accentuated by dysfunctions either at the symphysis pubis or more often the lumbosacral joint. Thus, when addressing sacroiliac joint dysfunctions, it behooves us to also address the lumbosacral and symphysis pubis joints to globally address the problem in sight.

LIGAMENTOUS ANATOMY

Much of the integrity of the sacroiliac joint depends upon ligamentous structures.

Iliolumbar Ligament

The iliolumbar ligament has been described in the chapter on the lumbar spine. The lower fibers of this ligament extend inferiorly and blend with the anterior sacroiliac ligaments. They limit anterior translation of the 5th lumbar vertebra and posterior rotation of the ilium.

Posterior and Anterior Sacroiliac Ligaments

The posterior sacroiliac ligaments have three layers. They are the short interosseous ligaments which is the deep layer and they run from the sacrum to the ilium. The intermediate layer runs from the posterior arches of the sacrum to the medial side of the ilium. The long posterior sacroiliac ligaments blend together and course vertically from the sacral crest to the ilium. Inferiorly, the posterior sacroiliac ligaments blend with the sacrospinous and sacrotuberous ligaments. All fibers of this ligament limit posterior seperation of the sacroiliac joint. The short fibers limit posterior rotation, internal rotation of the ilium and anterior movement of the sacral base. The long fibers limit anterior rotation of the ilium.

The anterior sacroiliac ligaments prevent anterior separation of the sacroiliac joints.

Sacrotuberous and Sacrospinous Ligaments

The sacrotuberous ligaments run from the inferior lateral angle to the ischial tuberosity above the sacrospinous ligament which runs from the inferior lateral angle to the ischial spine. These two ligaments contribute to the formation of the greater and lesser sciatic notches which are divided by the sacrospinous ligaments. The sacrotuberous ligaments limit anterior and posterior rotation of the ilium as well as sacral flexion. The sacrospinous ligament limits posterior rotation of the ilium and sacral flexion.

MUSCULAR ANATOMY

The musculature of the lumbar area are interdependent with the musculature of the pelvic area and hence are described together. This is for the fact that the mechanics of the two regions are essentially interdependent as well.

The musculature, as in the cervicothoracic complex, are classified as postural and phasic. Their primary functions are as described in the principles of management for they support alignment during function and absorb shock of activity. Their specific actions from an anatomical perspective is obvious, but their individual functions relevant to manual therapy is worth knowing. The postural and phasic muscles are elaborated as follows:[1]

Phasic

- Abdominals (transversus abdominis)
- Gluteus maximus
- Gluteus medius
- Quadriceps

Postural

- Iliopsoas
- Erector spinae
- Multifidus (transversospinalis)
- Piriformis
- Hip adductors/quadratus lumborum
- Hamstrings

Phasic Musculature

Abdominals

Currently, the transversus abdominis has gained attention in the core 'stabilization concept'.[2] Although earlier the rectus abdominus was stressed upon by way of 'curls' or 'crunches', currently 'sucking the abdomen in' is the mainstay of core stabilization, as this works the transversus abdominis as it has a cylindrical compressive effect on the lumbar spine and also reinforces the thoracolumbar fascia.

The primary function of the abdominals is described as the walls of a cylinder. This cylinder wall effect helps to contain the abdominal contents. By doing so it decreases the lever arm of the lumbar lordosis and minimizes its vulnerability to an anterior shear. It thereby maintains the lordotic curve of the lumbar spine.

This function prevents two possible dysfunctions. Theoretically, as the lordosis increases, the sacrum has a tendency to flex. If this is exaggerated due to weakness of the abdominal musculature, the risk of flexion dysfunctions of the sacrum arise as in a flexed sacrum or sacral anterior torsions. When the sacrum is restricted in a flexed position the lumbar segments are at the risk of nonneutral dysfunctions (ERS or FRS). Hence, strong abdominals help to prevent the above described dysfunctions.

The forward head and protracted shoulders posture is seen in patients with upper quarter pain. A weak abdominal wall is described as a contributing feature to this condition. A more caudal position of the sternum and chest results from a weak abdominal wall. This results in a compensatory forward head and protracted shoulders postures. Hence appropriate management of patients with upper quarter pain would include attention to the abdominal mechanism.

Gluteus Maximus

The gluteus maximus attaches to the fascia lata. The fascia has a hip and a knee attachment. Tension in the tensor fascia lata enhances stability at the hip and knee. This is brought about by effective contraction of the gluteus maximus.

It is also an important pelvic stabilizer. On weight bearing, with the foot on the ground, contraction of the gluteus maximus results in a posterior rotation of the pelvis. Hence weakness can result in anterior rotation dysfunctions of the innominate.

The posterior moment creates a flexion moment at the lumbosacral junction.

Flexion of the lumbosacral articulation decreases the lumbosacral angle and anterior shear stresses between the L5 and sacrum. Hence, the gluteus maximus should be strengthened for routine stability of the lumbopelvic complex and specifically for anterior innominate dysfunctions.

Gluteus Medius

Weakness of the gluteus medius is described as causing a 'Trendelenburg' gait. Due to weakness of this muscle, the pelvis on the opposite side tends to drop and hence has a tendency to increase stresses on the lumbar facet joints on the same side of the weakness.

The patient has a tendency to lean to the same side of the weakness and hence the stance time on the weak side tends to increase. This has a tendency to exaggerate the torsion position of the sacrum on that side resulting in torsional dysfunctions.

Hence as a routine for lumbar stability and specifically following correction of a sacral torsion, strengthening of the gluteus medius is recommended.

Quadriceps

Efficient contraction of the quadriceps is required in low back rehabilitation. This muscle should have sufficient girth in order to exert a 'pushing' effect to amplify tension within the fascia lata to enhance stability.

The rectus femoris, being a flexor of the hip tends to cause an anterior rotatory moment of the pelvis and an extension moment in the lumbosacral junction. The management principles are same as the iliopsoas and will be described in the next section.

Quadriceps strength is also essential for execution of proper body mechanics. Eccentric contraction of the quadriceps helps position the back with an intact lordosis to minimize the risk of injury during activity.

Postural Musculature

The postural muscles have a significance to dysfunction for the fact that they have a tendency to contract. Prolonged contraction can pull on their respective skeletal attachment and cause a change in alignment. Hence appropriate lengthening prior to strengthening is mandatory to correct and minimize the incidence and recurrence of a dysfunction.

Iliopsoas

In a weight bearing situation, contraction or contracted states of the iliopsoas can produce an anterior rotation of the ilium. This increases the lordosis in the lumbar area and predisposes the sacrum to flex as in weak states of the abdominals causing dysfunctions of sacral flexion and sacral anterior torsions. This may additionally predispose to nonneutral dysfunctions of the lumbar spine (ERS/FRS).

Hence, the iliopsoas needs to be lengthened if an anterior innominate dysfunction is identified and additionally in situations of a flexed sacrum or nonneutral lumbar dysfunction.

Conversely, weakness of the iliopsoas can cause the sacrum to extend predisposing to extension dysfunctions of the sacrum as in extension shears or sacral posterior torsions. This may additionally predispose to nonneutral dysfunctions of the lumbar spine (ERS/FRS).

Erector Spinae

These muscles have two sets of fibers, superficial and deep. The superficial group do not have a direct attachment to the lumbar spine. However, they exert a bowstringing effect over the posterior trunk. They pull the thorax posteriorly and create an extension moment over the lumbar spine. They also work by a lengthening contraction to control the trunk as forward bending is attempted. A more static contraction has a postural effect during function as this helps to stabilize the lower thorax over the pelvis. They also have a profound effect on sacroiliac joint mechanics. The inferior attachment of this muscle is to the sacrum. Its pull over the sacrum creates a flexion (nutation) moment on the sacrum. This stresses the extrinsic structures of the pelvis and creates a 'force closure'. Hence its weakness of the erector spinae can cause the sacrum to extend causing extension dysfunctions of the sacrum as in extension shears or sacral posterior torsions. However, being a postural muscle, excessive contraction of the erector spinae can increase the flexion moment on the sacrum and predispose to sacral flexion dysfunctions and sacral torsions. Conversely, weakness of the erector spinae can cause the sacrum to extend causing extension dysfunctions of the sacrum as in extension shears or sacral posterior torsions. These may additionally predispose to nonneutral dysfunctions of the lumbar spine (ERS/FRS). The deep group is concerned with sagittal plane stability and this is achieved by a cocontraction of the opposite iliopsoas.

Multifidus (Transversospinalis)

This is a bipennate muscle that originates from the mamillary process of the lumbar vertebra and the osseous and ligamentous structures of the pelvic complex. It also has attachments to the erector spinae. It traverses upwards and medially to attach to the spinous process of the lumbar vertebrae above.

Muscle spasm following injury is a protective mechanism. The muscle senses that further movement can aggravate the existing pathology and hence contracts as a reflex response to prevent further injury. The multifidus is capable of this protective feature. The muscle guarding of the multifidus can essentially cause ERS and FRS dysfunctions by virtue of their oblique attachment to individual vertebra, inhibition techniques like muscle energy techniques (MET) focus to contract or inhibit the multifidus muscle to correct a dysfunction. The multifidi also attach to the sacrum and can favor sacral extension. Contracted states of the multifidus, especially where there is muscle guarding can attribute to dysfunctions of the sacrum as well.

It is considered an inner muscle group. By virtue of being an inner muscle group, it functions as a stabilizer. So, while the prime movers of the spine work to move the spine as a single unit, the multifidus works to stabilize the individual segments in neutral alignment. Thus, following correction of lumbar dysfunctions be it an ERS or an FRS, subsequent strengthening of the multifidus minimizes the potential for recurrence of a dysfunction.

Piriformis

The piriformis muscle attaches to the lateral border of the sacrum and inserts into the trochanteric fossa bilaterally. By virtue of their attachment they favor sacral flexion leading to sacral flexion dysfunctions or sacral anterior torsions. Thus causing an extension moment at the lumbosacral junction leading to an ERS dysfunction.

The sciatic nerve passes close to the piriformis and in a smaller population through it. Hence dysfunctional states of the piriformis can irritate the sciatic nerve causing sciatic symptoms.

Overall, being a postural muscle, the piriformis has a greater tendency to tighten and is also extremely pain sensitive. Often times it is the source of the 'deep buttock pain' described by patients with low back pain. Optimal length and strength of the piriformis is essential to minimize the above described consequences. One often wonders as to why the piriformis is always hyperactive and tender. The hypothetical explanation may be the fact that the piriformis works harder, when the gluteus medius is weak, as it is an accessory abductor of the hip at about 60 degrees of flexion. This situation is worsened if the individual presents with hip flexor tightness or gluteus medius weakness.

Hip Adductors/Quadratus Lumborum

The hip adductors attach to the pubic and ischial rami and extend below to attach to the femur. When the foot is on the ground as in a weight bearing position, the adductor muscles can cause an inferior moment at the pelvis. Thus contributing to inferior or a 'downslip' of the pelvis. The adductors can also entrap the obturator nerve resulting in groin pain.

The quadratus lumborum attaches to the iliac crest and lumbar transverse processes and 12th rib. In contracted or shortened states, it can cause superior translations or an 'upslip' of the innominate. In addition the quadratus lumborum has been described to entrap the sciatic nerve and cause radicular symptoms.

Hamstrings

The hamstrings by virtue of their attachment to the ischial tuberosity control the amount of pelvic rotation during forward bending. Tightness of the hamstrings favors posterior rotation of the innominate. This can cause extension dysfunctions of the sacrum as in extension shears or sacral posterior torsions. As described earlier, extension dysfunctions of the sacrum tend to cause a flexion moment at the lumbosacral articulation leading to nonneutral dysfunctions of the lumbar spine. Hence appropriate lengthening or stretching of the hamstrings is recommended. In addition, the hamstrings have been described to entrap the sciatic nerve and cause radicular symptoms.

MECHANICS

The mechanics of the pelvis is complex owing to the several articulations working to maintain normal mechanics of a very complex function, walking. Dysfunctions of the pelvis are correlated to normalizing mechanics relevant to the walking cycle.[3] If the normal mechanics of the cycle of events that occur during walking is disturbed then dysfunctions result. The mechanics that occur in the pelvic complex during normal walking is described, however, the basic movements of nutation and contranutation will first be described.

Nutation or 'anterior nutation' is described as the anterior and inferior movement of the sacral base. Simple stated, despite all the controversies that exist in literature in this regard, it is considered as sacral flexion.

Contranutation or 'posterior nutation' is when the sacral base moves superiorly and posteriorly. Simply stated, it is sacral extension. In addition, the sacrum has the ability to side bend and rotate as well.

The ilia or innominates possess an ability to rotate forwards and backwards and is termed anterior and posterior rotation of the ilia. In addition, they also have the ability to turn inwards and outwards and is termed as an inflare/outflare or a medial/lateral rotation. A superior and inferior translatory motion occurs when the opposing surfaces are flatter and more parallel.

A combination of sacral and ilial movements is what occurs during the normal walking cycle.

WALKING CYCLE RELEVANT TO PELVIC MECHANICS

The axis of movement is the first important component that the clinician should understand. All movements in the human body occur in a diagonal plane as one would recollect concept of patterned motion that are taught in proprioceptive neuromuscular facilitation (PNF) courses. It is three-dimensional and is a combination of the frontal, sagittal and horizontal axes. The sacrum functions the same way and hence the movements of the sacrum as a combination of flexion side bending and rotation occurs in a hypothetical *oblique axis*. This axis is an imaginary line drawn from the superior aspect of one sacroiliac joint to the inferior aspect of the other. For example, the line of the axis running from the superior aspect of the left sacroiliac joint to the inferior aspect of the right sacroiliac joint is the left oblique axis, and vice versa for the right.

In the normal walking cycle, the events that occur are heel strike, foot flat or midstance, and heel/toe off. The cycle of events that are of greater clinical significance are the ones that occur during heel strike and midstance and are as follows:

Assuming the right leg is the one that is the leading leg, at right heel strike, the right innominate rotates posteriorly and the left innominate rotates anteriorly. The sacrum rotates to the right.

At right midstance, the right innominate begins to rotate anteriorly. The sacrum flexes forward and rotates to the right and side bends to the left.

In short, during one legged weight bearing the sacrum rotates to the same side of weight bearing and side bends to the opposite side in flexion.

This is what is known as a torsional movement. It then extends back to neutral and the same cycle of movement occurs during initiation of the left leg.

The other important component of this simplified version of the walking cycle is the movement occurring at L5. Remember as a rule that *when no restriction is prevalent in the facet joints, the L5 segment always moves in the opposite direction of the sacrum.*

Hence during the walking cycle, during one legged weight bearing or at midstance, if the sacrum rotates right and side bends left then L5 would rotate left.

To summarize the movement of the sacrum can be visualized as follows. Assume you have two obliquely horizontal crossbars in opposite direction and you are trying to cross them over. The two oblique crossbars represent a left oblique axis and a right oblique axis. Hence to cross over, one may have to flex and rotate over the crossbar and when this occurs a complementary side bending is happening to the opposite side. Then the individual will need to extend back to neutral and repeat the same activity to the right.

Point to note is that when the sacrum is restricted in a flexed position and does not extend to neutral during the gait cycle it is an anterior torsion. Vice versa, if the sacrum is restricted in extension and fails to flex it is a posterior torsion.

If for any reason the mechanics described above is altered then a dysfunction would result. So for example, assume that the individual is in left leg stance the sacrum is in a position of left rotation and right side bending. However, assume the sacrum is stuck or restricted in this position, then when the gait cycle reverses to right stance the ability of the sacrum to first extend back to neutral and flex, rotate right and side bend left is diminished. This can result in pain and dysfunction and this is what one is trying to identify and appropriately correct with manual therapy procedures. Hence a clinician addressing mechanical dysfunction in the lumbopelvic complex should primarily be concerned at restoring the normalcy of mechanics during the walking cycle.[4] The dysfunctions that may interfere with the normal mechanics of the walking cycle is described in the next section. The goal of treatment, hence, would be to identify these dysfunctions and correct them as appropriate to restore normal mechanics.

MECHANISM OF DYSFUNCTION

Dysfunctions in the pelvic complex occur in three regions. They occur either in the pubic symphysis, sacrum or ilium. Hence they are classified as pubic, sacral and ilial dysfunctions. The types, possible etiology, presentation and management are described below.[4,5]

Symphysis Pubis Dysfunction

Movements here are quite small. They occur during standing and during walking cycle. During gait, the symphysis pubis is the most stable joint in the pelvic girdle. It oscillates up and down in a sinusoidal curve but translates a little from side to side. There is a shearing movement during one legged standing and increases if this standing time is prolonged or when one lands hard on one leg supporting the body weight. This predisposes to a dysfunction. Also a pulling motion of one leg causes dysfunction especially if one is dragged by the leg. When two legged standing is maintained, the symphysis returns to symmetry.

Since the symphysis is the anterior joint of the innominates, a dysfunction tends to reduce the rotation movement of the innominates during walking, disturbing the mechanics of the walking cycle. It can also contribute to dysfunction of the posterior articulation of the innominates which is the sacroiliac joint. When the innominate translates up and down, or rotates anterior and posterior the pubic tubercles go up or down. For example, during anterior rotation of the innominate, the corresponding pubic tubercle rotate downwards. This brings the acetabulum lower and the leg on the same side appears longer. The reverse happens during posterior rotation of the innominates. It is then quite obvious that an upslip would cause the pubic tubercle to go upwards causing a short leg on the same side and vice versa for a downslip.

Pubic dyfunctions are very common secondary to muscle imbalances between the abdominals and adductors. Chronic overload on one leg accentuates the vulnerability. Restricted pubic motion disturbs symmetrical motion of the innominate bones during the walking cycle. Since there is an oscillatory motion of the pubis up and down the two possible dysfunctions of the pubis are:
1. Superior pubis.
2. Inferior pubis.

The above two dysfunctions occur at the symphysis pubis joint.

The causes for a superior pubic dysfunction is commonly a slip and fall on the ischial tuberosity. Hormonal influences as in pregnancy and postpartum pubic separation and weak pelvic stabilizers namely the gluteus medius are additional causes. Tightness of the iliopsoas with an posterior innominate rotation can cause a superior pubis. A posterior innominate dysfunction secondary to tight hamstrings is yet another cause.

An inferior pubis can also occur with hormonal influences as in pregnancy and postpartum pubic separation. Tightness of the adductors of the hip can cause an inferior descent of the pubis secondary to its pubic rami and femoral attachments.

The patient with a symphysis dysfunction typically complains of groin, medial hip and thigh pain. Local tenderness is usually evident over the hip adductors and groin area. There tends to be tenderness over the inguinal ligament. Pregnancy is yet another source for pubic and for that matter pelvic dysfunction as a whole.[6] Due to hormonal activity, the ligaments of the pelvic complex appear lax during pregnancy as the pelvic inlet is required to enlarge to accommodate the baby. Following childbirth the joint surfaces return back to their original states and this usually does not occur in symmetry and may predispose to faulty alignment and dysfunction.

Sacrum Dysfunction

Sacrum is probably the most important component of the pelvic complex and is often missed out in a sacroiliac dysfunction as the ilia receive more attention. The sacrum is the direct link of the lumbar spine to the pelvic complex and plays an important role in the walking cycle. The movements available in the sacrum are very limited for the fact that the center of gravity is located here and would make sense to have one that is stable. If this negligible movement of the sacrum is altered then a dysfunction would result. The sacrum has been described as a significant contributor to back pain and radicular pain. The reason being the close proximity of nerve structures to the sacroiliac joint, the ala of the sacrum and the piriformis muscle, as this muscle attaches to the lateral border of the sacrum. The mechanics of the sacrum has been described earlier in this chapter and significant to the walking cycle. This has to be maintained for normalcy from a mechanical perspective. It has to be reiterated that the sacrum has movements in three planes as for other major joints with movements of flexion (nutation)/extension (contranutation), side bending and rotation. A combination of all occurs in a hypothetical oblique axis. Hence, in all, dysfunctions of the sacrum occur as flexion and extension with a combination of side bending and rotation known as torsional dysfunctions.

One should remember that although a torsional dysfunction occurs as a combination of side bending and rotation, it does so in a flexed or extended position. Hence if side bending and rotation occur with flexion, it is a *anterior torsion*, and when it does so in extension it is termed as *posterior torsion*.

Torsional Dysfunctions

As described earlier, a torsion of the sacrum is a combination of side bending and rotation which can occur with flexion (nutation) or extension (contranuation). Thus torsions occurring in flexion are called anterior torsions and those occurring in extension are called posterior torsions (Figs. 11.2 and 11.3).

Anterior Torsion

The landmarks used as reference points for palpation are base and ILA.

Since a torsion is first a rotation, technically base and ILA on the same side move together. For example, if it is a left rotation, the left base and left ILA move posterior. This is followed by a side bending to the right. As this is occurring, the sacrum flexes or nutates on a *left oblique axis*. Since the rotation is to the left and the flexion is in a left oblique axis, it is called a *left on left sacral torsion*.

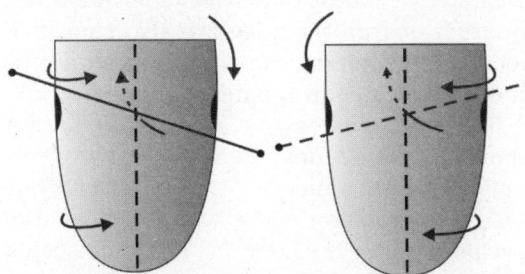

Fig. 11.2: Torsional positions of the anterior sacrum.

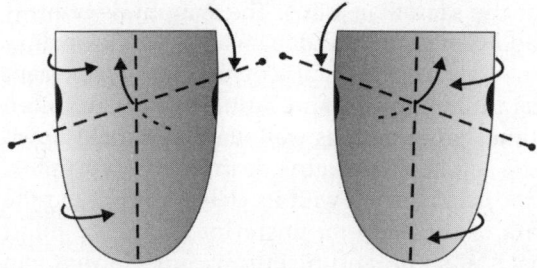

Fig. 11.3: Torsional positions of the posterior sacrum.

The exact reverse occurs in a *right on right sacral torsion*. Hence, there are two types of anterior torsions namely:
1. Left on left sacral torsion.
2. Right on right sacral torsion.

The clinician should recall that torsional movements are normal movements that occur in the sacrum during the gait cycle. Recall from the section on mechanics, that the sacrum goes into left torsional position on left stance but extends and moves into flexion and right torsional position on right stance. When restricted in left torsional position this reversal or its ability to extend (hence an anterior torsion) and go into a right torsional position is diminished, predisposing to a dysfunction.

Posterior Torsion

The reference points are as for an anterior torsion namely base and ILA.

Again, since a torsion is first a rotation, the base and ILA move in the same direction. For example, the left base and ILA move posterior and this is a rotation of the sacrum to the left. Then the sacrum side bends to the right. As this is occurring the sacrum extends or contranutates on a hypothetical *right oblique axis*. Since the rotation is to the left and the extension is on a right oblique axis it is called a *left on right sacral torsion*.

The exact opposite occurs in a *right on left sacral torsion*. Hence, there are two types of posterior torsions namely:
1. Left on right sacral torsion.
2. Right on left sacral torsion.

The clinician should recall that torsional movements are normal movements that occur in the sacrum during the gait cycle. Recall from the section on mechanics, that the sacrum goes into left torsional position on left stance but extends and moves into flexion and right torsional position on right stance. Now the sacrum has to extend to neutral and go into right torsional position on a right oblique axis, that is flex on a right oblique axis with right rotation and left side bending. Since this does not occur as the sacrum is stuck in extension and not flexing (hence a posterior torsion) it ends up extending or stays extended on this right oblique axis (in which it actually has to flex but cannot do so). Hence it is a left torsion but staying extended on a right oblique axis (left on right). The situation reverses for a right on left.

A left on left sacral torsion is most commonly seen among the torsions. Torsions can occur commonly due to alignment issues in the lower extremities or muscle imbalances. Nonneutral dysfunctions in the lumbar spine, limb length discrepancies, prolonged faulty postures can be predisposing factors. Weakness of the transversus abdominis, glutei or tightness of the piriformis and the erector spinae are causative factors. Again hormonal changes in pregnancy and postpartum women are at risk. Trauma as in falls, sudden jerky movement, etc. may also contribute to dysfunctional states.

The clinician should understand and remember that all sacral dysfunctions occur at the lumbosacral joints.

Innominates Dysfunction

As described earlier, the innominates oscillate up and down in a sinusoidal curve during the gait cycle. This up and down shearing movement tends to cause in dysfunctional states, what is known as an 'upslip' or a 'downslip' of the innominates.

Since the innominates rotate anteriorly and posteriorly during the gait cycle there is a tendency for the innominates to be restricted in one of these positions due to faulty mechanics. Thus in entirety, the innominates can either be restricted as an upslip or a downslip, and an anterior or posterior rotation. Some authors also describe restriction in internal and external rotation called inflares and outflares, however, it is not of a very big focus in this text from a diagnosis perspective. The causes for the innominates to be restricted in an upslip position is commonly a direct fall on the ischial tuberosity. Occasionally a tight unilateral quadrarus lumborum may predispose to an up lip. A downslip is less common than an upslip. Trauma may be a predisposing factor if the individual is dragged hard on one leg, however, instability in the form of muscle weakness or ligament laxity may be a causative factor.

Anterior rotation of the innominates are commonly seen when there is an evidence of tightness of the iliacus and the psoas major and minor. When an individual weight bears with a tight iliopsoas group, there is a compensatory hip hyperextension. This can cause a myriad of dysfunctions including an anteriorly rotated innominate, sacral flexion and nonneutral lumbar dysfunction. Unilateral weakness of pelvic stabilizers or an apparent or true long leg are also causative factors. The clinician can also consider a supinated foot creates an apparent long leg.

Causes for a posterior rotation are usually the reverse. Here the most common cause is tightness of the hip extensors. When an individual weight bears with a tight hip extensor group, there is a compensatory hip flexion. This can cause a myriad of dysfunctions including an posteriorly rotated innominate, sacral extension and nonneutral lumbar dysfunction. Again, unilateral weakness of pelvic stabilizers or an apparent or true short leg are also causative factors. The clinician can also consider a pronated foot creates an apparent short leg.

The innominates are susceptible to the following dysfunctions:
- Posterior rotation
- Anterior rotation
- Upslip
- Downslip.

The clinician must understand and remember that all innominate rotation dysfunctions occur at the sacroiliac joints. The symphysis pubis is additionally involved in an upslip or downslip.

Dysfunctions of the pelvic complex present as unilateral hip and buttock pain and often times groin pain as well. Radicular pain down the leg has its origins in the pelvic complex. The sciatic nerve with its close proximity to the ala of the sacrum, posterior sacroiliac joint, ischial spine and piriformis muscle that can be significantly irritated in dysfunctional states.

Sacral dysfunctions and innominate dysfunctions can effect this. The femoral nerve and the lateral cutaneous nerve anteriorly and the obturator nerve medially are also vulnerable.

The piriformis muscle attaches to the lateral borders of the sacrum and the lesser trochanter of the femur and serves to anchor the sacrum bilaterally in addition to externally rotating the hip. Sacral dysfunctions can stress this muscle as it may be stretched or be contracted. The sciatic nerve runs close to this muscle and in a small population runs through this muscle. This may irritate the nerve and predispose to radicular pain.

The ala of the sacrum is a bony landmark that can get closer to the nerve in faulty positions of the sacrum causing radicular pain. The capsule of the sacroiliac joint can be inflamed secondary to dysfunctional states and can throw off effusion on to the nerve causing radicular symptoms.

Additional causes for mechanical pain in the pelvis is enumerated in chapter 5 in the section on muscle weakness.

EXAMINATION

Examination of the pelvic complex firstly involves identification of the essential bony landmarks namely:
- Pubic tubercles.
- Posterior superior iliac supine (PSIS).
- Sacral base.
- Infero-lateral angles (ILA).
- Ischial spine.
- Iliac crests.

Examination procedures are in the order of the three regions, pubis, sacrum and ilium.

PELVIC COMPLEX SOMATIC DIAGNOSIS

Preceding all diagnosis in the pelvic complex, determination of the side of the dysfunction is important. The clinician is advised not to follow pain but rather the dysfunction as the side of pain does not necessarily determine the side of the dysfunction. The pain can very well be on one side with the dysfunction on the opposite side. Two simple tests are performed to determine the side of the dysfunction.[7]

PSIS Asymmetry and Sitting Flexion Test

The patient is seated and the clinician faces the patient from behind. The clincan palpates both PSIS and observes for asymmetry. The patient is then asked to place their hands between the knees and flex forward by pointing their hands towards the floor.

When flexion of the trunk is performed, the ilia rotate forward and hence the PSIS technically moves upward. Hence, as the clinician palpates both PSIS the side of the restriction is felt to *move upward first* (Fig. 11.4).

The side that moves first is considered to be the side of the dysfunction.

Stork Test

The patient is standing and the clinician faces the patient from behind. The clinician palpates both PSIS as in the sitting flexion test. Now the patient is asked to flex his hip by lifting the hip upwards (Fig. 11.5).

When the hip is flexed, the corresponding ilium tends to rotate backward, hence the PSIS technically should be felt to move downward. However, in situations of a restriction the PSIS is

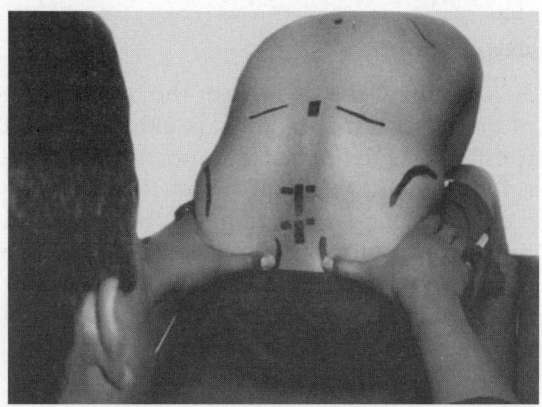

Fig. 11.4: Sitting flexion test.

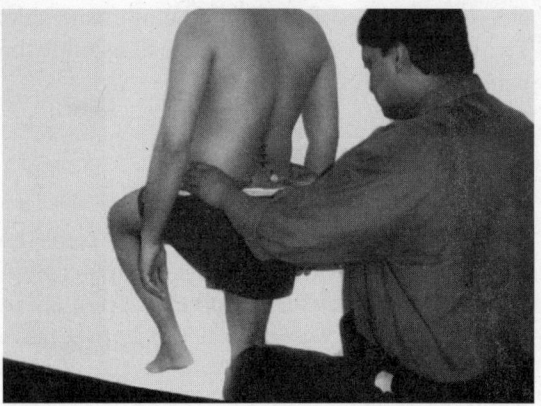

Fig. 11.5: Stork test.

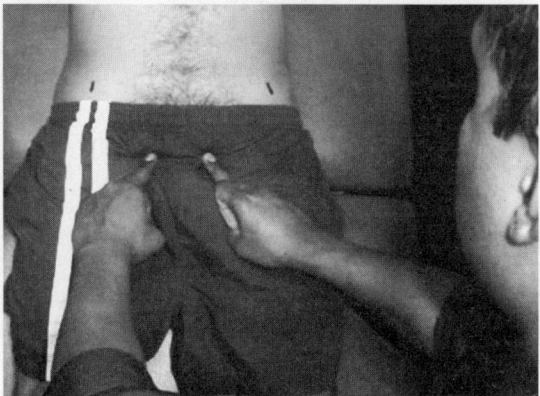

Fig. 11.6: Locating the pubic tubercles.

felt to *move upward* as the ilium does not rotate backward.

Thus, the PSIS on the side that is felt to move upward, rather than downward is considered the side of the dysfunction.[8]

Prone Prop Up Test

The patient lies prone and props up on the elbows with the chin resting on the hand. The clinician palpates the bases of the sacrum.

Assumption 1

Palpation of the base of the sacrum in prone prop up, if the base moves further anterior it is a flexed sacrum and more posterior it is an extended sacrum provided that sitting and standing flexion tests are positive on that side.

Assumption 2

Assume that on palpation of the base or *ILA* of the sacrum, if *both* appears either elevated (posterior) or depressed (anterior) on the same side. Then it is a torsional dysfunction.

Now on palpation of the base of the sacrum in prone prop up, if the base moves further anterior it is an anterior torsion and more posterior it is a posterior torsion provided that sitting and standing flexion tests are positive on that side.

Diagnosis of Pubis Dysfunction

The patient is lying supine and the clinician faces the patient from the side. The clinician places his palm on the abdomen and moves it down slowly until the heel of the hand contacts the superior aspect of the symphysis pubis/pubic rami. Moving laterally about 2 cm, the superior aspect of the pubic tubercles are palpated (Fig. 11.6).

The clinician looks to see if one pubic tubercle is higher or lower in comparison with the other to make a diagnosis of a superior or inferior pubis. The dysfunctional side is usually tender on palpation.

Diagnosis of Sacrum Dysfunction

The base and inferior lateral angle (ILA) of the sacrum are the two standard landmarks used for a diagnosis. The clinician faces the patient from the side and places the palm of the hand in the lower gluteal area. As pressure is applied upwards, the palm is felt to hit on the sacrococcygeal joint (Fig. 11.7). As the fingers are placed on the sacrococcygeal joint and moved laterally and upwards, the lower sacrum is felt to taper outwards. Now the thumbs of the clinician are brought to the superior surface and ILA is palpated (Fig. 11.8).

The Pelvic Complex

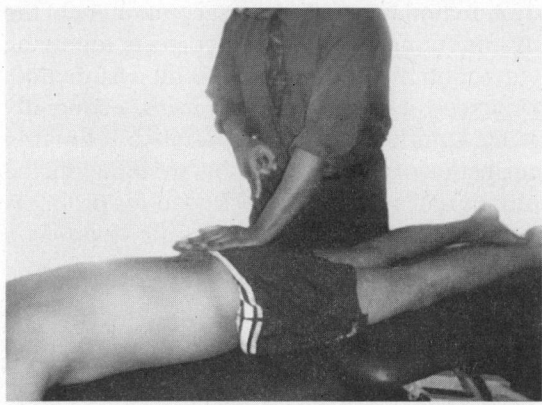

Fig. 11.7: Locating the inferior aspect of the sacrum.

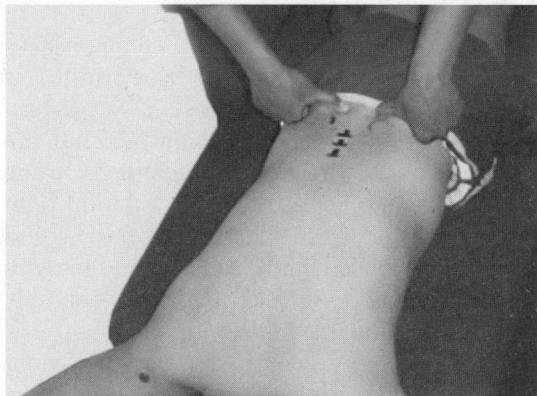

Fig. 11.9: Locating the base.

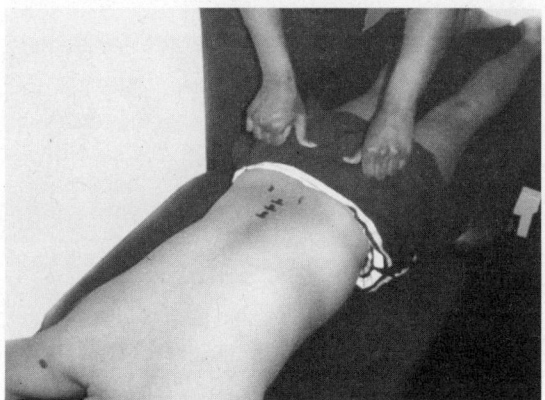

Fig. 11.8: Locating the ila.

The clinician then palpates the PSIS. The palpating thumbs are now moved 30° downward and medially to palpate the base (Fig. 11.9). This is a difficult landmark to palpate and requires a great deal of practice.

Torsional Dysfunctions

Left on Left Sacral Torsion

The patient is lying prone and the clinician faces the patient from the side. The palpation of landmarks are the same, being the base and ILA.

Assuming it is a left on left sacral torsion, the left rotation makes the base and ILA appear posterior (elevated) on the left.

On palpation of both ILAs, since a left on left torsion is a combination of left rotation and right side bending, ILA on the right appears inferior on palpation.

The right side bending tends to cause the pelvis to dip on the right and hence the acetabulum is lower. On palpation of the ischial tuberosity it is observed to be lower on the right. This tends to make the leg appear longer on the right.

The important thing to observe now is whether it is an anterior or a posterior torsion.

To confirm this, the patient is in prone lying. Now both bases are palpated and the patient is asked to prop up in extension (sphinx). *If the sacral base is felt to move more anterior (depressed) then it is considered to be an anterior torsion.*

Sitting and standing flexion tests are positive on the left.

Left on Left Sacral Torsion

Base	Posterior or elevated left
ILA	Posterior or elevated left
Leg length	Long leg right
Prone prop up (sphinx)	Sacral base moves further anterior (depressed)

The exact reverse occurs in a right on right sacral torsion, and the base continues to further depress anterior on prone prop up as it is an anterior torsion.

Left on Right Sacral Torsion

The patient is lying prone and the clinician faces the patient from the side. The base and ILA is palpated on both sides.

The clinician should remember that the objective findings in a left on right is the same as a left on left. For example, in a left on right sacral torsion, the base and ILA are posterior or elevated on the left with a long leg on the right, just as in a left on left sacral torsion. The only difference is that it is a posterior torsion.

Hence, determining whether it is an anterior or posterior torsion is the principle difference. This is done by using the prone extension test as described in the section on left on left sacral torsion.

The patient is lying prone and the clinician palpates both bases. Then, the patient is asked to prop up into extension (sphinx). *If the sacral base moves further posterior then it is a posterior torsion.*

Sitting and standing flexion tests are positive on the left.

Left on Right Sacral Torsion

Base	Posterior or elevated left
ILA	Posterior or elevated left
Leg length	Long leg right
Prone prop up (sphinx)	Posterior ILA moves further posterior (elevated)

The exact reverse occurs in a right on left sacral torsion.

The key for torsional dysfunctions is that on palpation of the base or ILA of the sacrum, *both* appears either elevated (posterior) or depressed (anterior) on the same side.

Secondly, the prone prop up test will determine if it is an anterior or posterior torsion.

Diagnosis of Innominate Dysfunction

Diagnosis of an innominate dysfunction involves application of a cluster of tests to determine the presence of a dysfunction.[9] An innominate dysfunction is usually the last component of the dysfunction. It usually self corrects following correction of a lumbar or a sacral dysfunction. However, if signs and symptoms, especially a leg length discrepancy persists following correction of a sacral or lumbar dysfunction, the innominates need to be assessed for probable dysfunction. The prediction rule involves a cluster of four tests:

1. PSIS asymmetry
2. Positive sitting or standing flexion test
3. Prone leg length discrepancy that corrects on knee flexion (Figs. 11.10 and 11.11)
4. Supine leg length discrepancy that corrects on coming up from supine to sit (Fig. 11.12).

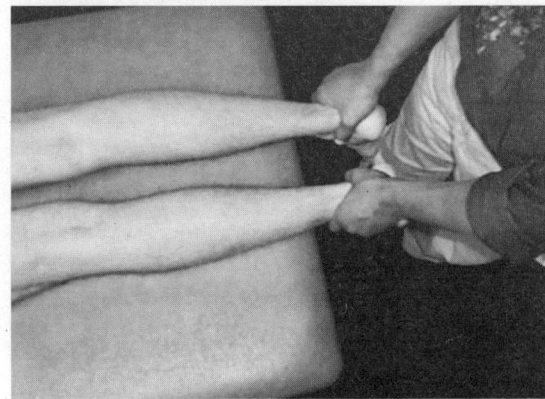

Fig. 11.10: Prone leg length assessment.

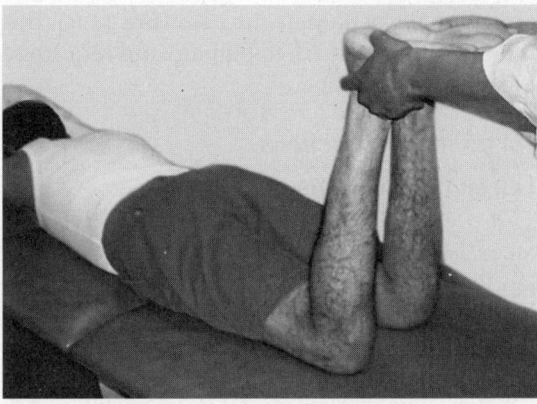

Fig. 11.11: Prone knee flexion.

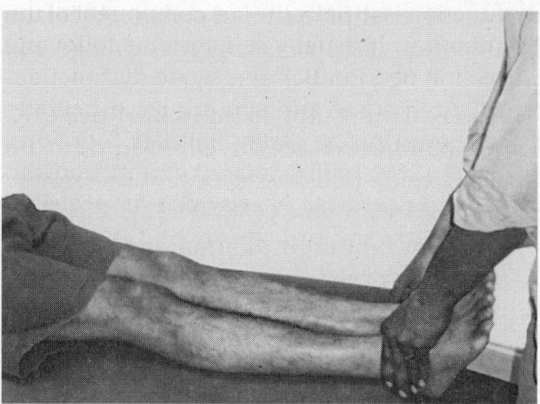

Fig. 11.12: Supine to sit.

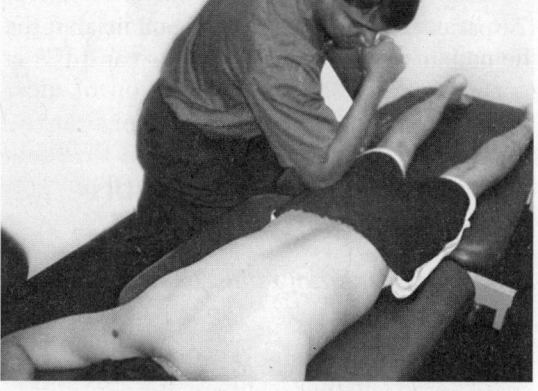

Fig. 11.13: Trigger point compression, gluteus medius and piriformis.

Posterior/Anterior Innominate

Assume the patient presents with PSIS asymmetry in sitting and has a positive sitting flexion test on the left. It is assumed then that the dysfunction is on the left side. Now, observe for leg length in prone and assume the patient presents with a long leg on the left. If the leg length returns to neutral in prone knee flexion, then it is an anterior innominate on the left as it goes with a long leg.

This can be further confirmed with the patient lying supine and the long leg on the left returns to neutral on supine to sit.

If the patient presents with a posterior innominate, then the same scenario is repeated. The side of the dysfunctions first determined, and a posterior innominate presents as a short leg on the same side which neutralizes on prone knee flexion and supine to sit.

Note: Leg length discrepancy holds well only for an apparent change. True changes in leg length occurring in the tibia, femur and the supratrochanteric region should always be ruled out.

Upslip and Downslip of Innominate

In an upslip, both ASIS and PSIS on the dysfunctional side appear higher along with the ischial tuberosity. Obviously then the leg on that side appears shorter.

Vice versa, in a downslip, both ASIS and PSIS on the dysfunctional side appears lower along with the ischial tuberosity. The leg on that side will hence appear longer.

TREATMENT

Treatment of the pelvic complex will sequence in correcting a lumbar dysfunction if any, first. Then pubic dysfunctions should be identified and corrected. This is followed by correction of sacral dysfunctions and lastly innominate dysfunctions are corrected.

Soft Tissue Inhibition

The patient is lying prone and the clinician faces the side to be treated. Two structures often irritable are piriformis and gluteus medius. Using the elbow, the clinician locates the piriformis half way between PSIS, ischial tuberosity and greater trochanter. A gentle compression is applied till tenderness is felt and the pressure is gradually increased (Fig. 11.13). The pressure is maintained for at least 60 seconds in this time the tenderness may decrease. A similar procedure is done for the gluteus medius which is located lateral and superior to the piriformis (see chart for myofascial tender points at the end of the chapter). This is usually done following inhibition of the soft tissue for the lumbar spine.

Deep frictions over the posterior sacroiliac ligament, sacrotuberous ligament and the iliolumbar ligament is also recommended. (Refer to section on palpation for location of these structures).

Treatment of Symphysis Pubis Dysfunction

Superior and Inferior Pubis: ("Shotgun Technique")

The patient is lying supine with the hips and knees flexed and the feet together.

The clinician stands by the side holding the patients knees together. The patient is first asked to abduct both legs and the clinician resists efforts in as in a static contraction. The clinician then places a forearm between the patients' knees (Fig. 11.14). The patient is then asked to statically adduct both legs which is resisted by the forearm placed between the legs. This distracts the pubis to correct the dysfunction (sometimes with an audible release).

Treatment of Sacrum Dysfunction

Left on Left Sacral Torsion

The patient is lying prone and flexion is induced by placing firm pillows under the abdomen (or flexing the treatment table). The clinician faces the patient from the side. Both legs of the patient are now abducted and internally rotated. This gaps both sacroiliac joints. The clinician now places the heel of the hand on the *left* lateral border of the sacrum *midway between base and ILA*.

The patient is now asked to inhale deeply. As the patient exhales the clinician takes up the slack and applies a downward pressure to hold the sacrum down (Fig. 11.15). This frees the sacrum into right rotation and *extension* as the lumbar spine is kept flexed with pillows under the abdomen, or by flexing the table. This encourages the sacrum to extend.

The exact reverse is done for a right on right sacral torsion and the patient position is the same.

Left on Right Sacral Torsion

The technique is the same as for a left on left sacral torsion except that the patient is in a prone prop up position.

The patient is lying prone and the clinician faces the patient from the left side. The patient is asked to prop up to the 'sphinx' position. The legs of the patient are now abducted and internally rotated to gap both sacroiliac joints. The clinician places the heel of the palm on the *left* lateral border of the sacrum *midway between base and ILA*.

The patient is now asked to inhale deeply. When this occurs the clinician takes up the slack and applies a downward pressure on the left lateral border of the sacrum to hold it down (Fig. 11.16). This frees the sacrum into right

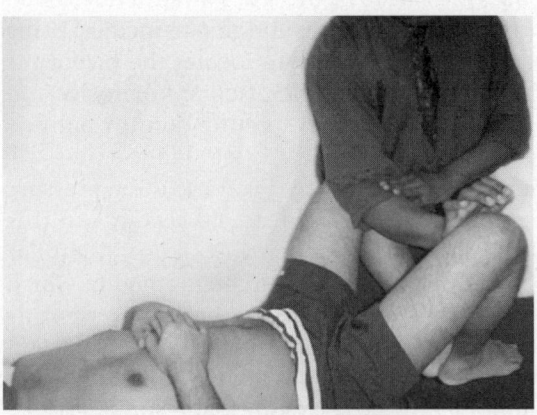

Fig. 11.14: Shotgun technique.

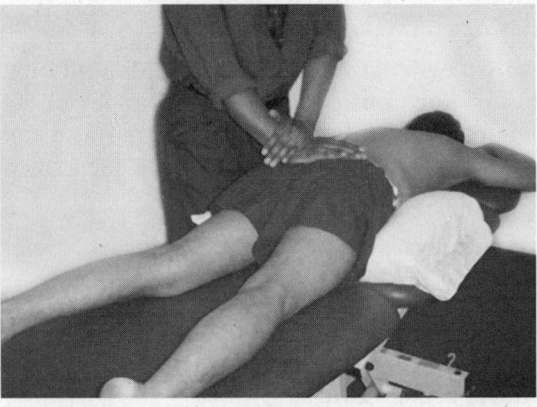

Fig. 11.15: Correction technique for anterior torsion.

rotation and *flexion* as the lumbar spine is kept extended by the prone prop up position. This encourages the sacrum to flex.

The exact reverse is done for a right on left sacral torsion and the patient position is the same.

Treatment of Innominate Dysfunction

Posterior Innominate

Assuming it is a left posterior innominate, the patient is then in right side lying and the clinician faces the patient from the face side. The clinician then rotates the trunk to the left till L5 begins to move. The left hip and knee is flexed and the foot is placed behind the right knee.

The clinician grips the iliac crest with the palm of the left hand and places the heel of the right hand on the ischial tuberosity of the patient. An anterior rotation of the left innominate is induced by an upward pressure on the ischial tuberosity with the right hand and simultaneously pulling the iliac crest inwards (Fig. 11.17).

Anterior Innominate

Assuming it is a left anterior innominate, the patient is then in right side lying and the clinician faces the patient from the face side. The clinician then rotates the trunk to the left till L5 begins to move. The left hip and knee is flexed and the foot is placed behind the right knee.

The clinician places the heel of the left hand anterior to the left iliac crest and the heel of the right hand posterior to the left ischial tuberosity. A posterior rotation of the left innominate is induced by a posteriorly directed pressure on the anterior aspect of the iliac crest and an anteriorly directed pressure on the posterior aspect of the ischial tuberosity (Fig. 11.18).

Upslip

The patient is lying supine and the clinician faces the patient from the leg side at the end of the table. The clinician then grasps the distal tibia and fibula above the ankle. The leg is in slight abduction and in internal rotation to stabilize the

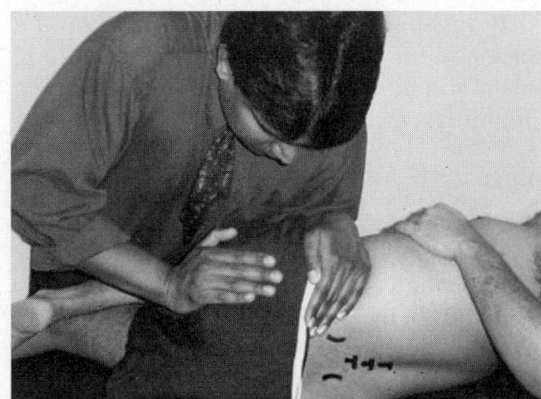

Fig. 11.17: Technique to correct posterior innominate.

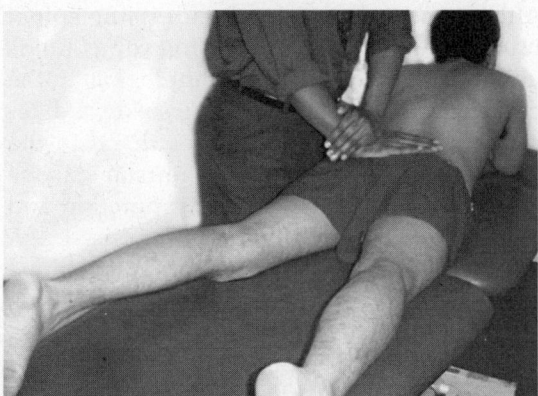

Fig. 11.16: Correction technique for posterior torsion.

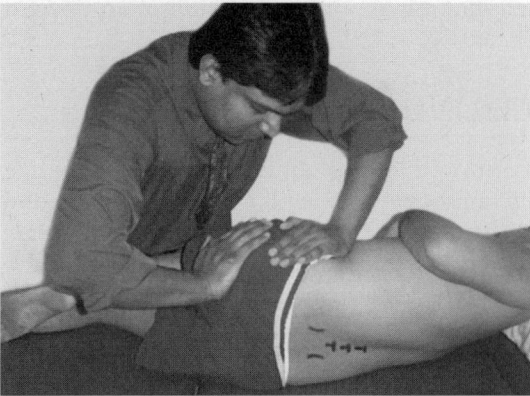

Fig. 11.18: Technique to correct anterior innominate.

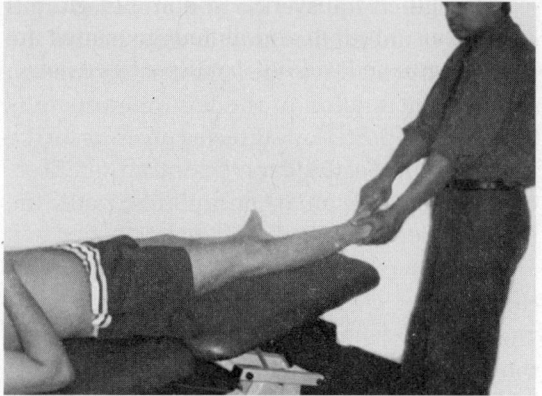
Fig. 11.19: Technique to correct upslip of innominate.

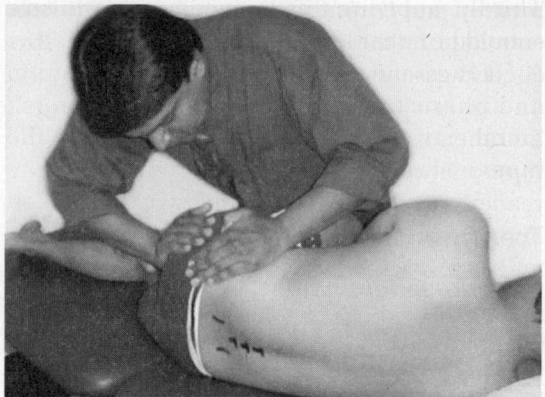
Fig. 11.20: Technique to correct downslip of innominate.

hip joint and gap the sacroiliac joint to localize the mobilization to the sacroiliac joint.

In this position, the clinician takes up the slack and imparts a short stretch in the long axis of the limb. This frees the corresponding innominate in an inferior direction (Fig. 11.19).

Downslip

The patient is right side lying assuming it is a left downslip. The left leg is flexed at the hip and knee and the foot is placed behind the right knee. The clinician faces the patient and the left hand stabilizes the left iliac crest and the heel of the right hand is placed on the left ischial tuberosity.

The clinician exerts a vertical and downward pressure (adduction) and imparts a sharp long axis stretch in a cephalic direction. This frees the left innominate in the direction of an upward shear (Fig. 11.20).

CEILING FAN ANALOGY

To conclude, the clinician should visualize the lumbopelvic complex as a ceiling fan. The suspending bar is similar to the lumbar spine, the cup to the sacrum and the blades to the innominates. Assume two sticks are hung from the blades, they would represent the legs. If the blades are tilted then a leg length discrepancy would result. A tilt in the suspending bar can throw off the alignment of the entire complex. If the suspending bar is tilted, the blades are tilted with one stick appearing long or short. Treatment should focus on tilting the suspending bar back to neutral. A wrong approach would be to tilt or adjust the blades to even out the sticks. Hence, the clinician is advised to address all dysfunctions of the lumbar spine first as the remainder might 'fall in place'. The sacrum is addressed second and the innominates last if the leg length continues to appear asymmetrical. Always evaluate for causes of true shortening as in a previous fracture or hip dysplasia.

PROPHYLAXIS

LumboPelvic Complex

Exercise Prescription

Although the principle of addressing spinal musculature as the supporting ropes holds good for the lumbopelvic complex (as in the cervicothoracic complex) there seems a difference with regards to the specificity. In the lumbopelvic complex, each muscle can be responsible for a particular dysfunction and hence should be individually addressed. A single dysfunction can occur due to combined dysfunction of a postural muscle (by tightening) and a phasic muscle (by weakening). Hence, knowledge of the appropriate muscle and its relevance to a certain dysfunction is first necessary. Secondly, the clinician must know whether the muscle is postural or phasic.

Thirdly, applying this knowledge the muscle should be either lengthened or strengthened.

It is essential then to first list the postural and phasic muscles of the lumbopelvic area and then list the dysfunctions occurring in the lumbopelvic area with their relevance to it. The reader may then infer the appropriate postural and phasic muscle relevant to the dysfunction and lengthen or strengthen it appropriately.

Postural Muscles
- Iliopsoas
- Hamstrings
- Hip adductors
- Erector spinae
- Piriformis
- Quadratus lumborum.

Phasic Muscles
- Transversus abdominis
- Multifidi
- Gluteus medius
- Gluteus maximus
- Quadriceps
- Pelvic floor.

Dysfunctions
Lumbar stabilization following correction of non-neutral dysfunction (ERS/FRS)
- Transversus abdominis, gluteals, multifidi, pelvic floor muscles.
- Functional length of iliopsoas, hamstrings, piriformis and iliotibial band.

Anterior Innominate Rotation
- Stretch iliopsoas, rectus femoris and hip adductors.
- Strengthen transversus abdominis, gluteus medius and maximus.

Posterior Innominate Rotation
- Stretch hamstrings
- Strengthen transversus abdominis, gluteus medius and maximus.

Sacral Flexion
- Stretch piriformis, iliopsoas
- Strengthen transversus abdominis, gluteus medius. Mutifidi and gluteus maximus are strengthened without excessive extension.

Sacral Extension
- Stretch hamstrings
- Strengthen lumbar paraspinals, multifidi, transversus abdominis, gluteus medius and maximus.

Superior Translation (Upslip) of Innominate

Stretch Quadratus Lumborum.

The clinician must remember that back pain is an entity that also involves the pelvic complex. Not just the innominates but the sacrum as well. More of the current philosphies are beginning to recognize the importance of addressing the sacrum and innominates as significant contributors of low back pain including radicular pain.

Indeed then should the stabilization component also address this deficit. Dynamic lumbopelvic stability is a group entity and as much as the transversus abdominis and multifidi have received attention in the past, the dynamic pelvic stabilizers may deserve a similar standing. Most importantly gluteus medius, gluteus maximus and pelvic floor muscles.

MYOFASCIAL TENDER POINTS

The concept of addressing myofascial tender points is to decrease actin and myosin cross-bridging and myofibrillar restriction. Their continued presence may encourage chemical accumulation, early fatigue and decreased muscle performance with accompanying pain and dysfunction. Their attachment to the spine can cause further alignment issues. They may be best treated with frictions and electrotherapy. Tender points secondary to aberrant gamma efferents may require an alternate positional release approach and the reader is encouraged further reading in the area of 'strain counterstrain' methods. The following are some common dysfunctional points of the lumbopelvic region (Figs. 11.21 and 11.22).

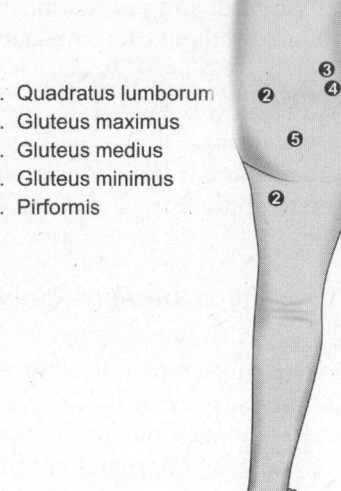

1. Quadratus lumborum
2. Gluteus maximus
3. Gluteus medius
4. Gluteus minimus
5. Piriformis

Fig. 11.21: Myofascial tender points: Lumbopelvic hip (posterior).

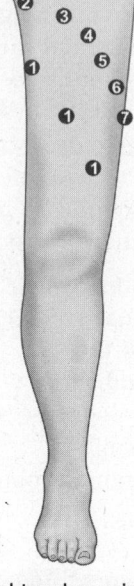

1. Sartorius
2. Tensor fasciaelatae
3. Pectineus
4. Adductor longus
5. Adductor brevis
6. Adductor magnus
7. Gracilis

Fig. 11.22: Myofascial tender points: Lumbopelvic hip (anterior).

REFERENCES

1. Porterfield JA, De Rosa C. Mechanical neck pain: Perspectives in functional anatomy. 1995, WB Saunders; Philadelphia.
2. Hodges P. Transversus abdominis: a different view of the elephant. Br J Sports Med. 2008;42: 941-4.
3. Greenman PE. Clinical aspects of sacroiliac function in walking. J Man Med. 1990;5:125-30.
4. Greenman PE. Syndromes of the lumbar spine, pelvis and sacrum. Phys Med Rehab Clin N Am.1996;7:773-85.
5. Nyberg R. S4 Course notes, 1993, St. Augustine, FL.
6. Sebastian D. The anatomical and physiological variations in the sacroiliac joints of the male and female: Clinical implications. Journal of Manual and Manipulative Therapy. 2000;8:127-34.
7. Magee DJ. Orthopedic physical assessment. 4th edn. 2002, WB Saunders; Philadelphia.
8. Hungerford BA, Gilleard W, Moran M, et al. Evaluation of the ability of physical therapists to palpate intrapelvic motion with the Stork test on the support side. Phys Ther. 2007;87:879-87.
9. Cibulka MT, Delitto A, Koldehoff RM. Changes in innominate tilt after manipulation of the sacroiliac joint in patients with low back pain. An experimental study. Phy Ther. 1988;68:1359-63.

Section 3

Extremity Manipulation

Chapter 12: Ankle and Foot
Chapter 13: Knee
Chapter 14: Hip
Chapter 15: Shoulder
Chapter 16: Elbow
Chapter 17: Wrist and Hand

Regional Application Extremity Manipulation

INTRODUCTION

Management of extremity joint dysfunction may vary from that of the spine in that all joints of the extremities do not function in weight bearing. The joints of the lower extremity, namely hip, knee, ankle and foot function in weight bearing. Proper arthrokinematics and muscle interplay is required to absorb the forces of weight bearing. If this is not present, dysfunction including mechanical orthopedic conditions result. Hence, their principles of management are essentially the same as the spine as in identifying alignment faults and subsequently stabilizing alignment with strong musculature followed by modification of function.

The upper extremities, although considered nonweight bearing from a gravity perspective is still subjected to compressive forces. These compressive forces are the powerful muscle contractions. A bowler that releases a cricket ball is subjecting the shoulder to significant compressive forces. A typist that types 5 to 8 hours a day is subjecting the wrist and fingers to compressive forces. As much as dynamic movement causes compressive forces, static postures do the same as well. An electrician or a painter positioning the shoulder and elbows and working with the hands and fingers is an example. Trauma of this type can be cumulative overtime.

Hence, mechanical dysfunction of the extremities may be occupational, sports related or single event traumas as in slips/falls or motor vehicle accidents. In all, dysfunctions or mechanical orthopedic conditions begin as a minor joint dysfunction, connective tissue strains or simply the process of aging. As the stresses continue to influence the vulnerable structures, a more serious condition results as in a tendonitis, bursitis, sprain/strain or nerve entrapment. Appropriate identification of the stressors is warranted which is invariably:
1. Faulty alignment/mechanics
2. Inadequate muscle length/strength
3. Poor functional mechanics.

If damage has already resulted as in a tendon/ligament rupture, or even a fracture, or in the physical therapy clinician following repair of such anatomical disruptions should continue to address the above 3 principles. This will help to prevent a second occurrence of the dysfunction and optimal return to function.

Dysfunctions in the lower extremity are more apparent in weight bearing, however, not an absolute rule. But it is of importance to know that in weight bearing, the alignment issues are determined by the position in which the ankle and foot contacts the ground. Dysfunctions are also determined by a similar concept. The reverse can occur, however, less common. Hence, the chapters are described starting with the ankle and foot for a better understanding of the dynamics of a lower extremity dysfunction. It is important to reiterate to the clinician again that these mechanical conditions are entities that should be considered only after ruling out the presence of a condition that is nonmechanical in origin. All other forms of investigation should be considered.

The manual therapy techniques per say can be used from a postimmobilization perspective, i.e. to restore mobility as taught in traditional physical therapy education. However, the basis of this altered arthrokinematic motion and faulty muscle mechanics form a basis for diagnosis of the 'cause' of the symptom.

In the upper extremity, the compressive forces are secondary to excessive muscle contraction forces rather than weight bearing as in the lower extremity. Often times the soft tissue component may be more involved than the arthrokinematic component. Hence, the basis for diagnosis will be altered tissue texture abnormality which is the third principle of the somatic diagnosis triad. Several theories exist as to why such a persistent soft tissue lesion can occur secondary to overuse. The three most common theories are as follows:

1. Prolonged and excessive contraction as would occur with overuse may induce fatigue in a muscle. The muscle contracts in response to fatigue and persists to create a local soft tissue dysfunction with localized tender point called 'trigger points'.
2. Excessive and faulty muscle contraction can cause injury to the myofibrils of the muscle bulk which may heal with scarring. This scarring can inhibit normal physiological contraction and deprive the area of nutrition and encourage chemical accumulation causing pain. In addition, possible nerve endings in the healed scar may also be pain sensitive.
3. Faulty activity can influence the muscle at an intrafusal level creating a constant aberrant gamma motor activity which renders the soft tissue dysfunctional.

Soft tissue irritability can aid in the diagnosis as it is obvious as palpable tender points. These tender points are seen in muscles, musculotendinous and tenoperiosteal junctions. Breaking down the scar or ischemic compression of trigger points are suggested forms of manual therapy in addition to restoring normal arthrokinematics. Routine electrotherapy is also advocated. Hence, this approach to musculoskeletal diagnosis is a component of conventional methods and not a cure all.

However, it is unique to the profession of physical therapy and a holistic approach with the arts of traditional medicine may result in a more effective outcome.

The diagnosis of mechanical dysfunction unique to this philosophy has been described in the section on principles of diagnosis. Hence, the joint play relevant to a specific neuromusculoskeletal pathology and the joint play required to correct and restore overall mobility in a motion segment will be described. The sections on somatic diagnosis will address pathology specific restrictions. The treatment sections hence will address treatment of mechanical dysfunction in the extremity joints as two categories:

1. Treatment for specific somatic dysfunction.
2. Treatment for overall improvement of range of motion.

Although there may be a considerable overlap in the treatment technique between the two categories the clinician must definitely understand the conceptual basis as to why they are differentiated and thereby use the technique in the most appropriate situations.

Prior to discussing regional application of the extremities, it is important for the clinician to be aware of the possible contraindications to manipulation of the extremities. It should essentially be the first thing that comes to mind before any treatment procedure is initiated. The major contraindications are listed, however, as most manual therapy gurus would advise:

"when in doubt, don't"

The clinician is hence advised to exercise sound clinical judgement prior to initiating treatment. The list is as follows, but not limited to:

- Ligament insufficiency
- Rheumatoid arthritis (with caution)
- Connective tissue disorders
- Recent fractures
- Osteoporosis
- Malignancy or tumors
- Instability
- Bone and joint disease
- Surgical or anomalous joint fusion
- Hemarthrosis
- Acute inflammation/muscle holding
- Joint replacement
- Anticoagulant therapy.

RATIONALE FOR JOINT MOBILIZATION TO IMPROVE RANGE OF MOTION REVISITED

Contemporary and critical reviews question the concept of gliding in joint mobilization.

Although the rationale is described in 'Principles of diagnosis' as a separation of normal joint 'roll and gliding' and 'passive gliding', this short note reiterates how best the clinician could possibly apply this rationale.

The concern of whether it is elongation of the capsule or gliding of the joint that restores range of motion remains elusive. The reason being, rolling and gliding are normal programed movements in a normally functioning joint. So one may argue then it is the lack of room or space for this normal roll and gliding to occur that results in a restriction. The structural cause for restricted mobility in a normal synovial joint is a tightness and shortening of the capsule. The contracted capsule is one, then, that limits the ability of the joint surfaces to normally 'roll and glide'. It may be the need then to focus intervention toward elongation of the capsule. Normal 'roll and gliding' will naturally resume as a programed function as long as the nervous system is intact. However, if the restriction has persisted long enough, passive gliding may assist with motor memory.

CHAPTER 12

Ankle and Foot

Ankle and foot complex are the most distal joints of the skeletal system from a weight bearing perspective. They function to appropriately distribute weight bearing stresses during function. Their normalcy in anatomy and mechanics is hence essential to minimize abnormal loading and predisposition to a dysfunction.

OSSEOUS ANATOMY

Ankle and foot by virtue of their function are divided into three regions, namely:
1. Rearfoot
2. Midfoot
3. Forefoot.

The rearfoot consists of the distal end of tibia, talus and calcaneus. The talus articulates with the tibia above to form the talocrural or ankle joint. The talus articulates with the calcaneus to form the subtalar joint. The alignment of the subtalar joint is an essential determinant for the assessment of foot dysfunction. The position of the rearfoot determines the mechanics of the mid foot and forefoot and overall load distribution in the foot.

The midfoot is made up of the navicular cuneiform and cuboid bones. Their articulation is known as the midtarsal joint. The midtarsal joint mechanics with relevance to function are in proportion to subtalar alignment. As the subtalar joint bears weight, the plantigrade foot position is achieved by the midtarsal joints modifying the forefoot in accordance to the rearfoot help to achieve a foot flat position.

The forefoot consists of the metatarsals and phalanges. The phalanges are also known as rays. These rays are described to be able to rotate longitudinally (twist) and this is done by a reciprocal movement of the 1st and 5th ray. This forefoot twist helps to accommodate the foot on the ground and it depends on the coordinated movement of the subtalar and midtarsal joints.

LIGAMENTOUS ANATOMY

Rearfoot

From a dysfunction perspective, the ligaments of the rearfoot are of importance owing to the incidence of strains. The inferior tibiofibular joints have anterior and posterior tibiofibular ligaments. The rearfoot has ligaments on the medial and lateral side. On the medial side of the talocrural joint is the deltoid or the medial collateral ligament which has four components, namely:
1. Tibiocalcaneal
2. Tibionavicular
3. Posterior tibiotalar
   These are superficial ligaments and resist abduction of the talus.
4. Anterior tibiotalar.
   These are deep ligaments and resist lateral translation and lateral rotation of the talus.

On the lateral side of the talocrural joint is the lateral collateral ligament which has three components namely:
1. Anterior talofibular
2. Posterior talofibular
3. Middle calcaneofibular.

The anterior talofibular ligament provides stability against increased inversion.

The posterior talofibular ligament resists adduction, medial rotation and medial translation of talus.

The middle calcaneofibular ligament resists maximum inversion.

The subtalar joint is supported by the lateral and medial talocalcaneal ligament. In addition, the interosseous talocalcaneonavicular- and cervical ligaments limit eversion.

Midfoot

The talocalcaneonavicular joint is supported by:
1. Dorsal talonavicular ligament
2. Bifurcated ligament
3. Plantar calcaneonavicular (spring) ligament.

The calcaneocuboid joint is supported by:
1. Calcaneocuboid ligament
2. Bifurcated ligament
3. Long plantar ligament.

MUSCULAR ANATOMY

The muscular function in the ankle and foot from a mechanical perspective is complex as they contribute to optimal arthrokinematics within the joint. They are hence important both to support alignment and minimize/distribute stresses within the joint surface.

Immediately following push off, the tibialis anterior assists in dorsiflexion of the foot to clear the ground.

On heel strike, to prevent the foot from plantar flexing excessively, the tibialis anterior contracts eccentrically along with the extensor hallucis longus and extensor digitorum longus. This function also prevents pronation of the forefoot during contact period.

As the forefoot makes contact with the ground, the tibialis posterior and gastrosoleus decelerate pronation of the subtalar joint.

During midstance, the tibialis posterior, soleus, flexor hallucis longus and flexor digitorum longus reduce the forward momentum of the tibia. The tibialis posterior and gastrosoleus reverse the deceleration of pronation mode and maintain stability at the midtarsal joint by increasing supination at the subtalar joint.

At heel off, the concentric and powerful contraction of the gastrosoleus and tibialis posterior activate push off, while the peroneus longus plantarflexes the first ray (assisted by abductor hallucis). The extensor hallucis longus and brevis and the flexor digitorum longus stabilize the first metatarsophalangeal joint and toes during propulsion.[1]

MECHANICS (NORMAL ROLL AND GLIDING)

The following is the normal sequence of occurrence in ankle and foot during the stance phase of the gait cycle[1]. Maintenance of this sequence is essential for optimal function of ankle and foot and minimal stresses on the supporting structures.

During heel strike at the rearfoot, the talus plantar flexes, adducts and the calcaneus everts. Tibial internal rotation is accompanied by this. As the midfoot moves to contact the ground, this is the shock absorption phase where the unlocking occurs. This is achieved by internal rotation of the navicular, cuboid and flattening of the cuneiforms.

The forefoot goes into a supination twist (1st ray dorsiflexion). As the foot moves into late midstance the foot has completed its shock absorption phase and is required to become a rigid lever for push off to occur. Hence, a reversal of pronation occurs for supination to take place. The talus begins to dorsiflex and abduct with external rotation of the navicular and cuboid and an elevation of the cuneiforms. Now since the weight bearing has shifted lateral and the medial aspect of the foot needs to make contact, the first ray plantar flexes to bring the great toe on the ground. The tibia externally rotates to complete the rigid lever. Now the foot is ready for propulsion/push off.

Fibula Mechanics

The fibular head at the superior tibiofibular joint has a significant contribution to movement by way of its very relevant joint play that occurs at this level. With talocrural dorsiflexion, the fibula glides in a superior direction. In addition, it also glides posteriorly and medially. The reverse occurs with talocrural plantarflexion where the fibula glides inferiorly with an additional anteriorly and laterally.

MECHANISM OF DYSFUNCTION

Mechanical dysfunction of the foot and ankle occurs if the above described mechanics is altered.[2] Mechanical dysfunction is obviously an acquired process and not congenital or disease related. They are usually classified as extrinsic (outside the joint) and intrinsic (inside the joint). The normal mechanics of the foot and ankle can be affected due to several factors and are commonly due to the following extrinsic causes:
- Malalignment of the pelvis, hip and knee.
- Muscle length imbalances.

Other factors may be in the category of overuse,[3] improper footwear and faulty training or functional mechanics.

Intrinsic causes are the arthrokinematic restrictions that occur within the joint as in a plantarflexed talus or pronated cuboid.

From a manual therapy perspective, it is the intrinsic factors that need to be diagnosed and addressed,[4] however, the extrinsic factors are also of equal importance and should also be addressed for stable functional outcomes.

Ankle

The two common dysfunctions that occur in the ankle are *pronation* and *supination*.[5] One needs to understand that these two conditions are normal movements that occur in the ankle and foot. Pronation helps the foot to adapt uneven terrain and supination helps to lock the foot as a rigid lever to be able to push off during gait. However, when these two positions are prolonged during the gait cycle as a result of one or more of the intrinsic or extrinsic causes described above, then a dysfunction results.

Pronation and supination are more clinically relevant in weight bearing and hence their components in weight bearing are described. They are both triplanar movements.

Pronation consists of calcaneal eversion, with adduction and plantarflexion of the talus. Supination consists of calcaneal inversion with abduction and dorsiflexion of the talus.

The talus is of importance in the ankle mortise. It has no direct muscle attachments and hence, the muscle action on the bones above and below determine its movement. Talar restriction from above or below significantly restricts ankle function. Structurally, it is narrower posteriorly and hence has a tendency to be restricted in plantarflexion. One should remember that the ankle is more stable in dorsiflexion.

The distal tibiofibular joint is quite stable and is associated with function of the proximal tibiofibular joint. These are in turn influenced by the movements of the tibia. Hence they should be first addressed before addressing dysfunctions of the ankle. They will be described in the section on the knee.

Foot

There are four *weight bearing* arches in the foot are as follows:
1. *Lateral arch:* Calcaneus, cuboid, 4th and 5th metatarsals, 4th and 5th toes.
2. *Medial arch:* Talus, navicular, 1st cuneiform, 1st metatarsal, 1st toe.
3. *Transverse arch:* Navicular, cuboid, 3 cuneiforms.
4. *Metatarsal arch:* Heads of the 5 metatarsals (although not a true arch).

The navicular and cuboid are the key to the function of the medial and lateral arches, respectively. They also function together to support the transverse arch, although the cuboid more than the navicular.

Dysfunction of the navicular is either pronated or supinated (internal or external rotation) restriction. Dysfunctions of the cuboid are the same as in pronated or supinated (internal or external rotation) restriction.

The cuneiforms support the transverse arch, and function differently from each other. The first cuneiform rotates internally and externally on the navicular. The rest have a gliding motion. They tend to be depressed or elevated in dysfunctional states and hence flatten the transverse arch.

The first tarsometatarsal joint also rotates in and out on the first cuneiform. Together they are called the first ray and are clinically significant. Their movement of dorsiflexion with inversion and plantarflexion with eversion probably gives them the ability to rotate in and out. In dysfunctional states, they tend to be restricted in plantarflexion compensating for a supinated foot or dorsiflexion favoring pronation, and resulting in a push off on a pronated foot.

The metatarsal heads form the metatarsal arch. They have the ability to glide up and down and the axis of the forefoot is the second metatarsal head. Interestingly, the area of restriction is commonly between the second and third metatarsal heads which untreated can restrict the rotation of the forefoot and stress the interosseous musculature resulting in pain.

Excessive pronation causes foot flattening. After the foot flat phase of gait, if the subtalar joint remains pronated and if the subtalar joint exhibits more than 30° of calcaneal eversion from foot flat to midstance, too much pronation is evident. This unlocks the foot even during stance where it technically needs to be locked, and renders the foot hypermobile or weak.

Excessive supination can occur if it remains at the phase of gait from heel strike to foot flat (where it technically needs to pronate to adapt on uneven ground). Since the foot is unable to adapt on uneven terrain, there tends to be a loss of alignment. Since the foot is supinated, the foot can buckle into inversion and possibly be the cause for repeated lateral ligament strains.

Common Pathologies Secondary to Mechanical Dysfunction

Plantar Fasciitis

The plantar fascia runs from the medial tuberosity of the calcaneus to the metatarsal heads. It covers all of the soft tissues on the plantar surface of the foot and supports the medial longitudinal arch. In a foot with excessive pronation and extension of the first MTP, the fascia is overstretched. When this abnormal loading continues, the fascia gets inflamed and a fasciitis results.[6]

Sprains

Lateral sprains are most common and is usually secondary to faulty alignment of the rearfoot. A rearfoot varus is usually a causative factor. This inverts the calcaneus and abducts the talus. Since the rearfoot is in varus, the forefoot pronates excessively to bring the foot flat on to the ground. This overall renders the foot with faulty alignment and a tendency to buckle inwards especially when landing on one leg (as in running or jumping). When this occurs, the lateral ligament is prone to be injured.[6]

The reverse can occur if the opposite mechanics is present and eventually stress the medial ligamentous structures, although less common.

Muscle Strain/Tendinitis

Prolonged pronation can cause a strain in the tibialis posterior tendon near the medial malleolus and the base of the medial calf bulk and predisposing to medial pain. The achilles tendon is also prone for strain as it inserts into the calcaneus. A pronation or supination can stress the tendon.

The peroneal tendon can be stressed over the lateral malleolus owing to a rearfoot varus or supination and is also seen in recurrent ankle sprains or instability.[7,8]

Neuromas

These are fibrotic proliferations of the tissue surrounding the neurovascular bundles between the metatarsals. The shearing that occurs between the metatarsal heads is the cause. The mechanical cause however, is the result of abnormal pronation during the propulsive phase of gait.

During abnormal pronation, the 1st, 2nd and 3rd metatarsal heads move laterally and upwards, while the 5th metatarsal head moves downwards and medially. This opposite movement of the metatarsal heads create a shear and irritate the tissue surrounding the neurovascular bundles resulting in fibrotic proliferations which are neuromas.

Stress Fractures

Stress fractures are usually a result of hyperpronation of the midtarsal and sub-talar joints. During the propulsion phase, the hyperpronation prevents the foot from locking. Hence, instead of the forces being transmitted up the kinetic chain, they are dissipated within the foot resulting in stress fractures.

Excessive supination can also cause stress fractures as the foot does not pronate and does not allow the forces to be absorbed well.

Anterolateral Impingement Syndrome

Excessive pronation can cause compression on the anterolateral aspect of the foot secondary to impingement on the soft tissue structures, commonly the capsule.

Nerve Irritation

Tarsal Tunnel Syndrome

This condition refers to an entrapment of the posterior tibial nerve and artery as they pass through a fibro at the osseous tunnel located-posteromedial to the medial malleolus. The roof of the tunnel consists of the lancinate ligament and the floor by underlying bony structures. The diameter of this tunnel can be reduced due to excessive pronation as this stretches the lancinate ligament.[9,6]

Superficial Peroneal Nerve

This nerve has been reported to be injured at the level of the fibular head but rarely at the ankle. The possible site of irritation is the distal portion of the lateral malleolus and the mode of injury is an inversion strain secondary to excessive supination. The mechanism of injury that results in a lateral ligament strain is hence the etiology for nerve injury at this site.[9,10]

Medial/Lateral Plantar Nerve

The medial plantar nerve is a branch of the tibial nerve and it passes beneath the spring ligament on the medial side of the foot. Excessive pronation can stretch this ligament and compress the medial plantar nerve below it. It is often termed a 'joggers foot'.

Excessive pronation can also stress and compress the lateral plantar nerve as it passes between the deep fascia abductor hallucis and flexor accessories muscles.[9,10]

ANKLE AND FOOT SOMATIC DIAGNOSIS

Subtalar Neutral

The patient is lying prone and the clinician faces the patient from the leg side. The clinician then grasps the lateral metatarsals with one hand, while the other hand palpates both sides of the subtalar joint (Fig. 12.1). The clinician alternately inverts and everts the foot and palpates both sides of the subtalar joint to look for symmetry in compression. When this is felt, the position of the heel in relation to the tibia is observed and maintained as neutral as possible. Alternately, a less qualitative way of assessment is to draw a straight line along the tibia and one along the calcaneus. Now the clinician holds the calcaneus on either sides and tries to align it with the tibia (Fig. 12.2). If the calcaneus does not align with the tibia, the rearfoot is supinated. If the calcaneus is in line with the tibia, the position of the first ray in relationship to the fifth ray is observed. If the first ray is higher than the fifth ray, then it is a forefoot varus. On weight bearing, when the forefoot is flat on the ground and a compensatory rearfoot valgus occurs. The result is a *pronated* foot.

Conversely, if the position of the heel is inverted and first ray is higher than the fifth ray. On weight bearing the weight bearing is on the lateral aspect of the foot. However, to bring the foot flat on the ground, the first ray will plantarflex. The result is a *supinated* foot.

Talus Plantarflexed

This is a common arthrokinematic dysfunction leading to restricted dorsiflexion in the ankle, in combination with a tight gastrosoleus. This dysfunction is seen in a pronated foot. Diagnosis of this dysfunction is done in two steps.

With the patient sitting, the clinician places the thumb on the neck of the talus and grips the foot with the palm of the hand. The clinician then passively swings the foot upward and a restriction may be noted (Fig. 12.3). This is compared with the other side. The neck of the talus is often tender.

A talus that is stuck in *plantar flexion* is a *pronated* foot.

A talus that is stuck in *dorsiflexion* is a *supinated* foot.

Calcaneus Inverted

The patient is lying prone and the clinician faces the patient from the leg side. One hand of the clinician holds and stabilizes the lower end of the tibia and fibula just above the level of the ankle joint. The other hand grasps the calcaneus

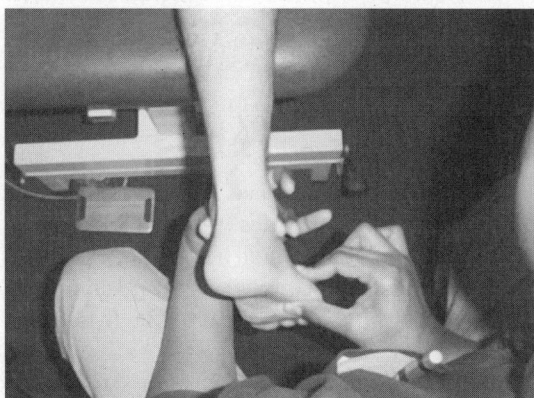

Fig. 12.1: Subtalar neutral assessment.

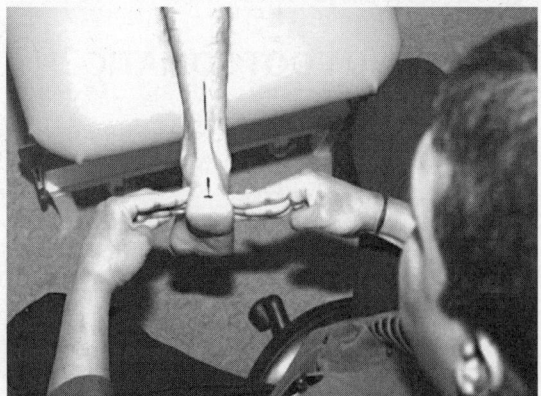

Fig. 12.2: Subtalar neutral assessment.

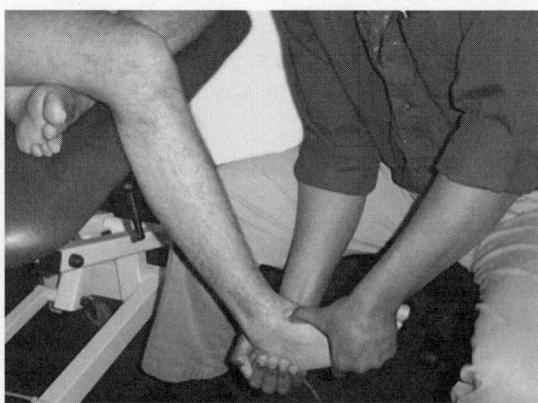

Fig. 12.3: Assessment of a plantarflexed talus.

Ankle and Foot

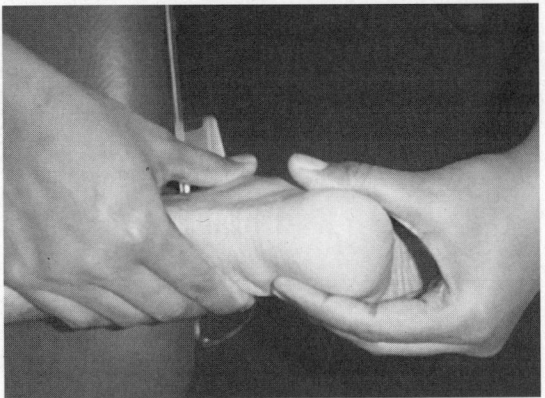

Fig. 12.4: Assessing calcaneal inversion and eversion.

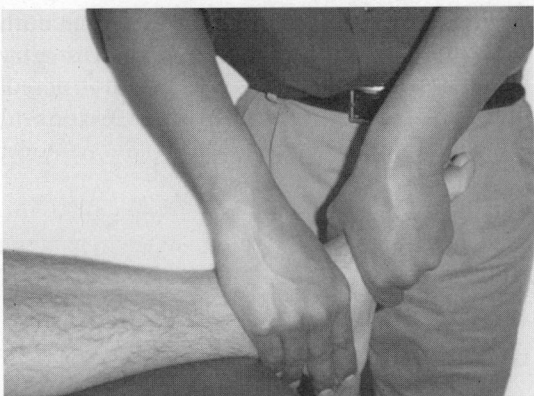

Fig. 12.5: Assessing midfoot internal and external rotation.

and move the calcaneus in and out sensing for restriction (Fig. 12.4). The calcaneus is mostly restricted in inversion resisting eversion.

A calcaneus stuck or restricted in *inversion* is a *supinated* foot.

Midfoot Pronated/Supinated/Internal/External Rotation

The patient is lying supine and the clinician faces the foot of the patient. One hand of the clinician grasps the talus and calcaneus to stabilize it. The web space of the other hand is placed on the navicular tuberosity and is firmly gripped with thumb and fingers. An internal and external rotation motion is imparted like opening and closing a door knob. The clinician senses for restriction as this movement is performed (Fig. 12.5).

A restriction in internal rotation is a pronated foot.

A restriction in external rotation is a supinated foot.

Elevated Cuneiforms

The patient is lying supine and the clinician faces the dorsum of the foot being examined. The index and middle finger firmly runs over the cuneiforms one at a time. An elevated position may be observed in comparison with the other foot. Elevation of the cuneiforms is the most

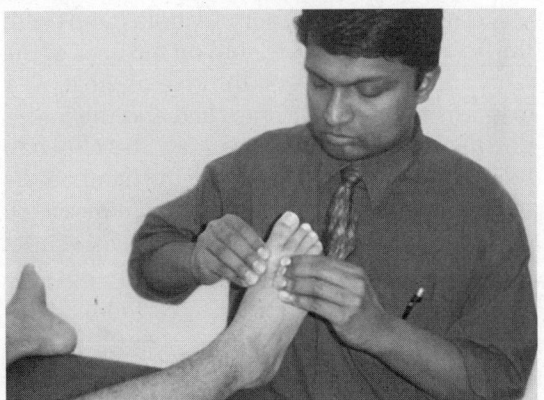

Fig. 12.6: Assessing first ray plantarflexion.

common dysfunction seen in this region and is usually seen in a rigid supinated foot.

First Ray Plantarflexed

The patient is lying supine and the clinician faces the sole of the foot. The thumb, index and middle fingers of one hand grasp the second metatarsal at the level of the intermetatarsal joint. The thumb, index and middle finger of the other hand grasps the first metatarsal at the level of the intermetatarsal joint. A gliding motion is imparted in a superior and inferior direction (Fig. 12.6). A sense of restriction in a superior direction will indicate the 1st ray stuck or restricted in plantarflexion. This is a common dysfunction seen in a supinated foot.

A plantarflexed 1st ray indicates a supination dysfunction of the foot. When the foot is supinated the weight bearing is more lateral elevating the medial side of the foot. As a compensation, to bring the foot flat on the ground plantarflexion of the first ray occurs.

TREATMENT

Treatment for Specific Somatic Dysfunction[2]

Talus Plantarflexed

Step 1: The patient is lying supine and the clinician faces the patient from the leg side. The clinician encircles the foot with both hands with the lateral border of the hand on the neck of the talus and the thumbs on the sole of the foot. A long axis traction is first applied and the foot is dorsiflexed till resistance is met. The clinician then using the lateral border of the hand on the neck of the talus imparts a mobilization stretch in an inferior direction and sustains it for at least 10 seconds (Fig. 12.7). The procedure is repeated 2 to 3 times.

Step 2: Posterior lateral glide of talus: The patient is lying supine and the clinician faces the foot from the side. One hand of the clinician stabilizes the distal end of the tibia and fibula just above the talus. The clinician grips the calcaneus and in a slightly plantarflexed position, imparts a gliding motion in a posterolateral (inferior) direction (Fig. 12.8).

Calcaneus Inverted

The patient is lying prone with the foot over the end of the table and the patient faces the patient from the leg side. One hand of the clinician grasps the lower end of the tibia and fibula to stabilize it. The other hand holds and stabilizes the calcaneus by holding the medial and lateral ends of the calcaneus with the thumb, index and middle fingers. In case of an inverted calcaneus, the calcaneus is stretched in eversion (Fig. 12.9).

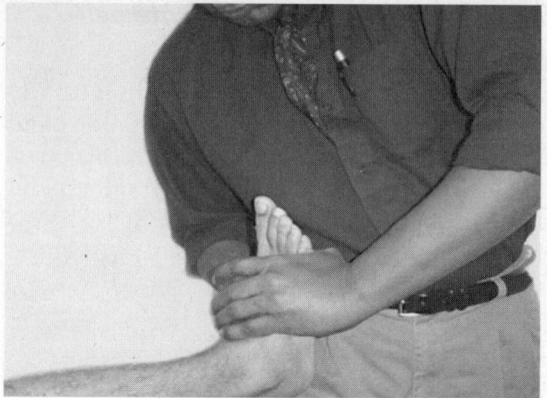
Fig. 12.7: Correction of a plantarflexed talus.

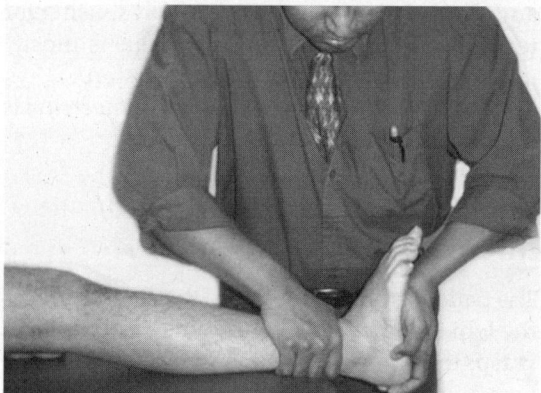
Fig. 12.8: Posterior lateral glide of the talus.

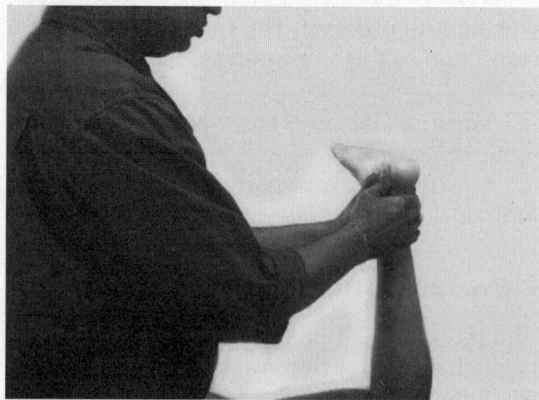
Fig. 12.9: Correction of an inverted calcaneus.

Midfoot Pronated/Supinated/Internal/External Rotated

Step 1: The patient is lying supine and the clinician faces the foot of the patient. One hand of the clinician grasps the talus and calcaneus to stabilize it. The web space of the other hand is placed on the navicular tuberosity and is firmly gripped with the thumb and fingers. The distal hand that supports the navicula with the web space 'wrings outward' for a restriction in internal rotation (Fig. 12.10).

Step 2: The reverse is done for a restriction in external rotation, however, with the patient lying prone. The clinician faces the patient from the leg side. The thumb is placed on the cuboid and the web space of the other hand encircles the medial aspect of the foot to reinforce the cuboid from the other side. The slack is taken up by plantarflexing the forefoot and the clinician imparts an inferiorly directed mobilizing force on the cuboid (Figs. 12.11, 12.12).

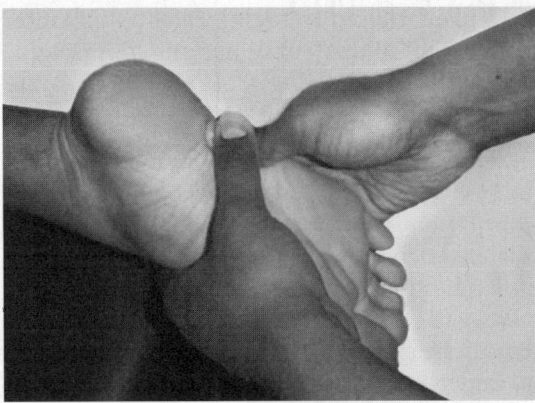

Fig. 12.11: Correcting midfoot external rotation restriction.

Elevated Cuneiforms

The patient is lying supine and the clinician faces the leg of the patient to be treated. The little fingers of the clinician are placed on the cuneiforms and the other fingers are interlaced over them. The thumbs are placed on the sole of the foot. The foot is taken into slight dorsiflexion and inversion (Fig. 12.13). A gentle distraction is

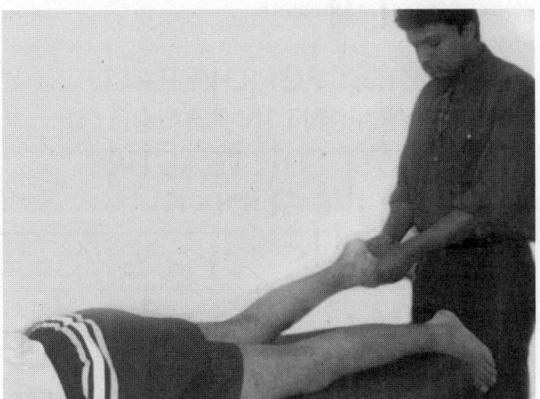

Fig. 12.12: Correcting midfoot external rotation restriction.

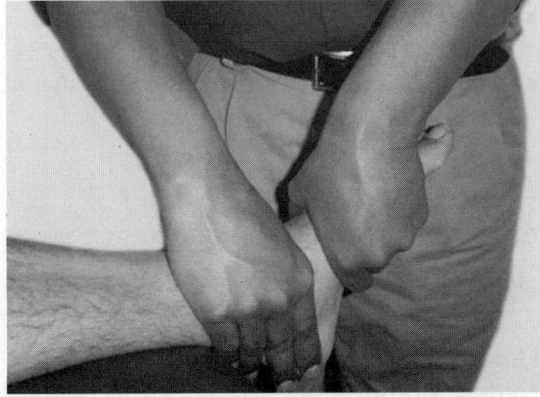

Fig. 12.10: Correcting midfoot internal rotation restriction.

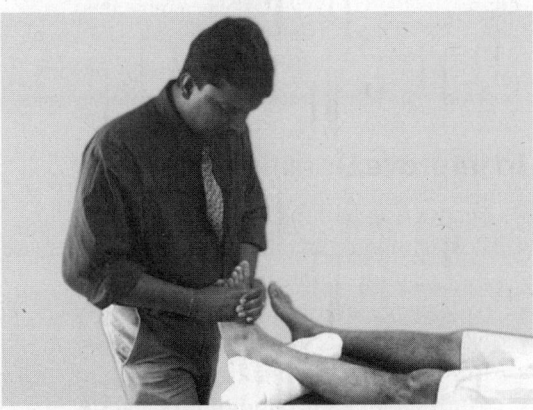

Fig. 12.13: Correcting elevated cuneiforms.

then applied in a long axis direction to depress the cuneiforms inferiorly.

First Ray Plantarflexed

The procedure is the same as for diagnosis. The patient is lying supine and the clinician faces the patient from the foot side. One hand of the clinician grips the intermetatarsal joints of second to fourth digits to stabilize it. The other hand grips the first intermetatarsal joint with the thumb, index and middle fingers and stabilizes it to impart a superior glide into dorsiflexion. The same procedure is done at the level of the first tarsometatarsal joint and the first cuneiform as they together comprise the first ray. For the first cuneiform, however, the technique for elevated cuneiforms is suggested.

TREATMENT FOR OVERALL IMPROVEMENT IN RANGE OF MOTION[11,12] (TJP: TRACTION AND PASSIVE GLIDING)

Joint Basics

Talocrural Joint

Type of joint	Diarthroidal hinge
Degrees of freedom	Dorsiflexion, Plantar flexion
Range of motion	Dorsiflexion: 0–20° Plantar flexion: 0–50°
Capsular pattern	Plantar flexion more than dorsiflexion
Loose packed position	10° of plantar flexion, midway between inversion and eversion

To Improve Dorsiflexion

- Distraction of talus
- Posterior glide of talus
- Lateral glide of talus
- Anterior/posterior (A/P) glide of fibula head
- Navicular/talus dorsal glide
- Cuneonavicular dorsal glide
- 4/5th metatarsal/cuboid dorsal glide

On completion, the tendoachilles should be appropriately stretched.

To Improve Plantar flexion

- Distraction talus
- Anterior glide of talus
- Medial glide of talus
- A/P glide of fibula head
- Navicular/talus plantar glide
- Cuneonavicular plantar glide
- 4/5th metatarsal/cuboid plantar glide

On completion, the anterior capsule should be appropriately stretched by simply sustaining osteokinematic plantar flexion stretch.

Joint Basics

Subtalar Joint

Type of joint	Diarthroidal bicondylar
Degrees of freedom	Pronation, supination
Range of motion	Inversion: 0–30° Eversion: 0–10°
Capsular pattern	Inversion (supination) more limited than eversion (pronation)
Loose packed position	Pronation

To Improve Inversion

- Distraction talus and calcaneus
- Inversion calcaneus
- Lateral glide talus

On completion, the joint is taken into osteokinematic inversion gently in the absence of contraindications.

To Improve Eversion

- Distraction talus and calcaneus
- Eversion calcaneus
- Medial glide talus

On completion, the joint is taken into osteokinematic eversion gently in the absence of contraindications.

Metatarsophalangeal Joints

Joint Basics

Type of joint	Diarthroidal condyloid
Degrees of freedom	Flexion, extension, abduction, adduction
Range of motion	Flexion: 0–20, extension: 0–70, abduction: 0–10
Capsular pattern	Greater limitation in extension than in flexion variable
Loose packed great position	10° extension great toe, 10° flexion than other toes

To Improve Flexion

- Distraction rotation
- Plantar glide
- Medial/lateral glide

To Improve Extension

- Distraction rotation
- Dorsal glide
- Medial/lateral glide

Pip/Dip Joints

Joint Basics

Type of joint	Diarthroidal hinge
Degrees of freedom	Flexion, extension
Range of motion	Pip flexion: 0-90, DIP flexion: 0–40, extension—neutral
Capsular pattern	Flexion more than extension
Loose packed position	Slight flexion

To Improve Flexion

- Distraction rotation
- Plantar glide
- Medial/lateral glide

To Improve Extension

- Distraction rotation
- Dorsal glide
- Medial/lateral glide

TECHNIQUE

Talocrural Joint

Distraction of Talus

The patient is lying supine and the clinician faces the leg of the patient to be treated. The little fingers of the clinician are placed on the talus and the other fingers are interlaced over the dorsum of the foot. The thumbs are placed on the dorsum of the foot. A gentle distraction is then applied in a long axis direction (Fig. 12.14).

Posterior Lateral Glide of Talus

The patient is lying supine and the clinician faces the foot from the side. One hand of the clinician stabilizes the distal end of the tibia and fibula just above the talus. The clinician grips the calcaneus and in a slightly plantarflexed position, imparts a gliding motion in a posterolateral direction (Fig. 12.15).

Anterior Medial Glide of Talus

The patient is lying prone and the clinician faces the foot from the side. One hand of the clinician stabilizes the distal end of the tibia and fibula just above the talus. The clinician grips the calcaneus and in a slightly plantarflexed position, imparts a gliding motion in an anteromedial direction (Fig. 12.16).

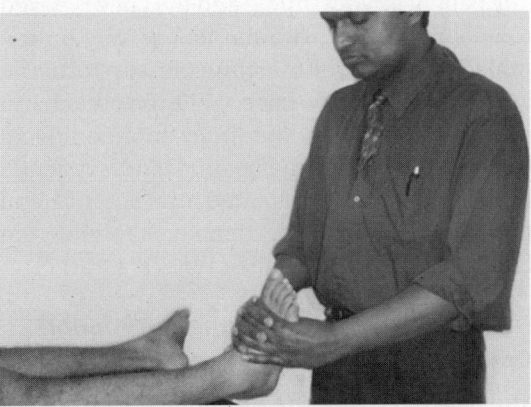

Fig. 12.14: Distraction of talus.

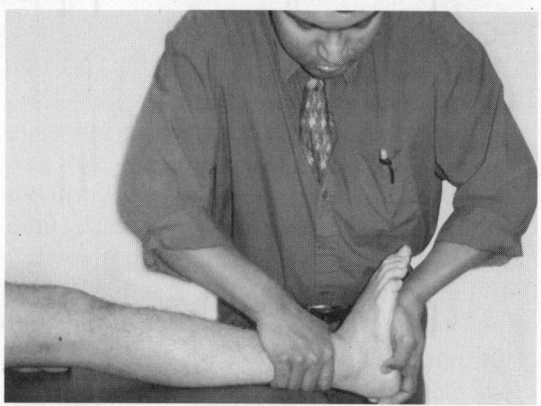

Fig. 12.15: Posterior lateral glide talus.

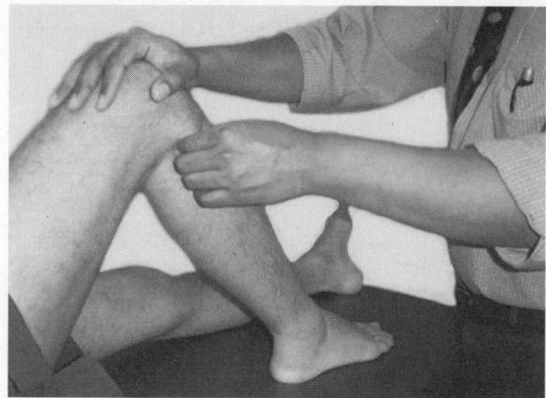

Fig. 12.17: Anterior/posterior (A/P) glide fibula head.

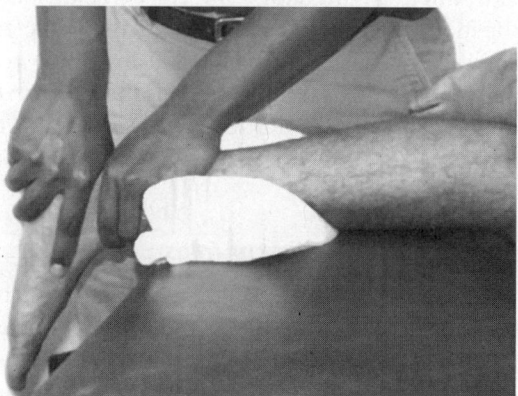

Fig. 12.16: Anterior medial glide talus.

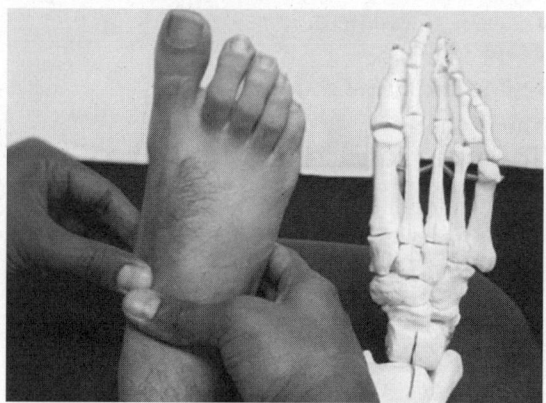

Fig. 12.18: Navicular talus dorsal and plantar glide

A/P Glide of Fibula Head

The patient is lying supine and the knee is flexed to about 70 to 90° with the foot resting on the table. One hand of the clinician supports the anterior aspect of the knee, while the other hand incorporates thumb and index/middle fingers to grip and stabilize the head of fibula. A gentle mobilization force is imparted in an anterolateral and posteromedial direction so as to glide the head of fibula in these directions (Fig. 12.17).

Navicular Talus Dorsal (Superior/Inferior) Glide

The patient is lying supine with the foot resting on the edge of the table or wedge. One hand of the clinician grasps the proximal foot at the talus. Thumb and index/middle finger grasps the superior and inferior aspects of the navicular. Stabilizing the talus with the other hand, the navicular is glided in a superior direction (Fig. 12.18).

Cuneonavicular Dorsal (Superior/Inferior) Glide

The patient and clinician position are the same as for a navicular dorsal glide. The stabilizing grip, however, extends down to the navicular. Thumb and index/middle fingers grip the 1st cuneiform. Stabilizing the navicular with the other hand, a gentle glide is imparted on the 1st cuneiform in a superior direction (Fig. 12.19).

Ankle and Foot

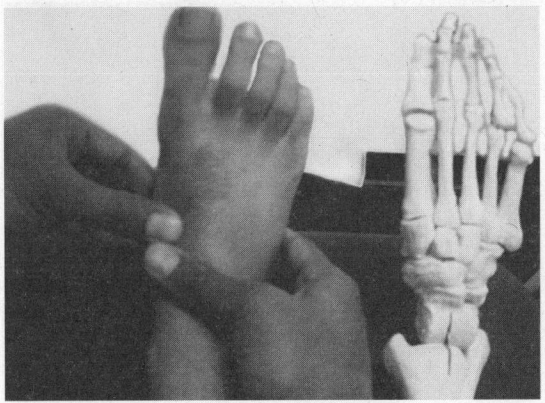

Fig. 12.19: Cuneonavicular dorsal and plantar glide.

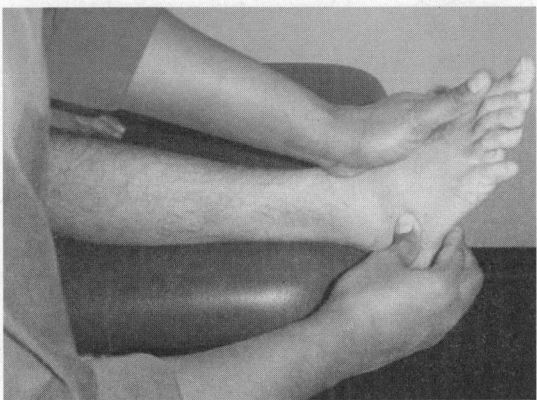

Fig. 12.20: 4/5th metatarsal/cuboid dorsal and plantar glide.

4/5th Metatarsal/Cuboid Dorsal (Superior/Inferior) Glide

The patient is lying supine with the knee flexed and the foot resting on the table/wedge. The clinician faces the foot from behind. One hand of the clinician stabilizes the talocalcaneal joint medially. Thumb and index/middle fingers of the other hand grip the superior and inferior aspects of the cuboid. Stabilizing the talocalcaneal joint, a gentle superior glide is imparted on the cuboid.

The stabilizing grip is then moved more distally and the cuboid is stabilized. Thumb and index/middle fingers are now placed on the superior and inferior aspects of the proximal 5th metatarsal. Stabilizing the cuboid, a gentle glide is imparted on the 5th metatarsal in a superior direction. The same procedure is adopted for the 4th metatarsal (Fig. 12.20).

Subtalar Joint

Distraction of Calcaneus

The patient is lying prone and the clinician is facing the leg to be treated. One hand of the clinician grips and stabilizes the distal tibiofibular joint, while the heel of the palm of the other hand is placed on the posterior inferior aspect of the calcaneus. While the hand supporting the distal tibiofibular joint offers counter-pressure. The heel of the palm of the

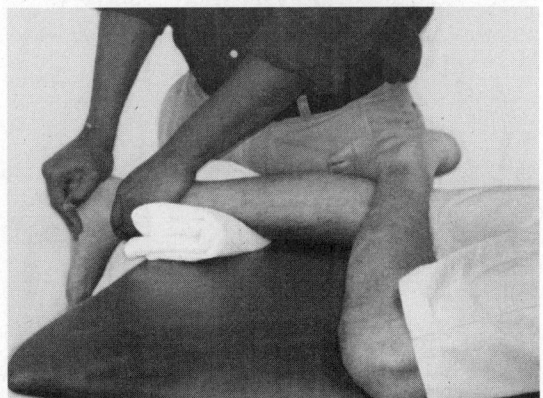

Fig. 12.21: Distraction of calcaneus.

other hand exerts a mobilization force downward to distract the calcaneus from the talus (Fig. 12.21).

Inversion/Eversion Calcaneus

The patient is lying prone with the foot over the end of the table and the clinician faces the patient from the leg side. One hand of the clinician grasps the lower end of the tibia and fibula to stabilize it. The other hand holds and stabilizes the calcaneus by holding the medial and lateral ends of the calcaneus with thumb, index and middle fingers. In case of an inverted calcaneus, the calcaneus is stretched in eversion. In case of an everted calcaneus, the calcaneus is stretched in inversion (Fig. 12.22).

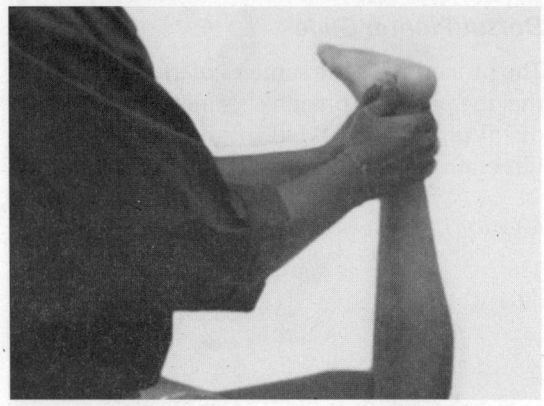

Fig. 12.22: Inversion/eversion of calcaneus.

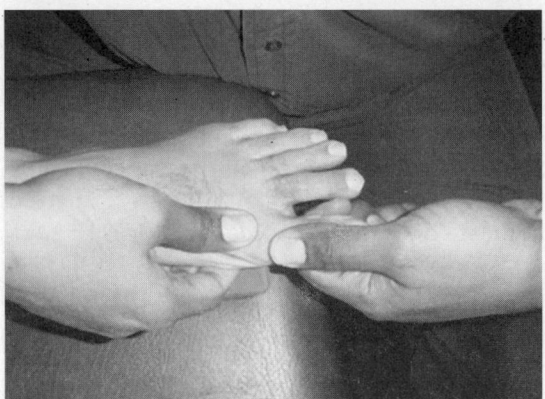

Fig. 12.24: Distraction and rotation MTP joint.

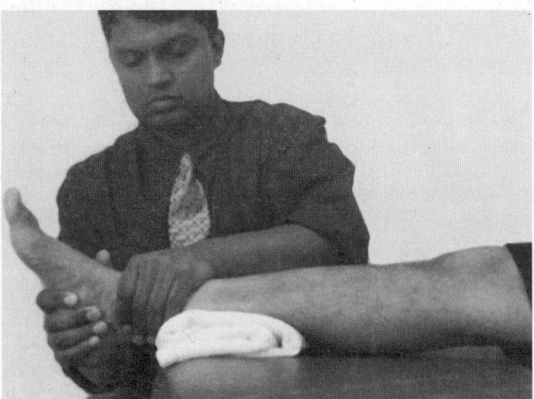

Fig. 12.23: Medial/lateral glide of talus.

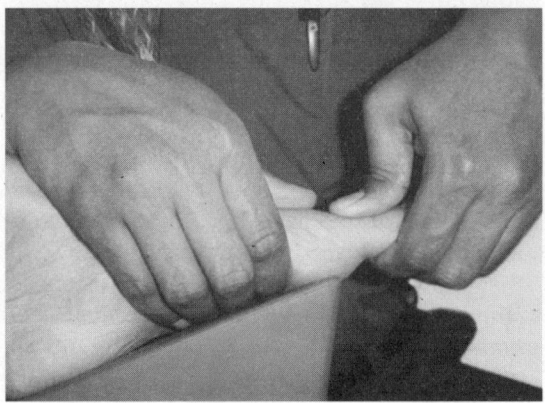

Fig. 12.25: Dorsal/Plantar glide MTP joint

Medial/Lateral Glide Talus

The patient is lying supine and the clinician faces the foot from the side. One hand of the clinician stabilizes the distal end of the tibia and fibula just above the talus. The clinician grips the talus and in a slightly plantarflexed position, imparts a gliding motion in a medial and lateral direction (Fig. 12.23).

Metatarsophalangeal Joints

Distraction and Rotation

The patient is lying supine and the clinician faces the foot to be treated. One hand of the clinician stabilizes the 1st metatarsal, while the other hand grips the superior and inferior aspects of the proximal phalanx of the great toe. Stabilizing the metatarsal, a distraction in the long axis direction is imparted via the proximal phalanx of the great toe. A gentle wringing motion is imparted in a medial and lateral direction so as to rotate the metatarsophalangeal (MTP). A similar procedure is done for 2nd to 5th metatarsals (Fig. 12.24).

Dorsal/Plantar Glide

The patient/clinician positions and the hand positions are the same as for a distraction. A gentle distraction is first applied and the proximal phalanx is glided in an superior/inferior direction. A similar procedure is repeated for the 2nd through 5th metatarsals (Fig. 12.25).

Medial/Lateral Glide

The patient/clinician position are the same except the hand positions which are now placed on the sides of the proximal phalanx of the toe. Stabilizing the metatarsal, the proximal phalanx is first distracted and a gentle glide is imparted in the medial and lateral direction (Fig. 12.26).

Proximal Interphalangeal/Distal Interphalangeal Joints

Distraction

The procedure is exactly the same as for an MTP distraction except that the proximal phalanx is stabilized, while the distal phalanx is distracted (Fig. 12.28).

Dorsal/Plantar Glide

The procedure is the same as of the MTP except that the proximal phalanx is stabilized, while the distal phalanx is glided in a superior/inferior direction (Fig. 12.29).

Medial/Lateral Glide

The procedure is the same as for a medial/lateral glide of the MTP except that the proximal phalanx is stabilized, while the distal phalanx is glided medial/lateral (Fig. 12.27).

PROPHYLAXIS

Muscle function within ankle and foot complex should be addressed not only from a dysfunction

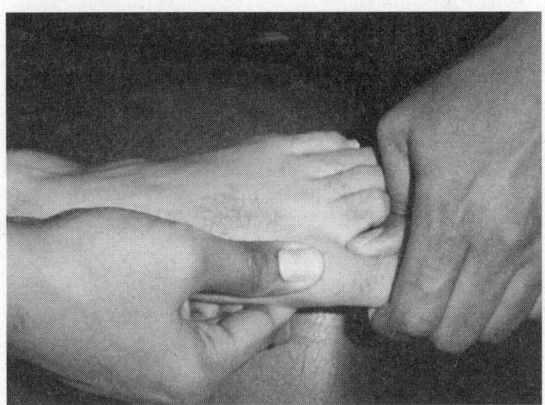

Fig. 12.26: Medial/lateral glide of MTP joint.

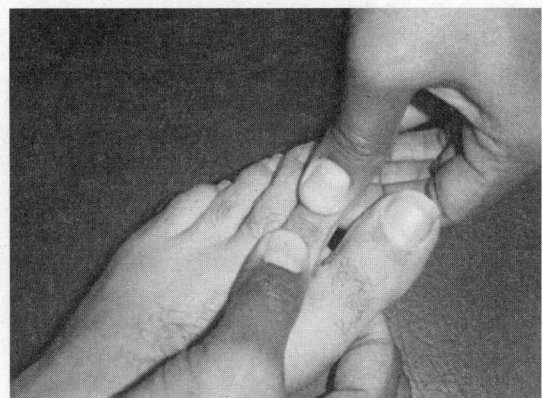

Fig. 12.28: Distraction of PIP/DIP joint.

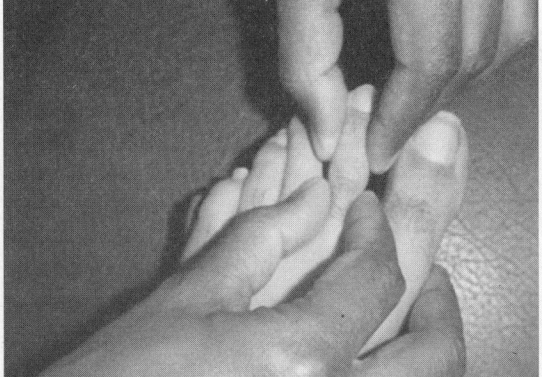

Fig. 12.27: Medial/lateral glide of PIP/DIP joint.

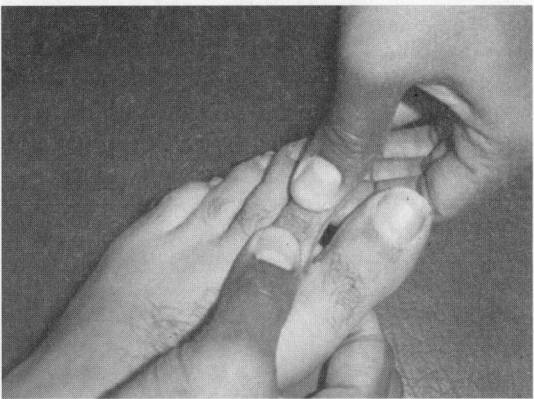

Fig. 12.29: Dorsal/plantar glide of PIP/DIP joint.

perspective but also from a functional perspective. As discussed, normal mechanics minimize and distribute weight bearing stresses within the joint complex, however, such a situation may best be achieved by strong specific supporting musculature. The key muscles that work during the gait cycle is to maintain normal mechanics are described.

The tibialis anterior works concentrically to help the foot clear the ground during the swing phase of gait. During the contact period of the gait cycle, the tibialis anterior contracts eccentrically to prevent excessive pronation of the forefoot. Hence, this muscle should be trained both eccentrically and concentrically in a pronation dysfunction.

During forefoot contact, the tibialis posterior and the gastrosoleus decelerate pronation and hence may be need to be trained both eccentrically and concentrically to prevent excessive pronation.

Pronation is a dysfunction that can cause tightness of the gastrosoleus and lengthening of the plantar fascia. The gastrosoleus should be stretched to minimize this situation with care not to overstretch the plantar fascia. This is usually accomplished by keeping the foot turned inward.

Supination can begin with a rearfoot varus which may render the peronei weak and the tibialis posterior tight. The plantar fascia can tighten if the rearfoot varus is compensated by a cavus which is caused by a compensatory pronation of the forefoot. A supination dysfunction will hence require strengthening of the peronei and stretching of the tibialis posterior and plantar fascia, if compensated.

The next elaborate area for prophylaxis in ankle and foot are corrective orthotics. The ankle and foot being highly dynamic and weight bearing structures require corrective support during all weight bearing situations. This is necessary if the symptom and the dysfunction is to be corrected. Orthotics, being a very elaborate area is beyond the scope of this book and may hence require additional reading. However, the clinician is reminded that the value of a comfortable and custom made orthotic is of prime importance and an adjunct that should not be overlooked.

MYOFASCIAL TENDER POINTS

The concept of addressing myofascial tender points is to decrease actin and myosin cross-bridging and myofibrillar restriction. Their continual presence may encourage chemical accumulation, early fatigue and decreased muscle performance with accompanying pain

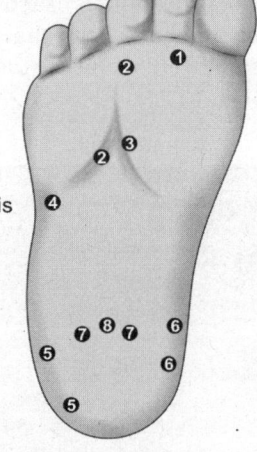

Myofascial tender points:

1. Plantar interosseous
2. Adductor hallucis
3. Flexor hallucis brevis
4. Flexor digiti minimi brevis
5. Abductor digiti minimi
6. Abductor hallucis
7. Flexor digitorum brevis
8. Quadratus plantae

Fig. 12.30: Myofascial tender points.

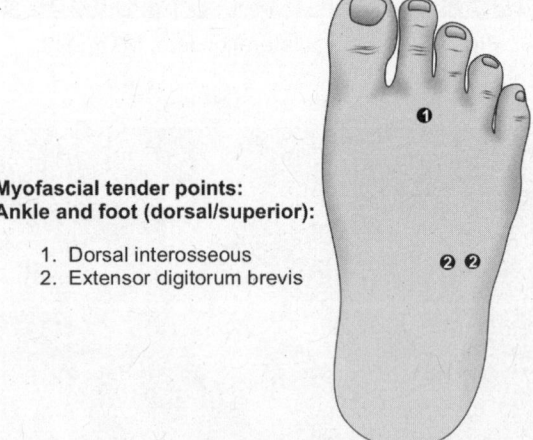

**Myofascial tender points:
Ankle and foot (dorsal/superior):**

1. Dorsal interosseous
2. Extensor digitorum brevis

Fig. 12.31: Myofascial tender points: Ankle and foot (dorsal/superior).

and dysfunction. They may be best treated with frictions and electrotherapy. Tender points secondary to aberrant gamma efferents may require an alternate positional release approach and the reader is encouraged further reading in the area of 'strain counterstrain' methods. The diagrams illustrate some common dysfunctional points of ankle and foot (Figs. 12.30 and 12.31).

REFERENCES

1. Donatelli R. The Biomechanics of the foot and ankle. 1990. FA, Davis Company, Philadelphia.
2. Greenman PE. Principles of Manual Medicine. 1996, Williams and Wilkins, Philadelphia.
3. Herring SA. Nilson KL. Introduction to overuse injuries. Clin Sports Med. 1987;6:225-39.
4. Heyman CH, et al. Mobilization of the tarsometatarsal and intermetatarsal joints for the correction of resistant adduction of the forepart of the foot in congenital club-foot or congenital metatarsus varus. J Bone joint Surg. 1958;40:299-309.
5. Botte RR. An interpretation of the pronation syndrome and foot types of patients with low back pain. J Am Podiatry Assoc. 1981;71: 245-53.
6. Saidoff DC, McDonough AL. Critical pathways in therapeutic intervention: Extremities and spine. 6th edn. 2002, St. Louis, Mosby.
7. Trevino S, Baumhauer JF. Tendon injuries of the foot and ankle. Clin Sports Med. 1992;11:727-39.
8. Lentell GL. Katzman LL, Walters MR. The relationship between muscle function and ankle stability. Journal of Orthopedic and Sports Physical therapy. 1990;11:605-11
9. Schon LC. Nerve entrapment, neuropathy, and nerve dysfunction in athletes. Orthop Clin North Am. 1994;25:47-59.
10. Norris CM. Sports Injuries: Diagnosis and management for physiotherapists, 1993, Butterworth-Heinemann: Oxford.
11. Patla CE, Paris SV. E1: Extremity manipulation and evaluation, course notes, 1996, Institute press: St Augustine.
12. Kaltenborn F. Mobilization of the extremity joints: Examination and basic techniques. 3rd edn. 1980: Olaf Noris Bokhandel A/S, Oslo, Norway.

CHAPTER 13

Knee

The knee forms the center point of the lower limb kinetic chain. The knee cap or the patella is also an important component of the knee complex from a manual therapy and dysfunction perspective. As described in literature, gait is a series of rotations and hence it may be of worthwhile to know that a significant proportion of this rotation occurs at the tibia.[1] Flexion and extension is commonly addressed in the knee complex but a greater attention to the internal and external rotation component of the tibia with relevance to the ankle and foot is suggested to minimize mechanical dysfunction at the knee.

OSSEOUS ANATOMY

The knee joint comprises the superior tibiofibular joint, tibiofemoral joint and patellofemoral joint. The tibiofemoral joint is formed by the distal femur and proximal tibia. The femur consists of two condyles, medial and lateral. The height of the lateral condylar wall is greater along the trochlear groove which helps to prevent lateral subluxation of the patella. The superior surface of the tibia has two asymmetric plateaus separated in the middle by the medial and lateral eminence. The contact surface of the medial surface is twice as large as the lateral surface.

The patellofemoral joint is the articulation between patella and femur. It is a triangular sesamoid bone. 'Tracking' is referred to the movement of the patella over the femur during flexion and extension of the knee. Optimal tracking is essential for normal mechanics and is considered normal if the apex of the patella is centered in the femoral trochlear groove through all degrees of flexion.[2] The patella functions to minimize friction and improve the leverage of the quadriceps mechanism and acts as a protective layer for the femoral condyle cartilage.[3]

The proximal tibiofibular joint comprises the articulation of the fibular head to the proximal tibia. The facet for the head of fibula faces laterally, posteriorly and inferiorly. The head of fibula hence faces medially, anteriorly and superiorly. These joints have an important part to play in the optimal function of the tibiofemoral joint. The fibular head glides posteriorly on the tibia on knee flexion and vice versa for extension. Hence a restriction of this motion can affect the mobility and mechanics at the knee.

LIGAMENTOUS ANATOMY

Primary Ligaments

Anterior Cruciate Ligament

This ligament arises from the posterior aspect of the medial surface of the lateral femoral condyle. It then travels anteriorly, medially, and distally to insert into the tibial plateau anterior and lateral to the anterior tibial spine. This ligament functions to resist anterior translation of tibia and tibial internal rotation/valgus stress.

Posterior Cruciate Ligament

This ligament arises from the posterior aspect of the tibial intercondylar region and travels anteromedially behind the anterior cruciate ligament (ACL) to the lateral surface of the medial femoral condyle. The posterior cruciate ligament (PCL) is considered is to be the strongest ligament in the knee. It functions to prevent posterior translation of the tibia on the femur. It additionally serves to prevent hyperextension at the knee, maintain rotatory stability and act as the knee's central axis of rotation.

Medial Collateral Ligament

This ligament originates at the adductor tubercle on the medial femoral condyle and advances distally to insert into the medial tibial diaphysis approximately 3 to 4 inches below the joint line inferior to the insertion of the pes anserinus. The deep layer of this ligament has an attachment to the medial meniscus.

The medial collateral ligament (MCL) and associated capsular structures are strong stabilizers of the medial aspect of the knee, offering protection against valgus stresses.

Lateral Collateral Ligament

This ligament originates from the lateral femoral condyle passes over the popliteus and inserts into the lateral fibular head. It serves to protect the knee from varus stresses and is rarely injured due to its high tensile strength.

MUSCULAR ANATOMY

The primary muscles that act at the knee are quadriceps, hamstrings, gastrocnemius and popliteus. The quadriceps is primarily a knee extensor and also a stabilizer of the patella. The hamstrings function as knee flexors and gastrocnemius besides being powerful plantarflexors of the ankle also act as flexors of the knee. In a weight bearing situation, however, gastrocnemius creates a posterior moment in the knee and helps to stabilize the knee. The popliteus[10] functions to unlock the knee during knee flexion and is also an internal rotator on the tibia. Their role during the gait cycle is enumerated in the next section.

MECHANICS (NORMAL ROLL-GLIDING)

During initial contact, the ankle is close to neutral and the subtalar joint is slightly supinated. The quadriceps begins to work eccentrically to allow the knee to flex. The popliteus muscle unlocks the knee and causes the tibia to rotate internally as the foot progresses to foot flat. The hamstrings initially work concentrically to extend the hip, however, as the knee flexes they no longer do so as the gluteals take over. The hamstrings contract to slide the tibia backwards. The biceps femoris portion of the hamstrings contract to glide the fibular head backwards. The initial part of midstance is the unlocking phase where shock absorption occurs with an internally rotated tibia and a pronated foot.

At late midstance the knee begins to extend with the quadriceps working concentrically. The tibia begins to externally rotate as the foot supinates in preparation for propulsion.

At the propulsion phase the knee reaches close to maximum extension. The tibia glides anteriorly via its quadriceps attachment at the tibial tubercle to facilitate extension. The quadriceps works eccentrically to control the knee. The calf works concentrically to actively plantarflex the ankle for propulsion, and by virtue of its attachment to the femoral condyles causes a posterior moment at the knee.

The neutral position of the knee is full extension. In full knee extension, no transverse plane motion occurs, but as the knee flexes, rotations occur. During the terminal ranges of knee extension, the tibia externally rotates to lock the knee (screw home). The fibula accompanies the tibia and glides anterior.

When knee flexion commences, initially rolling is the primary joint play. Gliding follows as the range of flexion increases and finally only gliding occurs. The medial condyle rolls only for the first 10 to 15° of flexion, while the lateral condyle continues until 20° of flexion. This is the most stable range of the knee as the part of the femoral condyles involved in the articulation is large. As the knee continues to flex beyond 20° this contact area decreases. This tends to result in the ligaments being more lax and subsequently favoring tibial rotation.

This tibial rotation is greatly determined by the position of the foot as described in the earlier chapter. During the initial contact phase the subtalar joint begins to pronate and this tibia internally rotates unlocking the knee. The biceps femoris which is the part of the hamstrings and a knee flexor, pulls the fibula backwards by virtue of its attachment to the head (and hence an accessory motion for knee flexion).

MECHANISM OF DYSFUNCTION

The bigger factor that determines the cause for mechanical dysfunctions at the knee is tibial internal rotation and will hence be described first. Tibial internal and external rotation are determined by the foot position as this is a response to weight bearing. As described earlier, at initial stance, the calcaneus everts with talar adduction and platar flexion. This is accompanied by the tibial internal rotation. During supination of the foot, the tibia rotates externally. However, when abnormal pronation occurs where the foot remains pronated throughout the stance phase, the tibia remains internally rotated and is arthrokinematically restricted in this position. This is a determinant for dysfunction.[4]

Common Pathologies Secondary to Mechanical Dysfunction

Patellar Compression

Internal rotation[5] of the tibia causes the lateral portion of the femoral trochlear groove to move anteromedially against the lateral patellar facet during weight bearing. Chronic irritation of the lateral patellar facet can result in lateral patellar compression syndrome.

Patellar Tracking

As the foot pronates abnormally beyond 4 to 6° and beyond 25% of the stance phase, the tibia is carried into excessive and prolonged internal rotation. This causes the femur to migrate into external rotation. The result is an increase in the Q-angle which is the quadriceps angle of pull in line with the femur superiorly relative to the pull of the patellar tendon inferiorly at the tibial tuberosity. When the Q-angle increases, there is a relative increase in the genu valgum angle and patella is pulled laterally resulting in lateral patellar tracking and patellofemoral pain.

Pes Anserine Bursitis

This condition is seen as inferomedial knee pain where the tendinous insertion of the gracilis, sartorius and semitendinosis are padded by this bursa. Prolonged internal rotation of the tibia can cause a hyperirritability of these muscles as they rotate the tibia inwards subsequently irritating the bursa beneath it. Tightness of the medial hamstrings can predispose to a similar condition.[6]

Iliotibial Band Friction Syndrome

The prolonged internal rotation that occurs secondary to abnormal foot pronation causes the femur to rotate externally and tibia internally. Internal rotation brings the Gerdy's tubercle on the lateral condyle of the tibia more prominent. This with the prominence of the lateral condyle of femur causes a tethering of the iliotibial (IT) band that crosses over it. Repetitive flexion and extension at the knee can cause the inferior portion of the band to rub on the relatively prominent lateral femoral condyle resulting in an iliotibial band friction syndrome and lateral knee pain.

Medial Ligament Strain

The effect of prolonged pronation and tibial internal rotation creates a genu valgum and opens the medial tibiofemoral joint space. This increases the tensile loading on the medial aspect of the knee resulting in stress on the medial ligament and medial capsule. This factor should also be considered when rehabilitating a medial ligament strain that has already occurred or partial tears.[7]

Lateral Ligament Strain

Supination has the exact reverse effect of pronation. It creates a varus stress opening the lateral joint space increasing the stress on the lateral ligament and possibly the iliotibial band.

Anterior Cruciate Ligament

The ACL functions is to resist tibial movement in the anterior direction, however, it has yet another function that is not frequently described. It also functions to resist tibial internal rotation and tibial valgum. Prolonged excessive tibial internal rotation and valgus of the tibia tends to cause a cumulative stress on the ligament increasing its vulnerability to injury. This should most definitely be considered when rehabilitating a reconstructed ligament or healing partial tears of the ACL.[5]

Nerve Compression

Superficial peroneal nerve: This nerve is superficial at the head of the fibula and can be irritated due to various causes. Varus stress test is that opens the lateral aspect of the knee joint, as described above can stress the superior tibiofibular articulation resulting in nerve irritation.

The peroneus longus, however, is a more common cause. This muscle works to plantarflex the first ray for foot propulsion. However, during excessive or prolonged foot supination, the first ray plantarflexes excessively to get the forefoot flat on the ground for propulsion. Hence, it may be restricted in a plantarflexed position. This results in contracted and hyperactive states of the peroneus longus and irritation of the nerve as it passes through this muscle.

A supination of the foot can cause an external tibial rotation. This in turn can displace the fibula head laterally due to a varus stress test and can cause an irritation of this nerve.

Saphenous nerve: This nerve is sensory and can be entrapped as it passes between the vastus medialis and adductor magnus. This nerve supplies the medial side of the knee and the calf and can cause pain in these areas.

Retinacular nerve: Lateral patellar tracking dysfunction can cause tightness of the lateral retinaculum and result in what is described as a lateral patellar hyper pressure syndrome. The retinacular nerve that is in close proximity can be irritated and is a source of lateral knee pain.

KNEE JOINT SOMATIC DIAGNOSIS

Tibia Internal/External

The patient is seated with the legs hanging to the side of the table and the knees flexed to 90°. The clinician grasps the foot and dorsiflexes maximally. The other hand fixes both condyles of femur in neutral. The lower end with the foot in dorsiflexion is turned in and out to sense for restriction in internal and external rotations (Fig.13.1). Comparison is made with the other side. An internal rotation of the tibia, as described in the section on mechanism of dysfunction, can predispose to dysfunctions ranging from patellar tracking to pes anserine bursitis. It is also commonly associated with a pronation dysfunction at the foot.

Restricted Superior Tibiofibular

The patient is lying with the knees flexed to about 60 to 70°. The clinician ensures symmetry by confirming that the knees and feet are close together and exactly adjacent. The clinician then

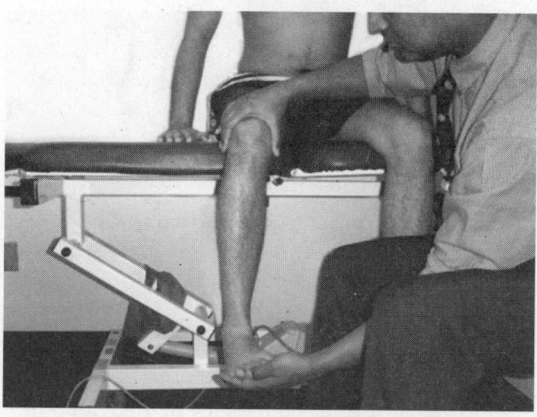

Fig. 13.1: Assessing tibial rotation.

palpates one fibular head at a time and grips it with index, thumb and middle fingers and notes for asymmetry (Fig. 13.2). A glide is applied in the anterior direction and the clinician senses for restriction and local tenderness (Fig. 13.3). Inability of the fibula head to glide anteriorly is the most common restriction seen. Dysfunctions of the fibula head can predispose to irritability of the peroneus longus and subsequently the peroneal nerve. It can also predispose to dysfunctions of the lateral collateral ligament and iliotibial band.

Femoral Head Posterolateral

Refer to Chapter 14 for a detail description.

Patella Superolateral

The patient is lying supine with the knee in slight flexion of about 5°. The clinician faces the knee to be examined from the other side. The clinician then grips the superolateral border of the patella with the fingers and gently stretches it in an inferior and medial direction (Fig. 13.4). Dysfunction is indicated by a painful sensation on the superolateral border. Comparison is made with the other side. A superolateral patella can indicate a patella tracking dysfunction, or a medial rotated tibia or a pronated foot.

Foot Pronation/Supination

Refer to Chapter 12 for a detail description.

TREATMENT FOR SPECIFIC SOMATIC DYSFUNCTION

Tibia Internal/External Rotation

The patient is lying prone and the clinician faces the leg to be treated. The knee of the patient is flexed to 90° and the foot is maximally dorsiflexed. The clinicians knee is placed on the posterior thigh of the patient, while the hand grips the ankle. The other hand holds and supports the foot. Using the knee of the clinician as leverage, the gentle traction is applied at the

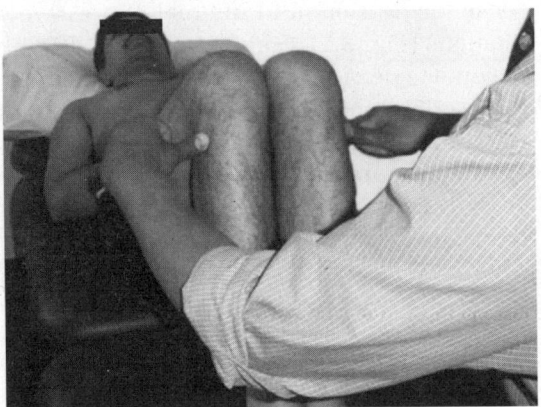

Fig. 13.2: Assessing fibular head symmetry.

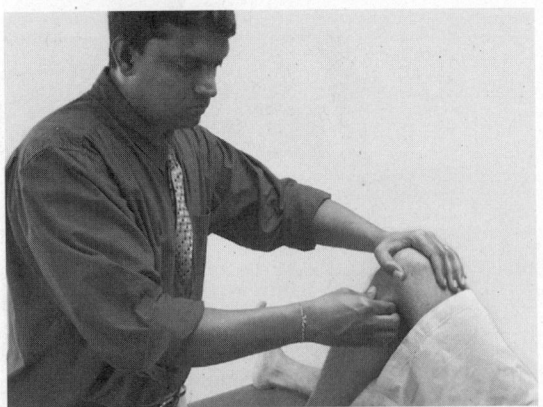

Fig. 13.3: Assessing mobility at the superior tibiofibular joint.

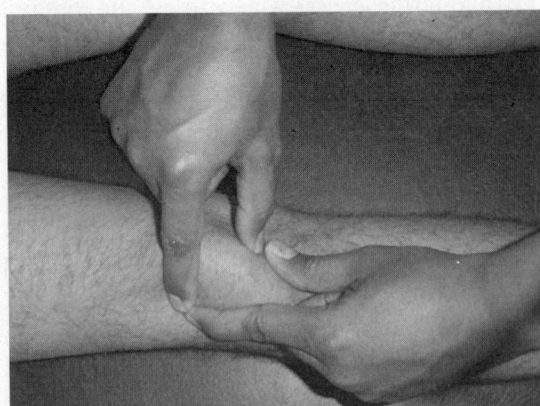

Fig. 13.4: Assessing superior lateral position of the patella.

ankle and the foot is gently turned outward as a stretch if the tibia is restricted in medial rotation (Fig. 13.5). The reverse is done for a tibia restricted in lateral rotation. Care must be taken to perform this maneuver gently especially if the patient has a meniscus pathology.

Restricted Tibiofibular

For an anterior dysfunction, the patient is lying supine and the clinician faces the leg to be treated. The knee is flexed to about 70 to 80° and the tibia is rotated medially by placing the foot pointing inward. One hand of the clinician cups and supports the superior aspect of the knee. The base of the thumb and thenar eminence of the other hand contacts the head of the fibula. A gentle mobilizing force is imparted in a posterior direction (Fig. 13.6).

For a posterior dysfunction, the patient is lying prone and the knee is flexed to about 70°. The clinician faces the leg from the other side. One hand of the clinician supports the ankle, while the thenar eminence of the other hand contacts the posterior aspect of the fibular head. A gentle mobilization force is imparted in an anterior direction (Fig. 13.7).

Femoral Head Posterolateral

Refer to Chapter 14 for a detail description of the technique of treatment.

Patella Superolateral

The technique is similar to the diagnosis. The patient is lying supine with the knee in slight flexion of about 5°. The clinician faces the knee to be examined from the other side. The clinician then grips the superolateral border of the patella with the fingers and gently stretches it in an inferior and medial direction. The stretch is maintained for about 5 seconds and repeated 3 to 5 times based on tolerance as this is painful in the presence of a dysfunction.

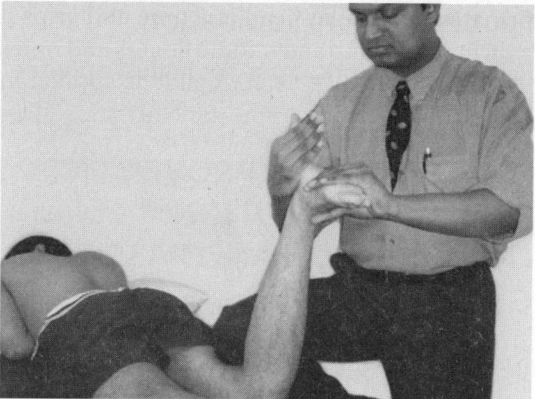

Fig. 13.5: Internal and external rotation of tibia.

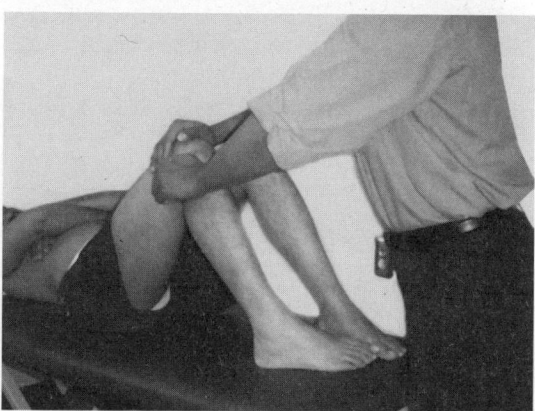

Fig. 13.6: Posterior glide fibula head.

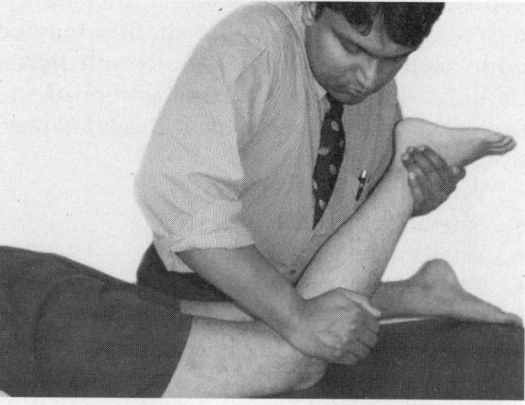

Fig. 13.7: Anterior glide fibula head.

Foot Pronation/Supination

Refer to Chapter 12 for a detail description of treatment techniques.

FOR OVERALL IMPROVEMENT IN RANGE OF MOTION[8,9] (TJP: TRACTION AND PASSIVE GLIDING)

Joint Basics

Type of joint	Diarthroidal ginglymus
Degrees of freedom	Flexion, extension, internal rotation
External	Rotation, abduction and adduction
Range of motion	Flexion: 0–135; Extension: 0–10; Tibial internal rotation: 0–30; Tibial external rotation: 0–40
Capsular pattern	Greater limitation of flexion than extension
Loose packed position	Slight to midflexion

To Improve Knee Flexion

Procedures are initiated by soft tissue mobilization of the retinaculum and the superior portion of the patella area in the absence of contraindication. Myofascial tender points described at the end of the chapter may be addressed as well. Additionally soft tissue mobilization of the inferior aspect of the sartorius is also recommended. This is followed by the following:
- Patella inferior glide
- Patella medial/lateral glide
- Patella medial/lateral tilt
- Tibia distraction
- Tibia posterior glide medial condyle
- Fibula anterior posterior AP glide

To Improve Knee Extension

- Patella superior glide
- Patella medial/lateral glide
- Patella medial/lateral tilt
- Tibia distraction
- Tibia anterior glide medial condyle
- Fibula AP glide

This is followed by the soft tissue mobilization of the posterior knee area and prone low load long duration extension stretch with ankle weights in the absence of contraindication.

TECHNIQUE

Patella Inferior/Superior Glide

The patient is lying supine with the knee in about 5° of flexion. The clinician faces the knee to be treated. The thumbs are placed on either sides over the inferior borders of the patella and the index and middle fingers are placed over the base. A gentle mobilization force is imparted in an inferior/superior direction (Fig. 13.8).

Patella Medial/Lateral Glide

The patient and clinician position are as for an inferior glide. Both thumbs are placed on the lateral border of the patella and the other fingers are placed over the upper tibia and lower femur to stabilize. A gentle mobilization force is imparted in the medial direction to glide the patella medially. The clinician changes position to the opposite side and changes the thumb positions medially for a lateral glide of the patella (Fig. 13.9).

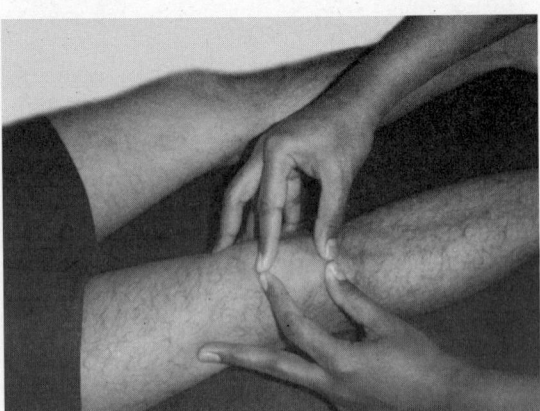

Fig. 13.8: Patella superior and inferior glide.

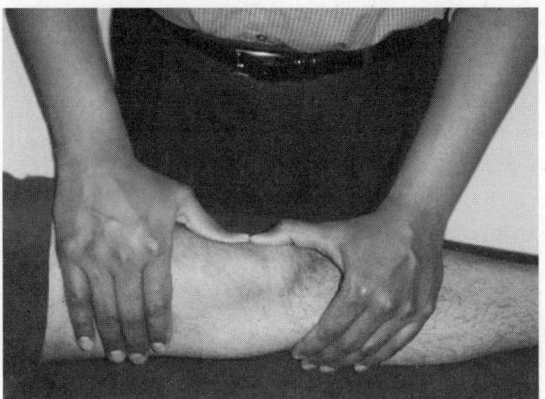
Fig. 13.9: Patella medial and lateral glide.

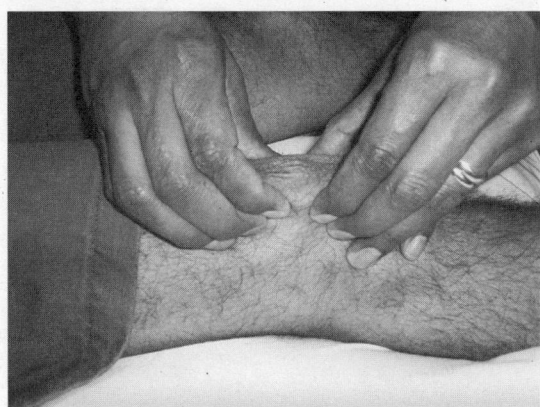
Fig. 13.10: Patella tilt.

Patella Medial/Lateral Tilt

The patient and clinician position are as for an inferior glide. Both index and middle fingers of the clinician are placed over the lateral aspect of the patella. The thumbs are placed medially. The patella is first glided laterally. A gentle superiorly directed pressure is applied over the lateral aspect of the patella to move the lateral border anteriorly and tilt the patella medially. The thumbs offer a counter pressure on the medial side. The reverse is done for a lateral tilt, however, the most common restriction seen in a medial tilt secondary to tightness of the lateral retinaculum (Fig. 13.10).

Tibia Distraction

The patient is lying supine with the leg by the side of the table and the clinician faces the leg to be treated. The knee of the patient is flexed to 90°. The clinicians' forearm is placed under the posterior thigh of the patient, while the hand grips the ankle. Using the forearm of the clinician as leverage, a gentle traction is applied at the ankle in a long axis direction (Fig. 13.11). If knee flexion is inadequate, then the procedure is done with available knee flexion range and not necessarily 90°.

Anterior Glide of Medial Tibial Condyle

The patient is lying prone and the knee is flexed to about 70°. The clinician faces the leg from the

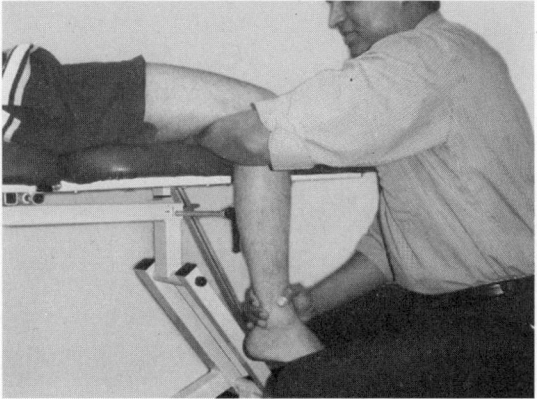
Fig. 13.11: Tibia distraction.

same side. One hand of the clinician supports the ankle, while the thenar eminence of the other hand contacts the posterior aspect of the medial tibial condyle. A gentle mobilization force is imparted in an anterior direction (Fig. 13.12).

Posterior Glide of Medial Tibial Condyle

The patient is lying supine with the knee flexed to about 5 to 10° and supported. The clinician faces the knee to be treated. The proximal aspect of the palm of the clinician is placed on the anterior medial and superior portion of the tibia. An inferiorly directed posterior force is imparted over the medial tibial condyle to glide it posteriorly (Fig. 13.13).

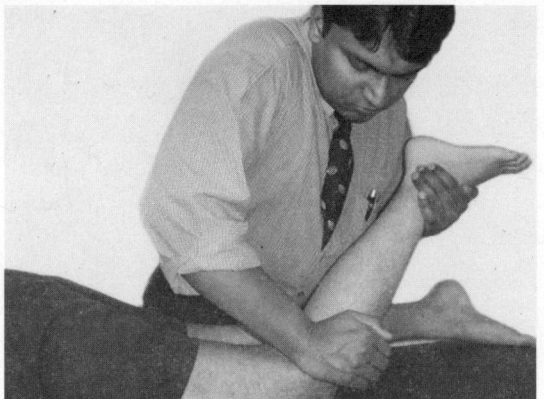

Fig. 13.12: Tibia anterior glide.

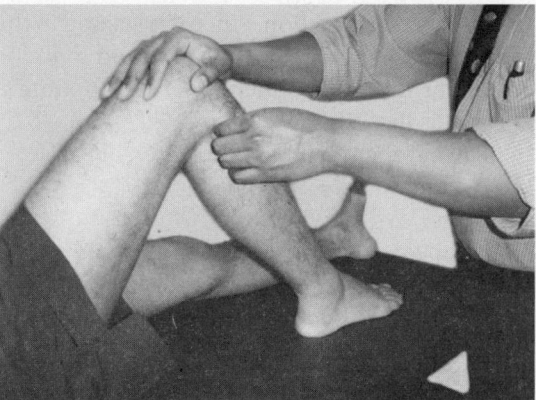

Fig. 13.14: Fibula glide.

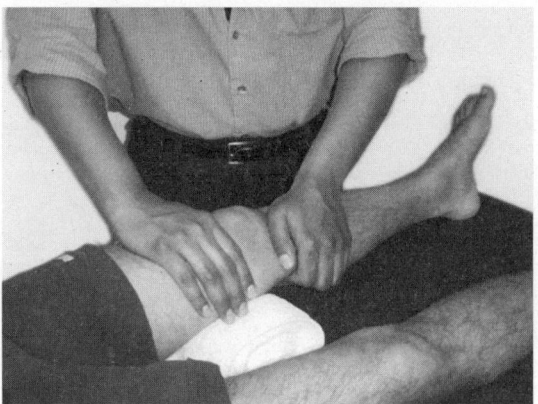

Fig. 13.13: Tibia posterior glide.

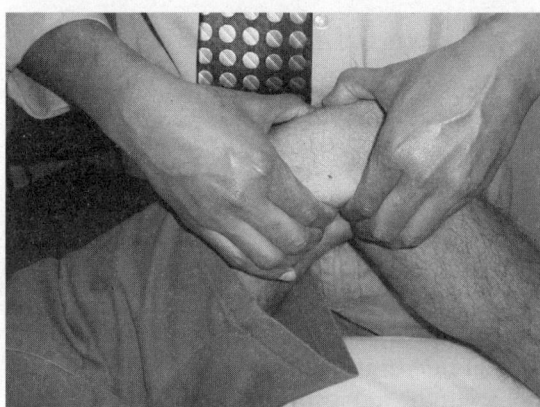

Fig. 13.15: Soft tissue mobilization of sartorius.

Fibula Anterolateral Glide/Posteromedial Glide

The patient is lying supine and the knee is flexed to about 70 to 90° with the foot resting on the table. One hand of the clinician supports the anterior aspect of the knee, while on the other hand incorporates thumb and index/middle fingers to grip and stabilize the head of fibula. A gentle mobilization force is imparted in an anterolateral and posteromedial direction so as to glide the head of fibula in these directions (Fig. 13.14).

Soft Tissue Mobilization of Sartorius

The sartorius is an anteriorly placed muscle and obliquely in line with the quadriceps. Hence, it has a tendency for shortening and potentially an inhibitor of knee flexion. Often, while flexing the knee of a patient with restricted knee flexion, the stretch discomfort is felt posterior to the knee joint. Recall, the tibia internally rotates on flexion taking the insertion of the sartorius more posterior. Soft tissue mobilization is achieved by placing the patient supine with the knee in the end range of available flexion. The index and middle fingers of both hands are placed on the medially place muscle bulk around the knee. Note that this area might be tender. Gentle frictions are applied in the transverse direction of the muscle fiber for 3 to 5 minutes (Fig. 13.15).

PROPHYLAXIS

The knee is yet another dynamic area that relies strongly on the muscular integrity to prevent and correct dysfunction. Since it is second in the weight bearing chain to the ankle and foot, the muscular mechanics including dysfunction in the foot is first addressed.

Patellar alignment is usually maintained (from a muscular perspective), by the vastus medialis obliquus (VMO) and the lateral retinaculum. The VMO should hence be routinely strengthened and the lateral retinaculum, including the iliotibial band, be routinely stretched. Following this, eccentric training of the quadriceps is warranted.

Tibial motion is also controlled by the muscular activity and can be taken advantage of. Anterior glide of the tibia occurs on contraction of the quadriceps and a posterior glide by the hamstrings. Medial rotation of the tibia by the medial hamstrings and lateral rotation by the lateral hamstrings. Hence the appropriate muscle must be trained for a specific dysfunction, as in training the quadriceps and lateral hamstrings if there is a medial rotation dysfunction of the tibia. Hence tightness is to be considered as the hamstrings are indeed prone for it and may lead to dysfunction.

Since tibial mechanics are controlled by ankle and foot motion, they should be addressed first. Foot orthotics are sometimes essential to address knee dysfunction. The reason being that knee dysfunction can be the result of a foot dysfunction or faulty foot mechanics. Regular footwear, if improper, should be considered as being possible aggravating factors. Especially those with excessively high or flat and hard heels or those lacking arch supports.

MYOFASCIAL TENDER POINTS

The concept of addressing myofascial tender points is to decrease actin and myosin cross-bridging and myofibrillar restriction. Their continual presence may encourage chemical accumulation, early fatigue and decreased muscle performance with accompanying pain and dysfunction. They may be best treated with frictions and electrotherapy. Tender points secondary to aberrant gamma efferents may

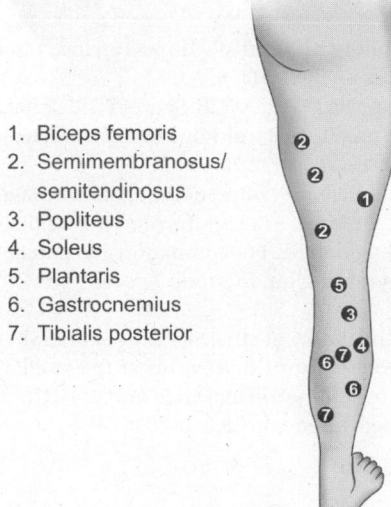

1. Biceps femoris
2. Semimembranosus/semitendinosus
3. Popliteus
4. Soleus
5. Plantaris
6. Gastrocnemius
7. Tibialis posterior

Fig. 13.16: Myofascial points: Knee (posterior).

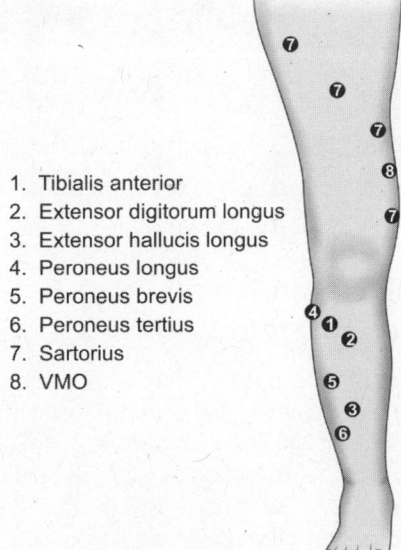

1. Tibialis anterior
2. Extensor digitorum longus
3. Extensor hallucis longus
4. Peroneus longus
5. Peroneus brevis
6. Peroneus tertius
7. Sartorius
8. VMO

Fig. 13.17: Myofascial tender points: Knee (anterior).

require an alternate positional release approach and the reader is encouraged further reading in the area of 'strain counterstrain' methods. The figures illustrate common dysfunctional points of the knee (Figs. 13.16 and 13.17).

REFERENCES

1. Hutter CG, Scott W. Tibial Torsion. J Bone Joint Surg.1949;31:511-8.
2. Zappala FG, Taffel CB, Scuderi GR. Rehabilitation of patellofemoral joint disorders. Orthop Clin North Am. 1992;23:555-66.
3. Mandelbaum BR, et al. Articular cartilage lesions of the knee. Am J Sports Med. 1998;26:853-61.
4. Klingman RE. Foot pronation and patellofemoral joint function. J Orthop Sports Phys Ther. 1999; 29:421.
5. Bufor WL, et al. Internal/external rotation moment arms of muscles at the knee: moment arms for the normal knee and the ACL-deficient knee. Knee. 2001;8:293-303.
6. Reilly JP, Nicholas JA. The chronically inflamed bursa. Clin Sports Med. 1987;6:345-70.
7. Ellenbecker TS. Knee ligament rehabilitation. Chapter 9. Rehabilitation after autgenic and allogenic anterior cruciate ligament reconstruction. New York: Churchill Livingstone, 2000:132-149.
8. Patla CE, Paris SV. E1,Course Notes: Extremity evaluation and manipulation. 1996, St. Augustine Institute press.
9. Kaltenborn F. Mobilization of the extremity joints: Examination and basic treatment techniques. 1980. 3rd edn. Olaf Norlis Bokhandel Universitetsgaten, Oslo,Norway.
10. Saidoff DC, McDonough AL, Duprey LP. Critical pathways in therapeutic intervention: extremities and spine. 2002. St. Louis .Mosby.

CHAPTER 14

Hip

The hip joint is a component of the lumbopelvic complex and hence is a determinant for dysfunctions within the complex. Since the walking cycle is determined by the normal overall function of the lumbopelvic hip complex, the hip is a significant contributor. Hip pain may hence not necessarily be a hip entity and so is back and pelvic pain. Attention to all vulnerable structures within the complex is essential.

OSSEOUS ANATOMY

The head of the femur forms the ball of the hip joint. The ilium, ischium and pubis fuse to form the acetabulum which is deepened by a labrum. The head of the femur articulates with acetabulum to form the joint. From a mechanical standpoint, the congruence of this joint is influenced by the alignment of several osseous structures.

From above, the lumbar vertebrae, especially L5, with the sacrum and innominates, and from below the angulation of the shaft of the femur and foot position. Alterations in the normal alignment of these structures can increase stress within the joint.[1,2]

LIGAMENTOUS ANATOMY

The hip is supported by three strong ligaments, namely:
1. Ischiofemoral
2. Iliofemoral
3. Pubofemoral

From a clinical perspective there is yet another ligament that runs anterior to the hip. It is more a ligament of the pelvic complex rather than the hip, and is called the inguinal ligament. The inguinal ligament runs from the ASIS to the pubic tubercles on either sides. These ligaments are irritated in dysfunctional states of the pubis or the innominates. They are usually tender to palpation and can cause anterior hip pain. Relief of symptoms are obtained by correction of the pubic or innominate dysfunction.

MUSCULAR ANATOMY

The musculature of the hip are elaborate and only the ones that are clinically relevant is described[3] as they help to control advancement, and stabilization of the leg during gait.

During initial contact, there is a marked contraction of the hamstrings and the gluteus maximus as they assist with hip extension. On progression to midstance the abductors, mainly the gluteus medius stabilize the pelvis and decrease compressive forces in the hip by distributing weight on both sides. The gluteus medius and minimus continue to provide lateral stability in terminal stance. Upon initiation of the swing phase, the muscles that are active are the iliacus, to flex the hip, and the anterior fibers of the tensor fascia lata. In the later part of the swing phase, the gluteus maximus and hamstrings are strongly active to decelerate hip flexion.

MECHANICS (NORMAL ROLL-GLIDING)

Movement in the hip should be interpreted as the movement of the femur relative to the pelvis although in a weight bearing (closed chain) situation it is interpreted as the movement of the pelvis over the femoral head. The reason for an interpretation of the femoral head over the pelvis is for easier understanding. The following is the normal sequence of events that occur in the hip during the eight phases of gait.[3] Upon initial contact, at about 30° of flexion the femoral head glides anterior on the acetabulum. During loading response, the hip assumes 30° of flexion, 5 to 10° of lateral rotation. This is the unloading phase accompanied by tibial internal rotation and pronation. On approaching midstance a posterior glide of the femoral head occurs and the head of the femur spins inward as in internal rotation, while the acetabulum spins outward. At midstance the gluteus medius contracts to stabilize the pelvis. The head of the femur continues to glide posterior and maximal internal rotation of the femoral head is maintained. At terminal stance which occurs at 10° of hip extension the femoral head glides anterior and as preswing is initiated, the femoral head begins to spin outward as in lateral rotation. During the swing phase, the hip returns to neutral flexion with maximal lateral rotation as in the femoral head begins to glide anterior and spins outward. 20 to 30° of flexion and 5° of abduction is maintained.

The important component of hip mechanics during the end of loading response and the midstance is hip extension and internal rotation which is the pattern of restriction exhibited in capsular tightness. Hip extension is therefore compensated by an excessive anterior rotation of the innominates, a subsequent pelvic and lumbar pathology.

Muscle weakness is yet another factor that can affect the mechanics at the hip joint and cause dysfunction. The dynamics are enumerated in the chapter on understanding mechanical dysfunction.

MECHANISM OF DYSFUNCTION

Mechanical dysfunction at the hip is closely associated with dysfunctions of the sacrum and the innominates. It also has a close relationship to the alignment of the lower extremity as well. In all it strongly depends on the line and distribution of weight bearing around the joint. Structural anomalies can occur and so do congenital anomalies and they are not considered in this discussion as with any other region described in this book. However, as possible causes for mechanical pain in the hip, pelvis and the lower extremity warrants attention.

When the walking cycle was considered in the chapter on the pelvic complex, the mechanics at the lumbopelvic area was described. Since the innominates undergo significant motion changes, the hip is well considered within the cycle as the acetabulum is a structure within the innominates. Hence a restriction in one of the articulations of the pelvis namely that involving sacrum and the innominates can predispose to increased stress in the hip and subsequently a dysfunction. The structures that are commonly involved in mechanical dysfunctions of the hip are cartilage and capsule within the joint, in association with the muscle, ligament and nerve outside of the joint.

Secondly, capsular restriction of the hip with lack of internal rotation and extension of the femur can alter the stance phase of the gait cycle (where most of the loading occurs) and result in musculoskeletal pathology.

Common pathologies secondary to mechanical dysfunction are as follows:

Osteoarthritis

The head of the femur forms two-third of a sphere and is completely covered with articular cartilage except for a slight depression to which yet another ligament, the ligamentum teres is attached. The cartilage is the thickest on the medial central surface where it makes contact with the acetabulum and is thinnest on the periphery. The head of the femur, hence, faces the acetabulum in a medial position. This medial congruence is alternated by lateral and medial rotation of the hip during the swing and the stance phases of gait. This way the load of weight bearing is distributed. This mechanism is lost during capsular tightening of the hip. The femoral head may then hypothetically stay restricted in lateral rotation and cause excessive shearing in that position as it does not alternate positions. In other words the load is not distributed and focused on the medial aspect which is where the articular cartilage is the thickest, predisposing to articular wear and tear and osteoarthritis.

Bursitis

Bursae are sacs of fluid interposed between soft tissue and bone to reduce friction. Faulty alignment or mechanics of the bony structures in combination with repetitive activity of the muscle coursing over it, or direct trauma can inflame the bursa resulting in pain.[6] The common precursor for this problem in the hip is the tendon sliding over bony prominences due to repetitive motion. This created a snapping sound and is conventionally diagnosed as a 'snapping hip syndrome'.[4] This can occur when the iliotibial band and gluteus medius glides over the greater trochanter resulting in trochanteric bursitis, or the iliopsoas tendon gliding over the iliopectineal eminence of the pubis resulting in iliopsoas or iliopectineal bursitis.

Trochanteric Bursitis

The mechanical causes for trochanteric bursitis may be faulty alignment or muscle weakness. Faulty alignment is more in the frontal lane. Any condition that causes leg length asymmetry can be a predisposition.[6] This can range from a dysfunction of L5 or sacrum or the innominates, etc. Hence a detail examination of the entire alignment of the lower extremity chain is essential.

Sacral torsions and anterior innominates can cause the leg to be longer on one side and it is usually the side of the long leg that is more prone for irritation. The reason being that the hip abductors on the long side are placed in a lengthened position (as weight bearing on a long leg creates a relative adduction on the same side and a pelvic dip on the opposite side) and subsequently an increase in compressive loading on the bursa as the pelvic dip causes the lengthened soft tissue to rub over the greater trochanter. A similar situation can occur when the pelvis dips due to weakness of the gluteus medius (trendelenburg gait).

Iliopsoas Bursitis

This occurs when the tendon of the iliopsoas rubs over the iliopsoas bursa over the iliopectineal eminence. This occurs in situations of an anterior pubis or a posterior rotation of the innominate which brings the iliopectineal eminence closer to the tendon. Repetitive activity can result in friction.

Hip Impingement

This condition is similar to a shoulder impingement that occurs secondary to a narrowing of the subacromial space, however, there is no tendon compromise, but rather a direct impingement of the anterior articular and ligamentous surface. The smooth gliding motion of the round femoral head within the acetabulum socket can be disturbed if there is a block or restriction to the normal hip motion. This can occur if the head of the femur is not entirely round causing jamming. This is known as cam impingement. If the anterior edge of the acetabulum is too prominent, a second type of impingement called pincer impingement occurs. In the presence of capsular tightness,[7] secondary to inadequate internal rotation, the femoral head stays lateral in the acetabulum increasing the risk of impingement.[8] This is further exacerbated if the gluteus medius is weak as this muscle in the absence of capsular tightness facilitates maximal internal rotation.

Soft Tissue Strains

Adductors

The adductors are commonly strained due to sudden stretching as in a slip and fall with the legs apart (on ice) or in sports due to a rapid change in direction where the adductors are used for propulsion. Strain is usually at the musculotendinous junction or at the tendo-osseous junction near the symphysis pubis. The adductors originate from the ischium and pubis and insert into the medial aspect of the femur. Dysfunctions of the innominate or the pubis and faulty alignment of the femoral shaft secondary to rotation as seen in capsular tightening and adductor tightness can alter the length tension of these muscles. With this, sudden movement or overuse can predispose to a strain.

Iliopsoas

The iliopsoas is often prone to tightening as it is a postural muscle. While the length tension is altered due to tightness, a sudden extension of the knee with the hip flexed as in a start for a sprint run can strain this muscle. Innominate dysfunctions as in an anterior rotation can predispose to a shortening. A posterior rotation, however, can predispose to a iliopsoas bursitis, and a tendonitis as the tendon is brought closer to the iliopectineal eminence.[9]

Piriformis

The mode of piriformis dysfunction has been described in the section on sacral dysfunctions. This often mimicks a hip pain due to its close proximity to the posterior aspect of the hip. The most common cause for piriformis dysfunction is secondary to sacral dysfunctions and a tight iliopsoas, as the piriformis muscle works as an abductor in hip flexion.

Nerve Irritation

Obturator

The obturator nerve runs downward from the lumbar spine to supply the adductors and are in close proximity to the iliopectineal eminence. Dysfunctions of the innominate, pubis and the iliopsoas can cause inflammation of the bursa. The nerve can be irritated in the process due the effusion from the inflammatory process and present as anterior hip and thigh pain. Additionally, a tight and dysfunctional pectineus muscle can irritate the nerve.

Sciatic/Superior Gluteal

The mechanism of sciatic pain secondary to a piriformis dysfunction has been described earlier. Another nerve that is in close proximity is the superior gluteal nerve, which passes between the piriformis and the inferior border of the gluteus minimus. A piriformis dysfunction can irritate this nerve as well giving rise to posterior hip or acute gluteal pain.[10]

Lateral Femoral Cutaneous (Meralgia Paresthetica)

The lateral femoral cutaneous nerve passes under the inguinal ligament close to the anterior superior iliac spine (ASIS). Dysfunctional states of the inguinal ligament, which occurs during innominate and pubic dysfunctions may irritate the nerve. The sartorius warrants attention as it may hypothetically contribute to a compression in contracted states owing to its close proximity to the inguinal ligament.

Ilioinguinal

This nerve also passes under the inguinal ligament and can also be stressed by dysfunctional states of the innominate and pubis. Since it passes through the transverse abdominus it can also be compressed by vigorous contraction or a spasm of this muscle. The symptoms are sensory, however, can extend upto the genitalia on that side.

Conventional diagnosis of osteoarthritis hip or hip bursitis or nerve palsy are essentially the end result of altered mechanics and a detail exam of all of the vulnerable structures is essential to rule out the cause.

Mechanical hip pain can be secondary to various factors and the most common are enumerated. Alignment changes of the sacrum has been described to cause dysfunctional states of the piriformis which spans over the posterior aspect of the hip joint. This causes a sensation of deep hip pain. Hyperactivity and dysfunction (including weakness) of the gluteus medius is a common associated feature and an alteration in the efficiency of its contraction can increase the compressive forces on the hip predisposing to wear and tear of the cartilage. If this compressive force is prolonged, then the trochanteric bursa can be irritated resulting in bursitis and hip pain. Piriformis dysfunction can irritate the superior gluteal nerve which passes through the piriformis and gluteus minimus leading to acute gluteal/hip pain. In addition, there is tenderness at the greater sciatic notch.

The innominates house the head of the femur and form the hip joint. Faulty alignment of the innominates can predispose to an alteration of the acetabulum/femoral head congruence leading to increased stress, wear and tear and subsequently pain.

Anteriorly, the innominates can cause a pubic dysfunction leading to anterior hip pain. This includes dysfunctional states of the inguinal ligament further predisposing to anterior hip pain. Pain that is of an osteoarthritic origin usually start as an anterior groin pain and hence a pubic or innominate cause should first be ruled out. The ischial bursa inferiorly and the psoas bursa anteriorly can be irritated due to faulty mechanics of the innominates and the sacrum, leading to ischial and psoas bursitis. Soft tissue strains of the tendons surrounding the hip area are also vulnerable to strain secondary to a mechanical dysfunction.

In all, osteoarthritis per say is secondary to altered congruency, mechanics and stability at the joint. Most of the factors described above can lead to it and hence should be addressed. Pain from a muscle (piriformis) or nerve (gluteal, sciatic) or from a bursa warrants attention as it may still cause hip pain and may be mistook for pain arising from within the joint. From a manual therapy perspective, restriction or altered mechanics at the hip joint may lead to localized stresses at the hip joint and examination will reveal a restriction of TJP (passive gliding) within the joint with an obvious asymmetry. Treatment procedures to improve TJP/alignment, and function is most definitely indicated. Rationally, however, it is important to understand that a restricted hip may cause increased activity in the joints of the pelvis and lumbar spine causing a dysfunction in those areas. Hence the joint play and mobility in the hip should be restored to distribute the stresses to the entire complex. Failing which the cartilage and surrounding soft tissue in the hip joint is predisposed to wear and tear and subsequently pain. In addition, it may lead to lumbopelvic dysfunction. Manual therapy has a significant role in this to restore normal TJP (passive gliding) and subsequently normal mechanics (roll and gliding) and alignment. The soft tissue and muscle integrity in terms of length and strength continually warrants attention.

However, it is pain that brings the patient to the clinic. The pain being in the hip is not necessarily due to restriction at the hip. It may be a restriction in a neighboring joint with faulty alignment/mechanics and irritation of a pain sensitive soft tissue around the hip (muscle, nerve, bursa, etc.). This still warrants effective manual therapy of the neighboring joints and soft tissue with correction of alignment to relieve the symptom and hip pain. Hence, a specific manual therapy diagnosis as to the cause for the hip pain is mandatory as it may involve a dysfunction of neighboring structures.

HIP JOINT SOMATIC DIAGNOSIS

Sacral Torsion

Examination of a sacral torsion is described in Chapter 11. The relationship of torsions to hip dysfunction and pain has been described earlier in the section on mechanism of dysfunction.

Innominate Anterior/Posterior

Examination of an anterior/posterior innominate is described in Chapter 11. The relationship of innominate dysfunctions to hip dysfunction and pain has been described earlier in the section on mechanism of dysfunction.

Superior/Inferior Pubis

Examination of a superior and inferior pubis is described in Chapter 11. The relationship of pubic dysfunctions to hip dysfunction and pain has been described earlier in the section on mechanism of dysfunction.

Femoral Head Posterolateral

The patient is lying prone with both legs internally rotated. The clinician faces the patient from the pelvic area. The clinician places both thumbs on either trochanters and observes for posteriority (Fig. 14.1). A more posterior trochanter may indicate a posterolateral dysfunction. Motion examination may reveal restriction in hip internal rotation and extension.

A posterolateral femoral head may disturb the internal rotation that occurs during the stance phase of gait.[11] This can disturb its medial congruence and increase compressive forces at the hip predisposing to wear and tear.

Hip Abduction Firing Pattern

The patient is in side lying. The inferior leg is flexed to 90° to stabilize the pelvis and the superior pelvis is kept straight. The main participants during hip abduction are the tensor fascia lata which is placed anterolaterally and the gluteus medius is placed posterolaterally.[12]

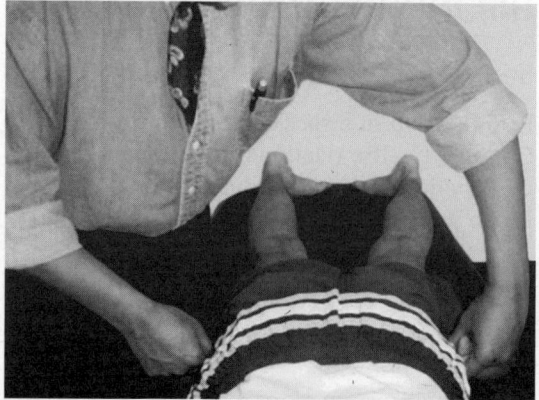

Fig. 14.1: Assessing femoral head posterolateral.

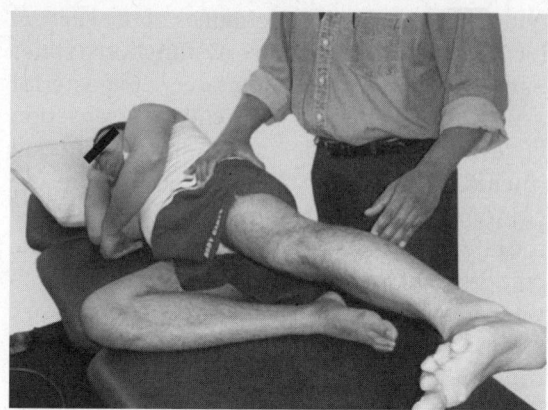

Fig. 14.2: Assessing hip abduction firing pattern.

The hands of the clinician simultaneously palpate both these structures, while the patient is asked to abduct his leg with the hip in slight extension and the knee is in full extension (Fig. 14.2). No flexion should be encouraged as the tensor fascia lata is empowered. Ideally the gluteus medius contracts first followed by the tensor fascia lata. If the reverse occurs there is an evidence of dysfunction and increased compressive forces at the hip and sacroiliac joint on the same side.

TREATMENT FOR SPECIFIC SOMATIC DYSFUNCTION

Femoral Head Posterolateral

This technique is primarily aimed at stretching the posterior capsule, however, the anterior capsule is addressed as well and hence is done in 2 stages.

Stage 1

The patient is lying supine and the clinician faces the leg to be treated. The patient's leg is held at the distal tibiofibular joint just above the ankle. The hip is in slight flexion, adduction, and the knee is fully extended. The clinician then imparts a gentle long axis distraction and internally rotates the hip to stretch the posterior capsule as shown in figure 14.3. This technique is *Strictly Contraindicated* for hip instability and total hip replacements. A regular piriformis stretch

Hip

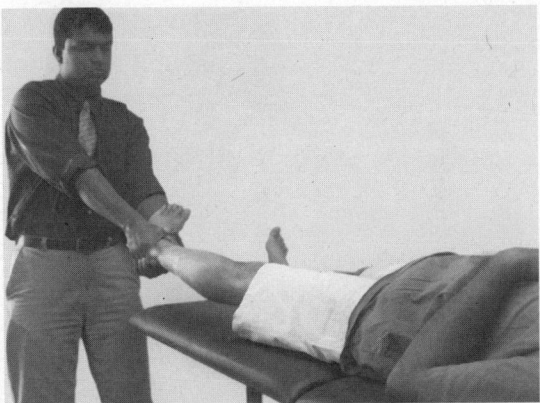

Fig. 14.3: Stage 1 femoral head posterolateral.

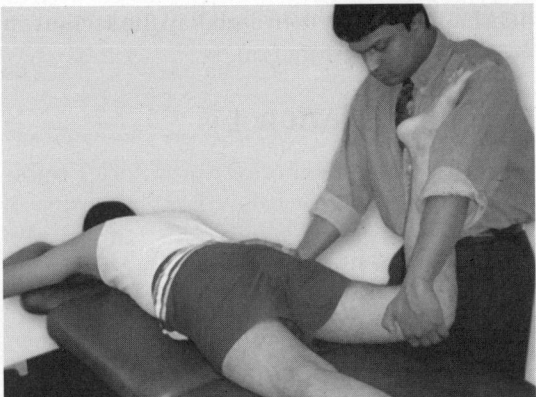

Fig. 14.4: Stage 2 femoral head posterolateral direction.

may assist in stretching the posterior capsule of the hip joint as long as there are no signs of an anterior impingement.

Stage 2

The patient is lying prone and the clinician faces the leg to be treated. One hand of the clinician cups the anterior aspect of the knee, while the forearm supports the lower leg of the patient. The other hand is placed on the posterior aspect of the gluteal area. An inferior pressure is applied to the gluteal area, while the other hand supporting the knee pulls it in a superolateral direction maintaining hip internal rotation (Fig. 14.4). Caution should be exercised depending on the irritability of the hip joint and existing clinical condition (e.g. instability, myositis, total hip replacement, etc.).

Sacral Torsion

Refer to Chapter 11 for a detail description of the treatment of sacral torsions.

Innominate Anterior/Posterior

Refer to Chapter 11 for a detail description of the treatment of innominate dysfunctions.

Pubis Superior/Inferior

Refer to Chapter 11 for a detail description of the treatment of pubic dysfunctions.

Hip Abduction Firing Pattern

This dysfunction will require routine strengthening of the gluteus medius and will be described in the section on prophylaxis.

FOR OVERALL IMPROVEMENT IN RANGE OF MOTION[13,7] (TJP: TRACTION AND PASSIVE GLIDING)

Joint Basics

Type of joint	Diarthrodial or spheroidal
Degrees of freedom	Flexion, extension, abduction, adduction, internal rotation, external rotation.
Range of motion	Flexion: 0–120 Extension: 0–30 Abduction: 0–45 Adduction: 0–30 Internal rotation: 0–45 External rotation: 0–45
Capsular pattern	Limitation of flexion, slight extension, abduction and maximally internal rotation
Loose packed position	30° of flexion and abduction with slight external rotation

Note that the femoral head is almost fully enclosed in the acetabulum and hence a true glide may not occur. The key is the capsular stretching and the distraction that accompanies the gliding technique.

To Improve Flexion

- Distraction
- Posterior glide.

To Improve Extension

- Distraction
- Anterior glide.

To Improve Adduction

- Distraction
- Lateral glide.

To Improve Medial Rotation

- Distraction rotation
- Posterior glide.

To Improve Lateral Rotation

- Distraction
- Anterior glide

TECHNIQUE

Distraction/Distraction in Medial Rotation

Distraction

The patient is lying supine and the clinician faces the leg to be treated. The patient's leg is held at the distal tibiofibular joint just above the ankle. The knee is fully extended and the hip is in slight lateral rotation. The clinician then imparts a gentle long axis distraction. Alternately with distraction maintained, a series of internal rotation stretches are applied in the absence of contraindications in the knee and hip (Fig. 14.5).

Posterior Glide

The patient is lying supine and the clinician faces the leg to be treated from the opposite side. The patient's hip is flexed to 90° and slightly adducted

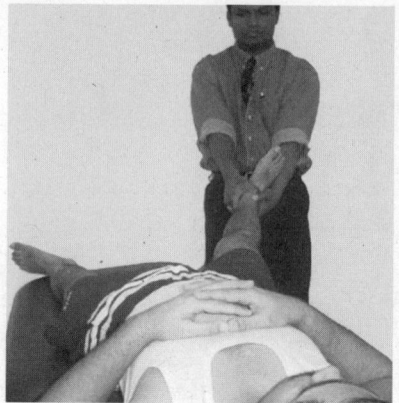

Fig. 14.5: Distraction.

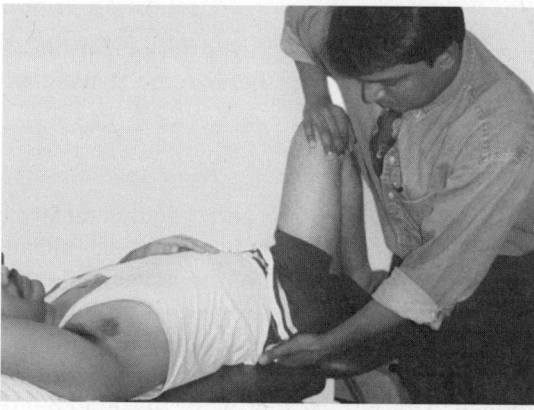

Fig. 14.6: Posterior glide.

and internally rotated. The knee is flexed fully. The clinician places both hands on the anterior knee area and imparts an inferiorly directed mobilization force (Fig. 14.6).

An alternate technique would be to keep the hip and knee in slight flexion and hip internal rotation. The position of the clinician is the same. The clinician supports the lower thigh with one hand. The other hand is placed on the superiolateral thigh area just below the greater trochanter. As the lower thigh is supported, it offers a counter pressure and the upper hand imparts a mobilization force in an inferior direction (Fig. 14.7).

Anterior Glide

The patient is lying prone and the clinician faces the leg to be treated. One hand of the

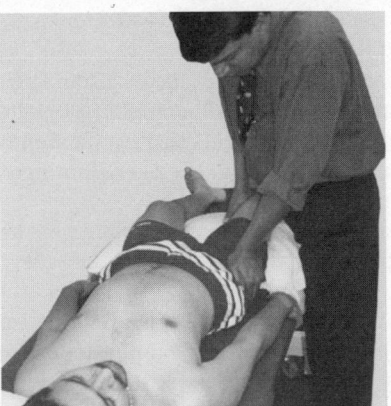

Fig. 14.7: Mobilization force in a inferior direction.

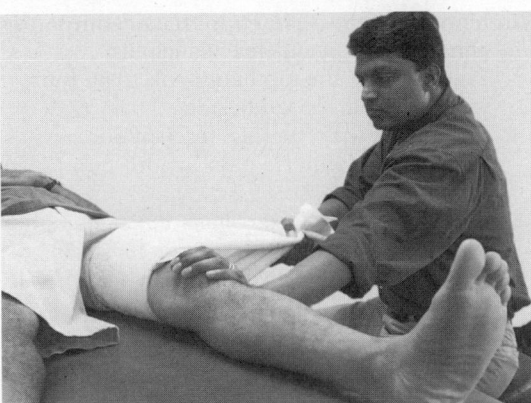

Fig. 14.9: Lateral glide.

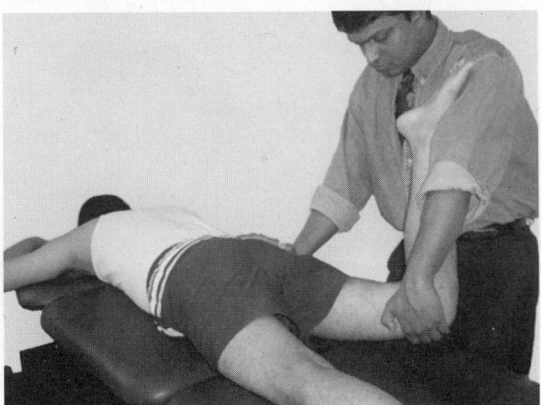

Fig. 14.8: Anterior glide.

clinician cups the anterior aspect of the knee, while the forearm supports the lower leg of the patient. The other hand is placed on the posterior aspect of the gluteal area. An inferior pressure is applied to the gluteal area, while the other hand supporting the knee pulls it superomedial direction (figureshows a slight lateral predisposition) (Fig. 14.8). Since anterior glide of the femoral head is an external rotation of the femur.

Lateral Glide

The patient is lying supine and the clinician faces the leg to be treated, from the opposite side. One hand is placed over the inferior lateral aspect of the femur, while the other hand holds a sheet wrapped around the mid shaft of the femur. A lateral mobilization force is exerted through the hand holding the sheet, while a counter pressure is applied over the inferior lateral thigh area. Alternately, with distraction maintained the patient is asked to internally rotate the thigh, while the clinician assists internal rotation with lateral pressure on the knee (Fig. 14.9).

PROPHYLAXIS

When considering prophylaxis for hip dysfunctions all factors that require stability of the innominates and sacrum should be considered.

The gluteus medius and the maximus requires attention and their importance in dysfunction has been described in the earlier sections. The tendency for anterior hip tightness should be appropriately addressed by stretching the iliopsoas, rectus femoris with the anterior capsule. In addition, flexibility of the posterior capsule with the lateral rotators including the piriformis is recomended. Strict contraindications should be observed especially in cases of the total hip replacement or other pertinent pathologies.

All factors to rule out an ankle, foot and knee dysfunction including prophylaxis should be addressed.

REFERENCES

1. Saidoff DC, McDonough AL. Critical pathways in therapeutic intervention: Extremities and spine, 6th edn, 2002, St. Louis, Mosby.

2. Magee DJ. Orthopedic Physical Assessment, 4th edn, 2002, WB Saunders.Philadelphia.
3. Fagerson TL. The hip handbook,1998, Butterworth-Heinemann Ltd.Boston.
4. Shbeeb MI, Matteson EL. Trochanteric bursitis (greater trochanteric pain syndrome). Mayo Clinic Proc. 1996;71:565-9.
5. Allen WC, Cope R. Coxa Saltans: the snapping hip revisited. J Am Acad Orthop Surg. 1995;3:303-8.
6. Moseley CF. Leg length discrepancy. Orthop Clin North Am. 1987;18:529-35.
7. Kaltenborn F. Mobilization of the extremity joints: Examination and basic treatment techniques, 3rd edn, 1980, Olaf Norlis Bokhandel Universitetsgaten, Oslo, Norway
8. Schaffer JL, Wilson MG, Scott RD. Capsular impingement as a source of pain following bipolar hip arthroplasty. J Arthroplasty. 1991;6:163-8.
9. Gose JC, Schweizer P. Iliotibial band tightness. J Orthop Sports Phys Ther. 1989;10:399-407.
10. Kopell HP,Thompson Wal. Peripheral entrapment neuropathies, 1976, Kreieger Huntington. New York.
11. Staheli LT. Rotational problems of the lower extremities. Orthop Clin North Am. 1987;18:503-12.
12. Donatelli R,Carlin PA,Backer GS et al. Isokinetic hip abductor to adductor torque ratio in normals. Isokinectics Exerc Sci. 1991;1:103-11.
13. Patla CE, Paris SV.EI Course Notes: Extremity Evaluation and manipulation.1996. St. Auguastine, Institute press.

CHAPTER 15

Shoulder

The shoulder joint (glenohumeral) is the primary attachment of the upper limb to the trunk and is often considered in isolation which only renders the treatment outcomes unfavorable. The shoulder joint is technically a complex and requires harmonious interplay of the following:
1. Sternoclavicular joint.
2. Acromioclavicular joint.
3. Glenohumeral joint.
4. Scapulothoracic articulation.
5. Thoracic spine.
6. Cervical spine.

OSSEOUS ANATOMY

The glenohumeral joint is the articulation between the glenoid fossa of the scapula and the head of the humerus. Since the glenoid fossa is much smaller (about one-third) than the head of the humerus it is extended by the glenoid labrum that is attached to the periphery. The joint is surrounded by a loose capsule and is twice as large as the humeral head. It is strengthened by the ligaments and rotator cuff.

The roof of the joint consists of an arch that is formed by the acromion process, bony coracoid and coracoacromial ligament. The space between these structures and the superior aspect of the humeral head is the subacromial space.

The acromioclavicular joint is formed by the articulation of the oval facet on the lateral end of the clavicle and on the oval facet on the acromion process. The joint capsule again is strengthened by ligaments and muscles. The movements of the acromioclavicular joints are strongly influenced by the scapula.[1]

The sternoclavicular joint is formed by the articulation between the medial end of the clavicle and the clavicular notch of the sternum and the adjacent edge of the first costal cartilage. The capsule of this joint is strengthened principally by ligaments. It is a ball and socket joint and essentially moves in opposition to the lateral end of the clavicle (concave/convex). The joint congruence is increased by the presence of a fibrocartilaginous disk.

The scapulothoracic joint is not a true synovial joint as it does not contain a capsule or a synovial tissue. The stability of this joint is important and as it is not a true synovial joint, it is considered a physiologic joint. Its stability is maintained by the atmospheric pressure and by strong muscular attachments. From a functional perspective there is a requirement of stability between scapula and thorax and mobility between scapula and humerus. The stability of the scapula is further enhanced by the acromioclavicular joint and sternoclavicular joint. The acromioclavicular joint is the only true bony joint attachment of the scapula.

LIGAMENTOUS ANATOMY

Sternoclavicular Joint

This joint is strengthened by four ligaments:
1. *Anterior sternoclavicular*: Strengthens the superior aspect of the joint.

2. *Posterior sternoclavicular*: Is weaker and is reinforced by the sternohyoid muscle.
3. *Interclavicular*: Runs between the two clavicles and offers attachment to the two clavicles.
4. *Costoclavicular*: Limits clavicular elevation and strengthens the inferior joint capsule.

Acromioclavicular Joint

This joint consists of the superior and inferior acromioclavicular ligaments that strengthens the capsule. The coracoclavicular ligament runs from the lateral end of the clavicle to the coracoid process. It consists of two parts:
1. The conoid ligament which resists forward movement of the scapula,
2. The trapezoid ligament which is stronger and restricts backward movement of the scapula.

Glenohumeral Joint

- The rotator cuff muscles (supraspinatus, infraspinatus, teres minor and subscapularis) act as active ligaments and blend with the lateral capsule.
- The anterior capsule is strengthened by the three glenohumeral ligaments.
- The coracohumeral ligament with the superior capsule supports the weight of the arm in the anatomical position.
- The transverse humeral ligament that runs from the lesser to the greater tuberosity converts the bicipital groove into an osseo-aponeurotic canal.
- The glenoid and capsular ligament attach to the circumference of the glenoid cavity. The glenoid ligament deepens the cavity for articulation and protects the edges of the bone. The capsular ligament is loose and lax, much larger and longer and allows freedom of motion while maintaining stability.

Scapulothoracic Joint

- The suprascapular ligament runs from the coracoid to the scapular notch. It converts the suprascapular notch into a foramen through which the suprascapular nerve passes. This nerve runs down to the infraspinous area through a ligament that runs between the inferior/lateral aspect of the scapular spine and glenoid called the spinoglenoid ligament.
- The subacromial arch is formed by a ligament along with the acromion and coracoid. This is the coracoacromial ligament and together they form the subacromial arch which is part of the impingement complex. This ligament also completes the vault formed by the coracoid and acromion process for the protection of the head of the humerus.

MUSCULAR ANATOMY

The muscles acting on the shoulder complex are as follows:[2]
- Muscles connecting the spine and trunk to scapula.
- Muscles connecting the spine and trunk to humerus.
- Muscles connecting the scapula to the humerus.

Their functions are described below:

Muscles connecting the spine and trunk to scapula:
- *Trapezius*: The upper fibers adduct, elevate and upwardly rotate the scapula and glenoid. The middle fibers adduct the scapula and glenoid and the lower fibers adduct depress and upwardly rotate the scapula and glenoid.
- *Rhomboids*: They adduct, elevate and downwardly rotates the scapula and glenoid.
- *Levator scapula*: This muscle adducts, elevates and downwardly rotates the scapula and glenoid. Acting unilaterally it rotates and side bends the cervical spine to the same side. Acting bilaterally, it extends the cervical spine.
- *Serratus anterior*: This muscle abducts and upwardly rotates the scapula. It also holds the scapula to prevent it from winging from the rib cage.
- *Pectoralis minor:* This muscle tilts the scapula anteriorly and downwardly rotates the scapula.

Muscles connecting the spine and trunk to humerus:
- *Pectoralis major*: The primary function is to adduct and medially rotate the humerus. The upper fibers flex and horizontally adduct the shoulder. The lower fibers depress the shoulder girdle.
- *Latissimus dorsi*: This versatile muscle medially rotates, adducts, extends and depresses the shoulder. Acting bilaterally, it extends the spine and tilts the pelvis anteriorly.

Muscles connecting the scapula to the humerus:
- *Deltoid*: The anterior fibers flex and medially rotate the shoulder. The middle fibers abduct the shoulder and the posterior fibers extend and laterally rotate the same.
- *Supraspinatus*: This muscle initiates abduction at the shoulder and is one of the primary external rotators of the shoulder. Acting with the deltoid, it helps to contain the head of the humerus into the glenoid cavity during the entire range of motion at the shoulder.
- *Infraspinatus*: Functions to laterally rotate the shoulder and depress the humeral head.
- *Teres minor*: Principally a lateral rotator and its function is synonymous to the infraspinatus.
- *Subscapularis*: This muscle medially rotates and depresses the humeral head.
- *Teres major*: It functions to medially rotate, adduct and extend the shoulder.
- *Biceps brachii*: This muscle flexes the elbow and with the elbow in extension, it assists to flex the shoulder. It is also a powerful supinator of the forearm and assists in adduction of the shoulder with the humerus in external rotation.

The supraspinatus, infraspinatus, teres minor, biceps brachii collectively depress the humeral head and stabilize it in the glenoid fossa.

MECHANICS (NORMAL ROLL-GLIDING)

The mechanics of the shoulder joint is elaborate and are broken down in components for each of the movements occurring in the shoulder. The four components of the shoulder complex require attention (but not limited to the cervico-thoracic spine).

The two primary areas that require attention in terms of mechanics are those laterally placed. Movements of the acromion (scapula) with the lateral end of the clavicle (acromioclavicular joint) and movements of the glenoid (scapula) to the head of the humerus (glenohumeral joint). In both cases the scapula is of importance as it stabilizes the humerus in the appropriate direction. Hence an understanding of the basic scapular mobility is required. The scapula[3] can elevate and depress, abduct and adduct, rotate upward and downward and in addition wing and tip anteriorly. However, the novice clinician may focus attention on two components, rotation and winging. The rotation will technically comprise the other components of the three plane motion as the concepts of diagonal motion would describe. Hence to avoid confusion of the elaborate mechanics of the shoulder described by many texts the basic force couples comprising the rotations are described as they comprise all three planes of motion. In addition, winging and tipping will also be addressed.

Acromioclavicular Joint

The scapula and clavicle move closely with each other and hence when considering mobility in either area either should be addressed. The scapula and clavicle (at the acromioclavicular joint) move in the same direction. Hence, when the scapula elevates the clavicle elevates and vice versa with depression. However, during protraction and retraction of the scapula there is an anterior and posterior movement as well. The orientation of the acromioclavicular joint is such that the arthrokinematic motion either occurs as a combination of anterior inferior and anterior rotation or a posterior superior and posterior rotation. Hence, the component arthrokinematic motion at the acromioclavicular joint is as follows:
- *Flexion*: Posterior, superior glide with posterior rotation.

- *Extension*: Anterior, inferior glide with anterior rotation.
- *Abduction*: Posterior, superior glide with posterior rotation.
- *Adduction*: Anterior, inferior glide with anterior rotation.
- *External rotation*: Posterior, superior glide with posterior rotation.
- *Internal rotation*: Anterior, inferior glide with anterior rotation.

Sternoclavicular Joint

The sternoclavicular joint is considered a ball and socket joint, however, the presence of a disk and the costoclavicular ligament heavily influence the joint mechanics. The concavity of the clavicle is oriented in an anteroposterior direction and hence a ball and socket joint, the movement of the lateral end of the clavicle will cause a movement at the medial end in the opposite direction (although there is much dispute regarding this theory). Hence all component motions described for the acromioclavicular joint will apply for the sternoclavicular joint in the opposite direction excluding rotation. Hence will be as follows:
- *Flexion*: Anterior, inferior glide.
- *Extension*: Posterior, superior glide.
- *Abduction*: Anterior, inferior glide.
- *Adduction*: Posterior, superior glide.
- *External rotation*: Anterior, inferior glide.
- *Internal rotation*: Posterior, superior glide.

Scapulothoracic Joint

The normal scapulohumeral rhythm has been described as being 2:1 of humeral and scapular motion. The rotation that occurs in the scapula is of functional significance and is described as a force couple[4] of interplay between muscles. It is clinically relevant and will be discussed in the next section, however, this motion during humeral elevation needs description.

During humeral elevation, the upper and lower trapezius and the serratus anterior rotate the scapula upwards. The lower fibers of the trapezius provide additional torque and the serratus anterior prevents the scapula from winging. The rotator cuff depresses the humeral head (Fig. 15.1). A pathological situation can occur when this is altered by the tightness in the levator scapula and pectoralis minor and weakness of the rhomboids and lower trapezius. A compromise at the subacromial space may occur leading to pathology.

Glenohumeral Joint

This is the bigger area of focus for manual therapists treating shoulder dysfunction which indeed is of importance provided the other joints of the shoulder complex are addressed. The glenohumeral joint is a concave/convex joint and follows the concave-convex rule. There is evidence of controversy about the relationship of the arthrokinematic motion to the osteokinematic motion. But it is well agreed that no matter the required direction, the need for normal arthrokinematics is obvious. The directions of joint play described are as follows:

Flexion: The head of the humerus glides posterior and inferior and the scapula rotates upward.

Extension: The head of the humerus glides anterior and the scapula rotates downward (retracts).

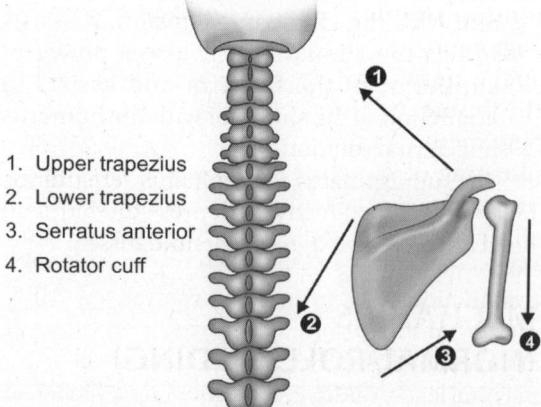

1. Upper trapezius
2. Lower trapezius
3. Serratus anterior
4. Rotator cuff

Fig. 15.1: Normal mechanics on shoulder elevation.

Abduction: The head of the humerus glides inferior and posterior and the humerus rotates externally during midrange for the greater tuberosity to clear the acromion.

External rotation: The head of the humerus glides anterior and the scapula retracts.

Internal rotation: The head of the humerus glides posterior and the scapula protracts.

MECHANISM OF DYSFUNCTION

Mechanical dysfunction of the shoulder is secondary to faulty mechanics including disturbances in muscle length and strength. Importance should be given to scapular mechanics including the humerus and appropriate attention to the acromioclavicular and sternoclavicular joints. In normalcy, the humerus is in a position where one-third of the humerus protrudes in front of the acromion. The antecubital creases face anterior and the olecranon faces posterior. The palms face the body. The scapula is in a position where the vertebral borders are about 2-2 1/2, inches from the spine and flat against the thorax between T2 and T7/8.

Impingement/Rotator Cuff Strains

The most common diagnosis of mechanical pain occurring at the shoulder is an impingement of tendon/s of the rotator cuff in the subacromial space.[5,6] This includes but not limited to the tendon, ligament and the bursa. Normal alignment described above maintains adequate space between acromion and the head of the humerus (subacromial space). Faulty alignment can narrow the space and cause a pinching of structures in this space resulting in impingement, tendinitis and bursitis. The clinician must remember that this is a very elaborate topic. Like all other upper extremity dysfunctions, the primary cause may be faulty muscular mechanics rather than aberrant arthrokinematics. Faulty muscular mechanics may still lead to faulty arthrokinematics, however, its restoration may only correct one component of the dysfunction and a bigger attention to the muscular dynamics may be warranted. Hence further reading is suggested to familiarize this area and to institute an appropriate mechanical diagnosis.[1,7,8]

The basic understanding is that during movement, especially those leading to elevation, the humerus glides posterior, inferior and rotates externally to clear the subacromial space. Medial rotation is adequate and not excessive during flexion. The scapula does not wing during movements and most importantly the scapula rotates upward during humeral elevation. There is adequate and not excessive protraction occurring during shoulder flexion.

When any component of the above described mechanics is disturbed, an alteration occurs in the subacromial space making the structures within this so called 'impingement complex' vulnerable to injury. The clinician is reminded that the above mentioned movement faults does not necessarily occur only with arthrokinematic restriction but also with faulty muscle mechanics secondary to weakness or tightness.

Instability

Faulty mechanics, overuse and restriction in joint play in the shoulder complex may produce compensatory movement by excessive overstretching of the joint capsule, ligaments and soft tissue structures. This can lead to instability. Instability can further lead to pathology including impingement that is secondary to the instability. Instability again is a very elaborate topic and the above theory is only one among the many theories that describe shoulder instability. Hence further reading is suggested in this area.[7, 6, 9]

Common Pathologies Secondary to Mechanical Dysfunction

Faulty Posture (include Bicipital and Rotator Cuff Tendinitis)
Faulty posture may be a predisposition to a compromise at the subacromial space. The origin is secondary to faulty scapular mechanics in

combination with faulty humeral mechanics. As decribed in the earlier section on the scapular force couple, a tightness of the levator scapulae and pectoralis minor with weakness of the rhomboids can predispose to dysfunction. This is commonly seen in people with a forward head posture, who perform long periods of desk work, typing, etc.

Tightness of the levator scapula causes the scapula to rotate downward bringing the acromion closer to the humeral head. In addition, weakness of the rhomboids will protract the scapula with anterior tipping secondary to a tight pectoralis minor. The resulting rounded shoulders will in turn internally rotate the humerus. Hence, here are multiple reasons as to how the subacromial space may be compromised. The supraspinatus tendon is one that is predominantly involved. Description of other causes and structures of the rotator cuff that may be impinged are beyond the scope of this chapter and may require further reading.

The biceps tendon is also a vulnerable structure for impingement and usually occurs secondary to a rotator cuff pathology. The biceps tendon passes between the supraspinatus and subscapularis. Its intimate association with the cuff has extended its partnership to assist in humeral head depression which is one of the important functions of the cuff. The missing downward force of the cuff during dysfunctional states results in a further upward displacement of the humeral head causing an impingement of the coracoacromial arch on the biceps tendon. The other cause for bicipital tendinitis due to humeral internal rotation is a primary bicipital tendinitis and is less common than a secondary bicipital tendinitis that accompanies a rotator cuff pathology.

Subacromial Bursitis

The incidence of this problem secondary to a mechanical dysfunction is the same as mentioned above. Note that the subacromial bursa is the intervening structure between the acromion and supraspinatus and is one the first structures to be compromised.

Snapping Scapula

This is an unusual condition and is seen in following surgery or in females after skeletal maturity. The trapezius, levator scapula and rhomboids are involved and are a source of scapular pain. This is seen during excessive shearing of the scapula which occurs due to restriction at the glenohumeral joint with excessive compensatory motion of the scapula. This over works the above mentioned muscles producing pain and dysfunction.

Acromioclavicular joint degeneration/impingement/strain: All conditions described above are relevant to a forward head and rounded shoulders posture that favors protraction and tipping of the scapula (and in some cases winging), can increase compressive forces in the acromioclavicular joint. The coracoclavicular ligament and the joint capsule are vulnerable to strain. Additional strain factors would be repetitive pushing and also during throwing maneuvers.

Nerve Entrapments

Suprascapular Nerve Impingement

The suprascapular nerve passes through the suprascapular notch to reach the supraspinatus fossa. The nerve is held there by the transverse scapular (suprascapular) ligament. This area may become stenotic or excessive protraction of the scapula as seen in a forward head posture may cause a traction on the nerve. This may result in weakness and pain of the supraspinatus and infraspinatus as it supplies these muscles and mimic a rotator cuff pathology.[12] Sensory changes in the acromioclavicular joint and weakness of the supraspinatus and infraspinatus with tenderness in the suprascapular notch and spinoglenoid area may be indicators of an irritation. This nerve is also vulnerable in people who do excessive overhead activity as in painters, electricians, playing badminton, volleyball, etc.

Axillary Nerve Entrapment (Quadrilateral Space Syndrome)

The axillary nerve can be irritated as it passes through the quadrilateral space formed by the teres major and minor, the triceps and medial humerus. This is seen often with hypertrophy of the teres minor muscle but it can very well occur with scapular dysfunctions namely protraction.

Thoracic Outlet

The pectoralis minor can be contracted in a forward head and rounded shoulders situation and cause protraction and tipping of the scapula. Anteriorly, this can compress the lower trunk of the brachial plexus against the second rib resulting in symptoms.

The sternoclavicular joint forms the lower border of the costoclavicular space. Dysfunctions of the sternoclavicular joint with an elevated first rib can compress the subclavian structures and the lower trunk of the brachial plexus resulting in pathology.

Radial Nerve Entrapment (Triangular Interval Syndrome)

The radial nerve can be irritated as it passes through the triangular interval formed by the teres major and minor, the triceps. This is seen often with hypertrophy of the triceps and teres major muscle but it can very well occur with scapular dysfunctions namely protraction. Prolonged faulty postures of scapular protraction and humeral internal rotation, or punching in the air as seen in martial arts are some causes.

Myogenic Headaches and Cervical Pathology

There is a significant proportion of patients with rotator cuff pathology that experience myogenic headaches. Recall chapters from the section on the cervical spine where dysfunctions of the subcranial spine can be a predisposing cause. Their relationship to a shoulder pathology is with the scapula. The scapula offers attachment to the levator scapulae and the trapezius which have origins in the subcranial spine and the occipital protuberance, respectively. Altered scapula mechanics can affect the length tension of these muscles which may cause a traction in the subcranial area owing to their attachment and trigger a myogenic headache.

SHOULDER JOINT SOMATIC DIAGNOSIS

Mechanical diagnosis at the shoulder is classified under the following categories:
- Arthrokinematic
- Soft tissue related

Although these categories are closely related, they are described separately owing to the strong muscular influence on the mechanics of the shoulder. Essentially, both tend to cause the same dysfunction but the cause may be arthrokinematic or soft tissue related, or a combination of both. They are found in the scapula and humerus.[2]

Humerus

Anteromedial (Arthrokinematic)

This dysfunction is characterized by a relative anterior migration of the humeral head with a medial rotation. These two directions may be complementary due to the protraction nature of the scapula.

The patient is seated and the clinician faces the patient from the back and above (superior view). The clinician then observes, palpates and firmly holds the head of the humerus. The other hand palpates the acromion and the spine of scapula. Once all landmarks are firmly held, the distance between the head of the humerus and the acromion is palpated or observed (Fig. 15.2). No more than one-third of the head of the humerus should protrude in front of the acromion. If more than one-third of the head of the humerus protrudes in front of the acromion, it is an anterior dysfunction of the head of the humerus. This is further enhanced by a decrease in posterior glide of the humeral head. Comparison is made with the other side.

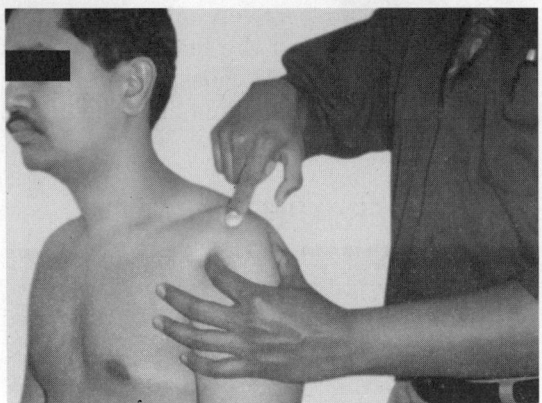

Fig. 15.2: Assesing humeral head position.

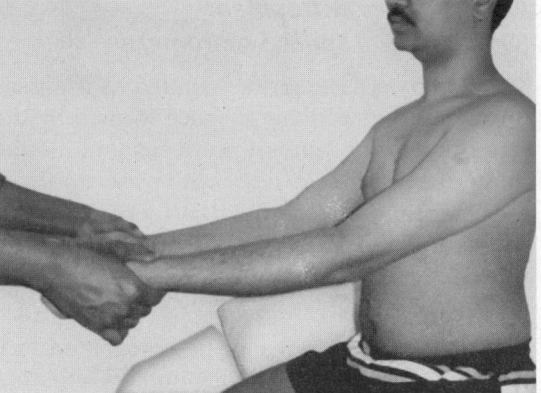

Fig. 15.3: Assessing humeral rotation.

In the next step the patient is seated and the clinician faces the patient. The hand of the clinician grips the patients wrist and the patients elbow is extended. The humerus is then rotated externally with a supination movement of the clinicians upper extremity (Fig. 15.3). The clinician senses for restriction and if present, denotes a medial rotation dysfunction of the humerus. Comparison is made with the other side.

Anteromedial (Soft Tissue)

In this dysfunction, there tends to be an excessive anterior motion of the head of the humerus into the anterior joint capsule. Two possible causes can lead to this dysfunction and should be examined which are as follows:
1. Weakness or lengthened subscapularis and teres major.
2. Tightness of the short scapulohumeral lateral rotators.

Anterior dysfunctions of the humerus may be suggestive of and predispose to instability. There is also a possibility of excessive stress on the biceps tendon in this dysfunction.

The next hallmark of this dysfunction is that there is insufficient lateral rotation of the humerus. The possible dynamic causes to this dysfunction are tightness of the axiohumeral medial rotators namely pectoralis major and the latissimus dorsi.

A medial rotation dysfunction of the humerus can delay external rotation of the humerus during abduction resulting in an impingement and a painful arc on abduction. It can also lead to anterior impingement of the subscapularis and biceps and stress on the transverse humeral ligament. It favors tightness of the pectoralis minor and predispose to a thoracic outlet (hyperabduction syndrome) and possible anterior tipping of the scapula with further impingement. Restricted or lack of adequate external rotation may also predispose to instability.

Superior (Arthrokinematic)

The patient is lying supine and the clinician faces the shoulder to be examined. One hand with metacarpal of the index finger blocks the infraglenoid tubercle of the scapula. The other hand grasps the lower condyles of the humerus and imparts an inferior glide and senses for restriction (Fig. 15.4). A decrease in the inferior glide denotes a superior dysfunction.

Comparison is made with the other side.

Superior (Soft Tissue)

In this dysfunction, there is excessive superior movement of the head of the humerus against the acromion. The possible causes are:
- Weakness of the supraspinatus, infraspinatus, teres minor and subscapularis (rotator cuff).
- Weakness of the biceps brachii.

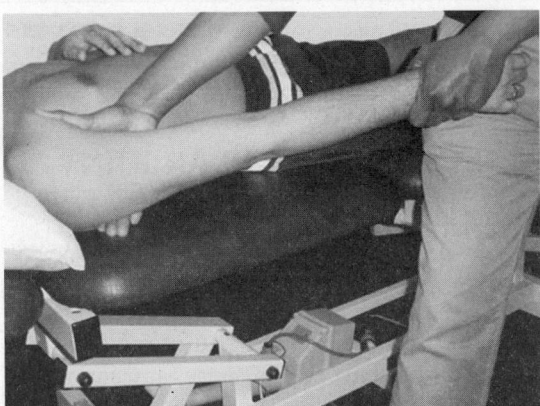

Fig. 15.4: Assessing superior dysfunction of the humerus.

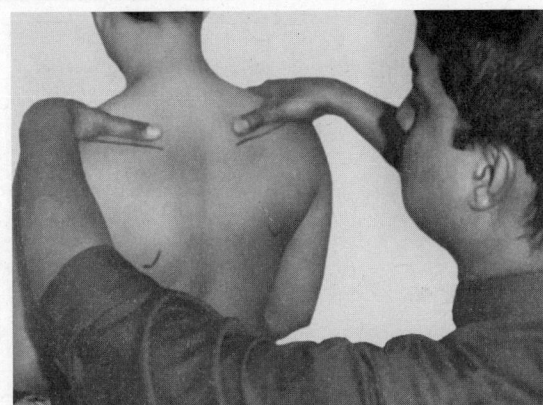

Fig. 15.5: Assessing scapular downward rotation.

A superior dysfunction of the humerus may compromise the subacromial space and predispose to impingement, rotator cuff tendonitis and subacromial bursitis. The biceps tendon can also be predisposed to a secondary impingement.

Scapula

Winging (Soft Tissue)

This can be of two types. Winging can occur due to weakness of the serratus anterior and is obvious on shoulder flexion and a push up. However, winging can also occur during return from flexion back to midline. This obviously is not due to weakness of the serratus but due to a timing problem. The possible cause is that the scapulohumeral muscles do not relax as rapidly as the axioscapular muscles. Additionally, the scapulohumeral muscles are stronger than the axioscapular muscles.

Scapular winging can compromise the subacromial space and also predispose to compression at the acromioclavicular joint.

Adducted/Downward Rotation (Arthrokinematic)

The patient is seated and the clinician faces the patient from behind. The clinician locates the spines of the scapula bilaterally and then places both thumbs in line with the superior border of the spine of the scapula (Fig. 15.5). The angles of both thumb placements are observed. If one thumb appears relatively more horizontal than the other then that scapula is considered to be in downward rotation.

In this dysfunction, the scapula rotates downward during the initial phase of shoulder abduction instead of the normal upward rotation after the initial setting phase.

The possible causes for this dysfunction are:
- Tightness of levator scapulae.
- Insufficient activity of the lower trapezius.

Again, during the last phases of humeral elevation, the scapula fails to rotate upward.

The causes for this dysfunction are as above but also due to tightness of the pectoralis minor.

A downward rotation of the scapula can compromise the subacromial space predisposing to impingement. If the cause is due to as tightness of the pectoralis minor, then dysfunction is due to tight pectoralis minor, as described in the earlier section, can occur. A dysfunction of the levator scapula and the upper fibers of the trapezius can predispose to myogenic headaches.

Abducted/Protraction (Arthrokinematic)

The patient is lying prone in an anatomical position, hence will be lying with his palms facing down, cubital fossa facing anterior and

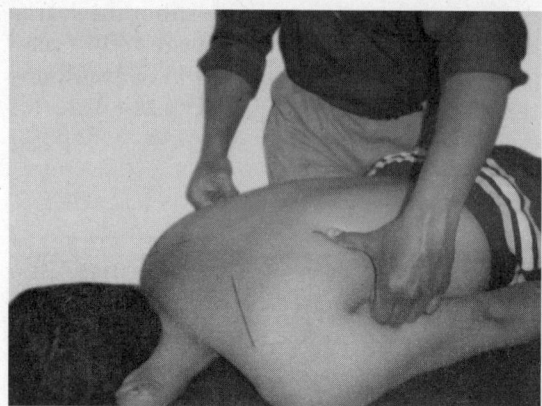

Fig. 15.6: Assessing scapular protraction.

the olecranon facing posterior. The clinician uses the palm of his hands to locate the inferior angles and then places both thumbs on them to mark their location. Their distance from the midline (spinous process of T7,8 is observed). Next the spines of the scapula are located and their medial borders are palpated. The clinician observes for their distance from the midline. If both, the spine and the inferior angle of the scapula is further from the midline on one side, then that scapula is considered to be protracted (Fig. 15.6).

Abducted/Protraction (Soft Tissue)

In this dysfunction, the scapula protracts excessively during shoulder flexion. The possible causes for this dysfunction are:
- Tightness of the pectoralis minor, pectoralis major and serratus anterior.
- Weakness of the scapular retractors.

A protracted scapula predisposes to a forward head posture and rounded shoulders. This primarily compromises the subacromial space causing impingement and also increases compression at the acromioclavicular joint. It can also predispose to irritability of the rhomboids and by virtue of their attachment to the thoracic spine, cause thoracic dysfunctions. Protraction can also cause tightness of the pectoralis minor causing a compromise of the thoracic outlet. A protracted scapula can also cause traction on the suprascapular nerve causing symptoms. It can also compromise the quadrilateral space and triangular interval causing an irritation of the axillary and radial nerves, respectively.

ACROMIOCLAVICULAR JOINT

Anterior Superior Dysfunction

The patient is lying supine and the clinician faces the patient from the side of the shoulder that is being examined. One hand of the clinician supports the head of the humerus and acromion, while the other hand grips the subcutaneous lateral border of the clavicle. The clavicle is then glided upwards and posterior and downwards and anterior as the clinician senses for restriction (Fig. 15.7). A decrease in the superior posterior glide will denote an anterior inferior dysfunction of the acromioclavicular joint. Comparison is made with the other side.

The causes for pain and dysfunction in the acromioclavicular joint are either due to direct injury or due to dysfunctions of the scapula (winging, protraction, tipping). They are commonly sprains or eventually degeneration. But it would be of worth to remember that the vulnerability of these joints may increase if faulty mechanics persists. It may also be important to know that in many situations this joint may be hypermobile which may call for correcting hypomobility in the other joints within the complex.

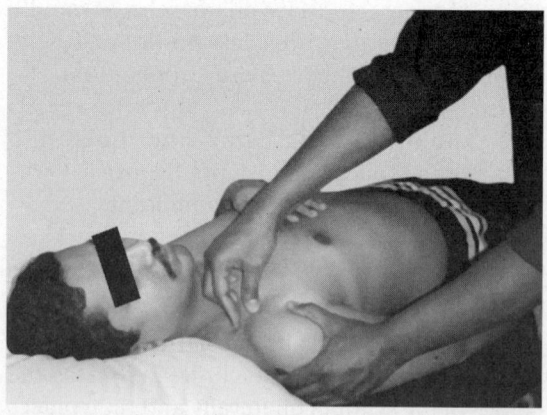

Fig. 15.7: Assessing acromioclavicular mobility.

STERNOCLAVICULAR JOINT

Superior Posterior Dysfunction

The patient is lying supine and the clinician faces the patient from the head side. The thumbs of the clinician are placed on the superior part of the medial border of the clavicle immediately next to the clavicular fossa. The clinician should note for asymmetry as in the landmark being slightly superior in comparison to the opposite side. This would denote a superior posterior dysfunction (Fig. 15.8).

Mechanical dysfunctions of the sternoclavicular joint are relatively rare. The one implication is that it forms a boundary of the costoclavicular space with the first rib. Hence it may compromise the outlet. This is, however, rare and more often occurs secondary to an elevated first rib. A superior dysfunction is often seen and if persistent can affect acromioclavicular mechanics and subsequently the overall mechanics of the complex. Hence, it warrants attention and appropriate intervention.

SUBCRANIAL SPINE/ MIDCERVICAL SPINE

Routine examination of the subcranial and midcervical spine for mechanical dysfunction is advocated. Owing to their influence on the scapula, they can significantly affect shoulder mechanics and lead to pathology. Hence, correction of mechanical dysfunctions of the cervical area especially subcranial area is warranted. The reader is suggested to refer Chapter 8 for a detail description of examining the subcranial and midcervical spine for mechanical dysfunction.

FIRST RIB ELEVATED

An elevated first rib can compromise the costoclavicular space leading to symptoms of a thoracic outlet. The reader is suggested to refer Chapter 9 for a detail description on examination of the first rib.

THORACIC SPINE

Mechanical dysfunction of the thoracic spine can also influence mechanics of the scapula. Mechanical dysfunctions of the thoracic spine especially T2 through T7, 8 is important due to their more intricate relationship to the scapula. The reader is suggested to refer Chapter 9 for a detail description of examining the thoracic spine for mechanical dysfunction.

TREATMENT FOR SPECIFIC SOMATIC DYSFUNCTION

Humerus Anterior and Medially Rotated

The patient is lying supine with the arm slightly abducted and rotated internally. The clinician stands by the side of the shoulder to be treated. One hand of the clinician is placed under the scapula and the fingers support and stabilize the spine of the scapula. The proximal thenar and hypothenar eminence of the other hand is placed on the humeral head and upper shaft. As the spine of the scapula stabilized from below, the other hand gently imparts a glide in the posterior direction (the direction is inferior as the patient is lying supine) (Fig. 15.9).

In the next step, the clinician blocks the infraglenoid tubercle of the scapula with one hand and grips the lower end of the humerus with the other. The clinician then glides the humerus in the inferior direction so as to first

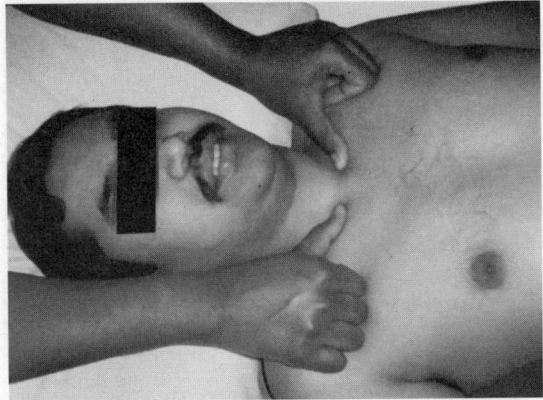

Fig. 15.8: Assessing sternoclavicular mobility.

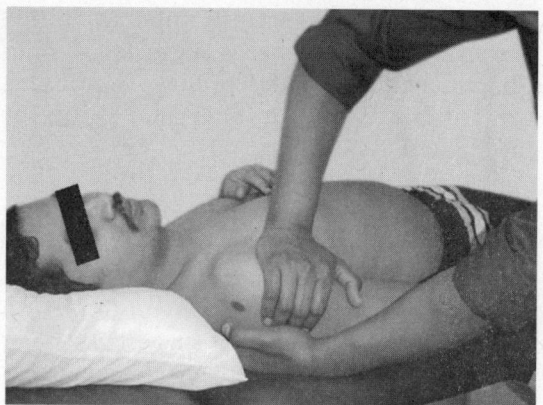

Fig. 15.9: Posterior glide of humerus.

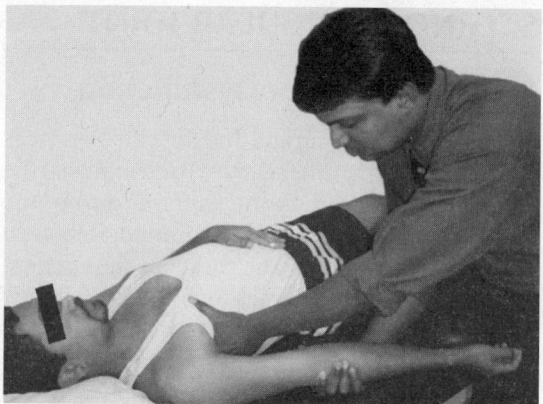

Fig. 15.10: Humerus external rotation.

distract the joint. The humerus is then extended to stretch the anterior capsule and then rotated externally by a pronation motion of the clinicians hand (Fig. 15.10). They are repeated about five to six times in a slow sustained fashion.

This is followed up by strengthening the subscapularis and external rotators.

Humerus Superior

The treatment technique is the same as for the somatic diagnosis. To sustain the effect the glides are imparted about five to six times in a slow and sustained fashion. It is followed up by strengthening the rotator cuff and biceps brachii.

Scapula Downward Rotated

The patient is in side lying and the clinician stands facing the patient. One hand of the clinician is placed on the spine of the scapula. The other hand is brought under the humerus and the fingers are placed on the inferior and medial border of the scapula. The patients trunk is brought closer to the abdomen of the clinician to stabilize (a pillow may be used in between). Stabilizing the spine of the scapula in an inferior direction, the inferior medial border of the scapula is slightly distracted and directed in a superior direction to rotate the scapula upward and outward (Fig. 15.11). The procedure is followed up by strengthening exercises for the lower trapezius.

Protracted

The patient is lying prone. The thumbs of the clinician stabilize the spine of the scapula and hook on to the superior medial border of the scapula. The other fingers of both hands are taken over the scapula and hooked on the lateral border of the scapula. The clinician then imparts an upward and inward stretch over the lateral border of the scapula (Fig. 15.12).

Winged

This is more of a dynamic dysfunction rather than a structural dysfunction and the strength of the relevant musculature need to be addressed. Prolonged dysfunctional states can also cause tightness of the muscles on the lateral border of the scapula and hence the technique for a

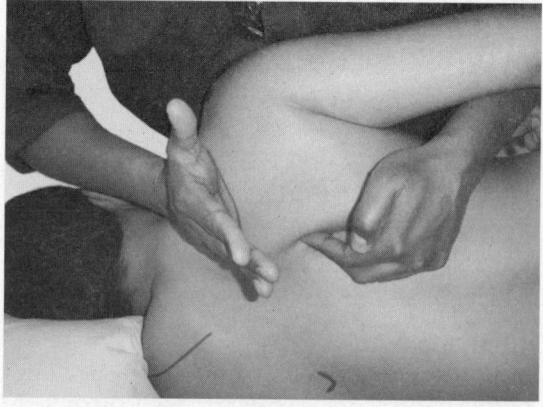

Fig. 15.11: Scapula upward rotation.

Shoulder

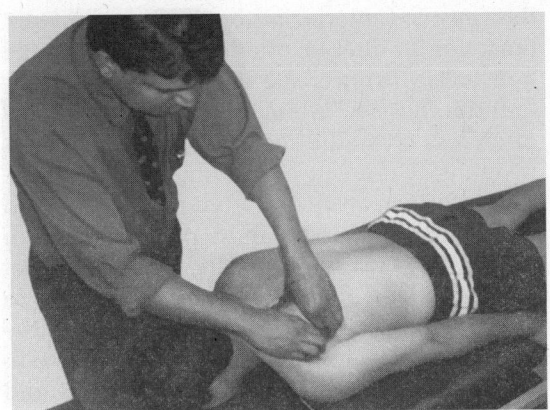

Fig. 15.12: Scapula retraction.

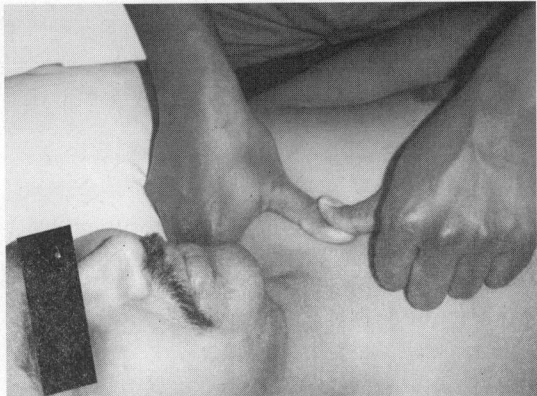

Fig. 15.14: Superior and posterior glide of sternoclavicular joint.

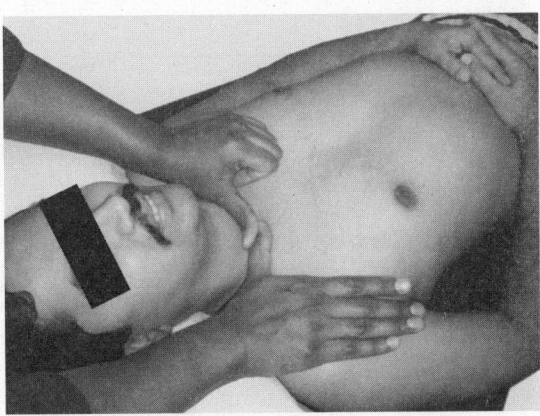

Fig. 15.13: Inferior anterior glide of sternoclavicular joint.

protracted scapula can be used to mobilize the structures in the lateral border. This is followed by strengthening of the serratus anterior.

Acromioclavicular Inferior Anterior

The technique is the same as for a somatic diagnosis, except that the focus in a posterior superior direction. The clinician should be aware of a hypermobile situation and if so vigorous mobilization should be avoided.

Sternoclavicular Superior Posterior

The patient is lying supine and the clinician faces the patient from the head side. The thumb of one hand is placed on the superomedial end of the clavicle. The thumb of the other hand reinforces this thumb. The clinician imparts an inferiorly directed force to mobilize the joint in an inferior and anterior direction. The reverse is done for a inferior anterior dysfunction except the mobilizing force from the other hand is from the hypothenar eminence rather than the thumb (Figs. 15.13 and 15.14).

FOR OVERALL IMPROVEMENT IN RANGE OF MOTION[10,11]
(TJP: TRACTION AND PASSIVE GLIDING)

Joint Basics

Type of joint	Ball and socket, diarthrosis, spheroidal
Degrees of freedom	Flexion, extension, abduction, adduction, internal rotation, external rotation
Range of motion	Flexion–180°, extension–60°, abduction–180°, internal rotation–110°, external rotation–90°
Capsular pattern	External rotation, more than abduction more than internal rotation
Loose packed position	60° of abduction and 30° of horizontal adduction

To Improve Flexion

- Scapula distraction
- Scapula upward rotation
- Acromioclavicular superior posterior glide
- Sternoclavicular inferior anterior glide
- Glenohumeral distraction

- Glenohumeral posterior glide
- Glenohumeral inferior glide.

To Improve Extension

- Scapula distraction
- Scapula downward rotation
- Acromioclavicular inferior anterior glide
- Sternoclavicular superior posterior glide
- Glenohumeral distraction
- Glenohumeral anterior glide.

To Improve Abduction

- Scapula distraction
- Scapula upward rotation
- Acromioclavicular superior posterior glide
- Sternoclavicular inferior anterior glide
- Glenohumeral distraction external rotation
- Glenohumeral anterior glide
- Glenohumeral inferior glide.

To Improve Scaption

- Scapula distraction
- Scapula upward rotation
- Acromioclavicular superior posterior glide
- Sternoclavicular inferior anterior glide
- Glenohumeral distraction
- Glenohumeral inferior glide.

To Improve External Rotation

- Scapula distraction
- Acromioclavicular superior posterior glide
- Sternoclavicular inferior anterior glide
- Glenohumeral distraction external rotation
- Glenohumeral anterior glide.

To Improve Internal Rotation

- Scapula distraction
- Scapula upward rotation
- Acromioclavicular inferior anterior glide
- Sternoclavicular superior posterior glide
- Glenohumeral distraction
- Glenohumeral posterior glide.

All techniques are initiated by heating the capsule and followed up by active stretching of the capsule (anterior for external rotation and posterior for internal rotation). Caution should be exercises to not create an instability especially anterior. Passive osteokinematic stretching is often less favorable secondary to the obvious involuntary protective guarding that is evident. The inferior capsule is often most neglected in a tight shoulder. It can be palpated deep in the axilla as it runs from the superior aspect of the humerus to the infraglenoid tubercle. In the supine position, the arm is abducted to the available range and deep pressure is applied to the posterior superior aspect of the axilla and gentle frictions are applied in the transverse direction (Fig. 15.15).

TECHNIQUE

Scapula Distraction

The patient is in side lying and the clinician stands facing the patient. One hand of the clinician is placed on the spine of the scapula. The other hand is brought under the humerus and the fingers are placed on the inferior and medial border of the scapula. The patients trunk is brought closer to the abdomen of the clinician to stabilize (a pillow may be used in between). The clinician now retracts the shoulder by an anteriorly directed stabilizing force at the abdomen and using the fingers on the medial border of the scapula, gently distracts the scapula from the thoracic cage (Fig. 15.16).

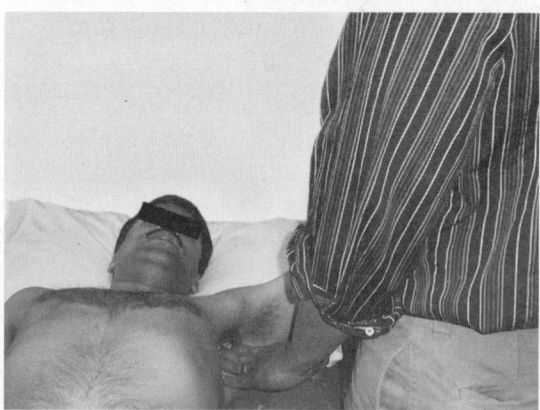

Fig. 15.15: Soft tissue mobilization of the inferior capsule.

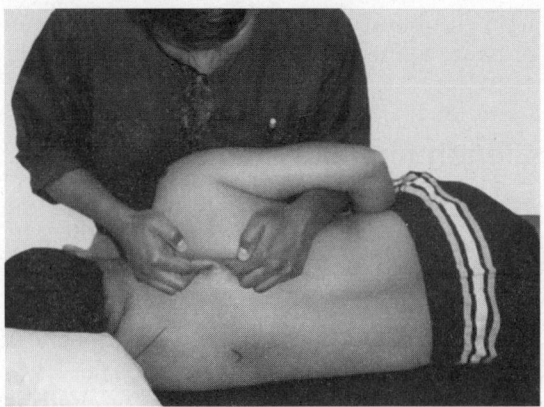

Fig. 15.16: Scapula distraction.

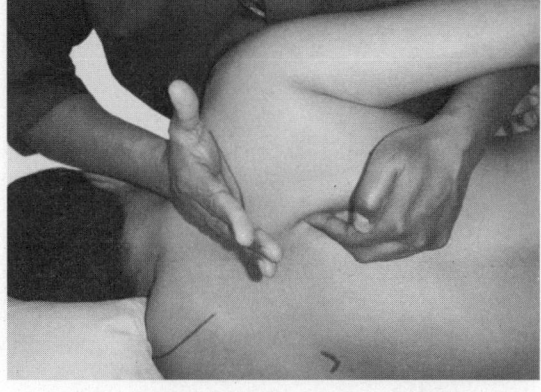

Fig. 15.17: Scapula upward rotation.

Scapula Upward Rotation

The patient is in side lying and the clinician stands facing the patient. One hand of the clinician is placed on the spine of the scapula. The other hand is brought under the humerus and the fingers are placed on the inferior and medial border of the scapula. The patients trunk is brought closer to the abdomen of the clinician to stabilize (a pillow may be used in between). Stabilizing the spine of the scapula in an inferior direction, the inferior medial border of the scapula is slightly distracted and directed in a superior direction to rotate the scapula upward and outward (Fig. 15.17).

Acromioclavicular Superior and Posterior Glide/Inferior and Anterior Glide

The patient is lying supine and the clinician faces the patient from the side of the shoulder that is being examined. One hand of the clinician supports the head of the humerus and acromion, while the other hand grips the subcutaneous lateral border of the clavicle. A glide is imparted in the superior posterior and inferior anterior directions respectively (Fig. 15.18). Note that this is often an area of instability or excessive motion and hence, the clinician is cautioned of encouraging hypermobility.

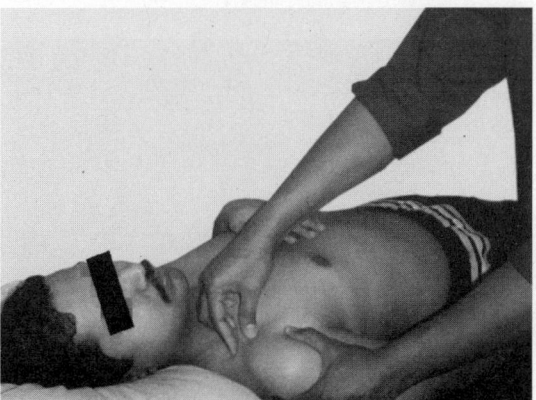

Fig. 15.18: Acromioclavicular superior and posterior and inferior and anterior glide.

Sternoclavicular Inferior and Anterior Glide

The patient is lying supine and the clinician faces the patient from the head side. The thumb of one hand is placed on the superomedial border of the clavicle. The thumb of the other hand reinforces this thumb. The clinician imparts an inferiorly directed force to mobilize the joint in an inferior and anterior direction (Fig. 15.19).

Sternoclavicular Posterior and Superior Glide

The patient is lying supine and the clinician faces the patient from the head side. The thumb of one

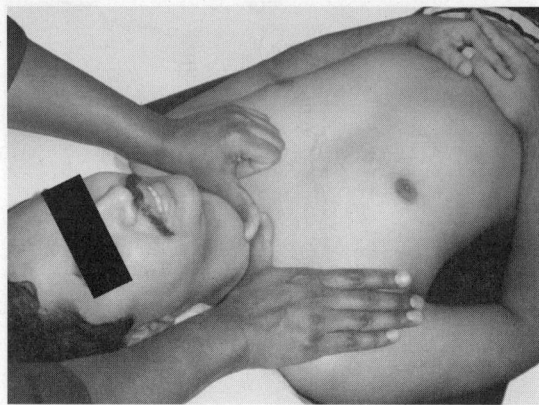

Fig. 15.19: Sternoclavicular inferior and anterior glide.

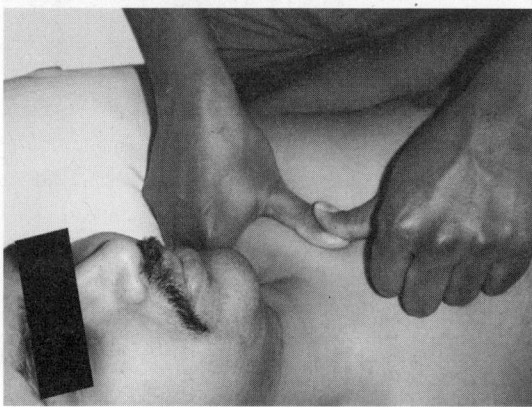

Fig. 15.20: Sternoclavicular superior and posterior glide.

hand is placed on the inferior medial border of the clavicle. The hypothenar eminence of the other hand reinforces this thumb. The clinician imparts a superiorly directed force to mobilize the joint in a superior and posterior direction (Fig. 15.20).

Glenohumeral Distraction

The patient is lying supine and the clinician faces the patient from the side of the shoulder to be treated. One hand of the clinician is placed under the axilla with the palm firmly gripping the superior portion of the humerus. The other hand stabilizes the inferior and lateral portion of the elbow joint. A gentle distraction is now applied with the hand under the axilla and counter pressure at the lateral aspect of the elbow (Fig. 15.21).

Glenohumeral Distraction and External Rotation

The patient is lying supine with the arm slightly abducted and rotated internally. The clinician stands by the side of the shoulder to be treated. The clinician blocks the infraglenoid tubercle of the scapula with one hand and grips the lower end of the humerus with the other. The clinician then glides the humerus in the inferior direction so as to first distract the joint. The humerus is then extended to stretch the anterior capsule and then rotated externally by a pronation motion of the clinician's hand (Fig. 15.22).

Glenohumeral posterior glide: The patient is lying supine with the arm slightly abducted and rotated internally. The clinician stands by the side of the shoulder to be treated. One hand of the clinician is placed under the scapula and the fingers support and stabilize the spine of the scapula. The proximal thenar and hypothenar eminence of the other hand is placed on the humeral head and upper shaft. As the spine of the scapula stabilized from below, the other hand gently imparts a glide in the posterior direction (the direction is inferior as the patient is lying supine) (Fig. 15.23).

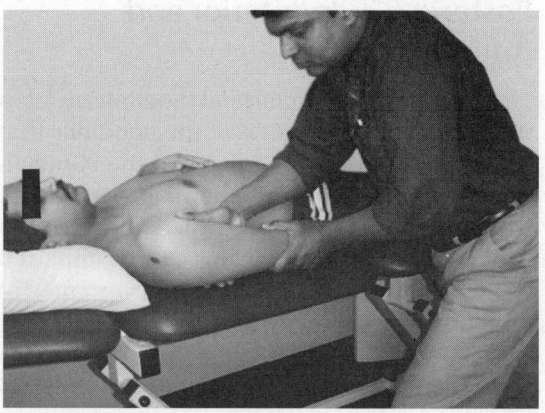

Fig. 15.21: Glenohumeral distraction.

Shoulder

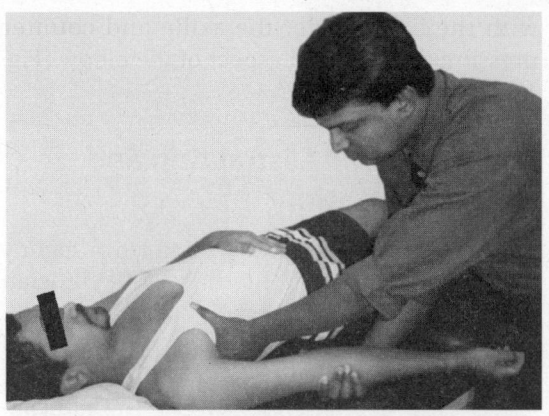

Fig. 15.22: Glenohumeral distraction and external rotation.

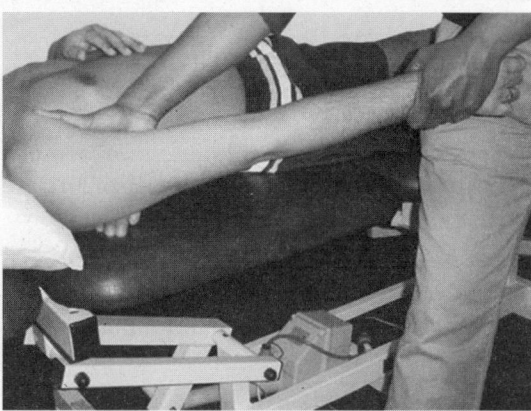

Fig. 15.24: Glenohumeral inferior glide.

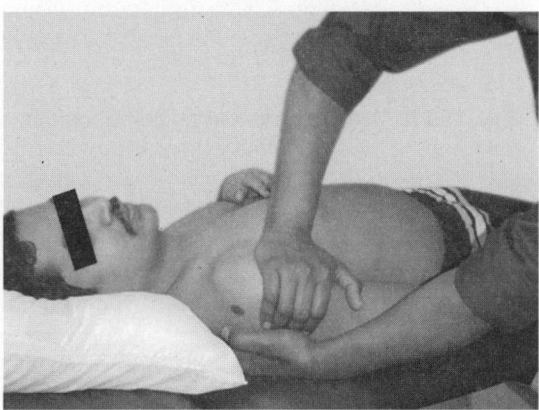

Fig. 15.23: Glenohumeral posterior glide.

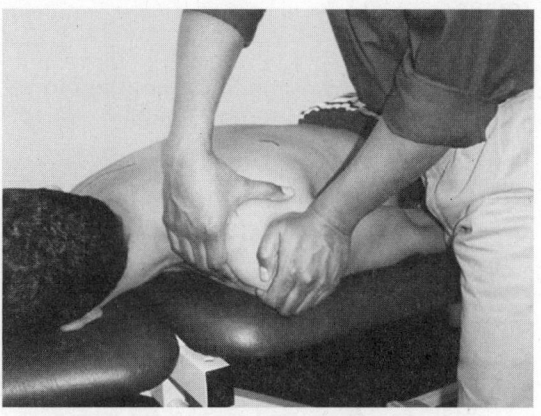

Fig. 15.25: Glenohumeral anterior glide.

Glenohumeral inferior glide: The patient is lying supine and the clinician faces the shoulder to be examined. One hand with metacarpal of the index finger blocks the infraglenoid tubercle of the scapula. The other hand grasps the lower condyles of the humerus. While the hand under the infraglenoid tubercle offers counter pressure, the hand grasping the lower condyles of the humerus gently imparts an inferior glide (Fig. 15.24).

Glenohumeral anterior glide: The patient is lying prone with the arm by the side and the palm facing downward. A folded towel can be placed on the anterior aspect of the shoulder just medial to the joint line. The clinician stands by the side of the shoulder to be treated. One hand of the clinician is placed over the spine of the scapula and the fingers encircle and support the shoulder girdle. The proximal thenar eminence of the other hand is placed on the posterior aspect of the humeral head and upper shaft. As the spine of the scapula and the shoulder girdle are stabilized, the other hand gently imparts a glide in the anterior direction (the direction is inferior as the patient is lying prone) (Fig. 15.25).

All mobilization procedures are followed by osteokinematic movement. One should understand passive stretching of osteokinematic motion often causes an inability of the patient to relax. The clinician is advised to incorporate a more active approach.

PROPHYLAXIS

Exercise prescription of the shoulder is very dysfunction specific. As the clinician may peruse the described dynamic components of somatic diagnosis of the shoulder the appropriate exercise therapy is obvious. They are as follows:

Anterior and medial rotation of humerus: Stretch or strengthen as appropriate the subscapularis and teres major. Stretch scapulohumeral lateral rotators. Stretch latissimus dorsi and pectoralis major.

Superior humerus: Strengthen rotator cuff and biceps brachii.

Winged scapula: Strengthen serratus anterior and lower trapezius.

Downward rotated scapula: Strengthen lower trapezius and stretch levator scapulae.

Protracted scapula: Strengthen scapula retractors namely lower trapezius and rhomboids and stretch pectoralis major, pectoralis minor and teres major.

Additional muscles that require attention are the scalenes, subclavius. They are frequently tight and increase overall vulnerability to dysfunction. The cervicothoracic component also warrants attention. However, for overall stability of the shoulder complex the rotator cuff muscles and the lower trapezius warrant attention. Also, always consider contraindications before exercise prescription.

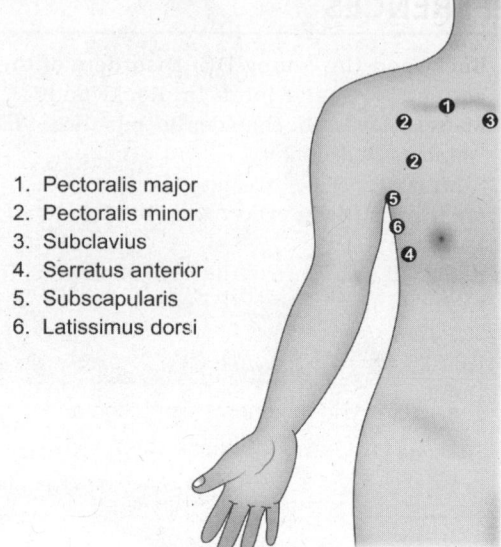

1. Pectoralis major
2. Pectoralis minor
3. Subclavius
4. Serratus anterior
5. Subscapularis
6. Latissimus dorsi

Fig. 15.26: Myofascial tender points: Shoulder (anterior).

MYOFASCIAL TENDER POINTS

The concept of addressing myofascial tender points is to decrease actin and myosin cross-bridging and myofibrillar restriction. Their continual presence may encourage chemical accumulation, early fatigue and decreased muscle performance with accompanying pain and dysfunction. They may be best treated with frictions and electrotherapy. Tender points secondary to aberrant gamma efferents may require an alternate positional release approach and the reader is encouraged further reading in the area of 'strain counterstrain' methods. The figures Figs. 15.26 and 15.27 illustrate some common dysfunctional points of the shoulder.

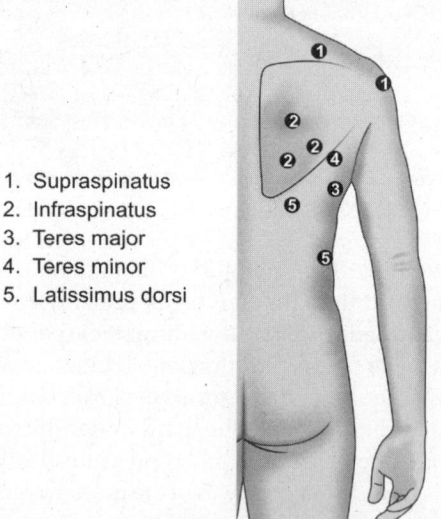

1. Supraspinatus
2. Infraspinatus
3. Teres major
4. Teres minor
5. Latissimus dorsi

Fig. 15.27: Myofascial tender points: Shoulder (posterior).

REFERENCES

1. Rockwood CA, Young DC. Disorders of the acromioclavicular joint. In: Rockwood CA, Matsen FA, eds. The shoulder. 3rd edn. 1990, WB Saunders, Philadephia.
2. Sahrmann S. Diagnosis and treatment of movement impairment syndromes, 2002, St Louis, Mosby
3. Kibler WB. The role of the scapula in athletic shoulder function. Am J Sports Med. 1998;26: 325-37.
4. Palastanga N, Field D, Soames R. Anatomy and Human Movement, 1989, Heinemann medical publishers, Oxford.
5. Hawkins RJ, Hobeika PE. Impingement syndrome in the athletic shoulder. Clin Sports Med. 1983;2: 391-405.
6. Stroh S. Shoulder impingement. J Manual and Manipulative Ther. 1995;3:59-64.
7. Donatelli RA. Physical Therapy of the Shoulder. 1996. Churchill Livingstone, New York.
8. Tovin BJ, Greenfield BH. Evaluation and treatment of the shoulder: an intergration of the guide to physical therapist practice, 2001, FA Davis Company, Philadelphia..
9. Magee DJ. Orthopedic Physical Assessment, 4th edn, 2002. WB Saunders, Philadelphia.
10. Patla CE, Paris SV. EI Course Notes: Extremity Evaluation and manipulation.1996. St. Auguatine, Institute press.
11. Kaltenborn F. Mobilization of the extremity joints: Examination and basic treatment techniques, 3rd edn, 1980, Olaf Norlis Bokhandel Universitetsgaten, Oslo, Norway.
12. Butler D. Mobilisation of the nervous system. 1991 Churchill Livingstone. Melbourne.

CHAPTER 16

Elbow

The elbow joint is the intermediate joint of the upper extremity and functions to help bring the hand to the face and closer to the body. It also functions to lengthen the arm during an extended reach. Maximum compression of the cartilage occurs during flexion and hence full flexion is required to maintain adequate nutrition of the cartilage besides the function described above.[1] The mechanics at the elbow is greatly determined by its more distal counterpart, wrist and hand. Hence management should address both components of the functional chain.

OSSEOUS ANATOMY

The elbow consists of the humeroradial, humeroulnar and superior radioulnar joints. The capitulum of the humerus articulates with the upper surface of the head of the radius and the trochlea of the humerus articulates with the trochlear notch of ulna to form the humeroradial and humeroulnar joints, respectively.

All three joints are of clinical significance and hence appropriate attention is to be addressed. Coordinated mechanics of all three articulations in addition to the inferior radioulnar and wrist joints determine the overall joint compression and tissue tensile stress occurring at the elbow joint.

LIGAMENTOUS ANATOMY

The ligaments of the elbow joints in accordance with their clinical significance are here:

Ulnar Collateral

This ligament arises from the medial epicondyle of the humerus. It has three bands: Anterior, posterior and intermediate. The anterior band attaches to the coronoid process of ulna and the posterior band attaches to the olecranon process. These two ligaments are joined together by the intermediate fibers.

The ligament has a close relationship to the ulnar nerve, flexor digitorum superficialis, flexor carpi ulnaris and triceps.

Radial Collateral

This ligament arises from the lateral epicondyle of the humerus and attaches to the annular ligament of the radial head. It diverges out and splays structurally.

This ligament has a relationship to the extensor carpi radialis brevis (ECRB) and the supinator.

Annular Ligament

The annular ligament is a ligament of the superior radioulnar joint. Annular, denoting 'ring shaped' describes this ring like ligament that encircles the radial head and offers attachment to the radial collateral ligament.

MUSCULAR ANATOMY

The muscles of the elbow that are of clinical significance are described below. Some of them are not muscles that effect movement at the elbow but are relevant to the elbow as they cause pain around the joint.

Pronator Teres

This muscle arises as two heads, one from immediately above the medial condyle and the other from the inner side of the coronoid process of ulna. They insert into the outer surface of the shaft of the radius and function to pronate the forearm and when the radius is fixed, it assists in flexing the forearm. The median nerve enters the forearm between the two heads of the pronator teres.

Supinator Brevis

This muscle arises as two heads from the lateral epicondyle of the humerus and inserts into the bicipital tuberosity and the posterior and external surface of the shaft of the radius. It functions to supinate the forearm. The posterior interosseous branch of the radial nerve passes through the two heads of the supinator brevis in an area called the *arcade of Frohse*.

Flexor Carpi Ulnaris

This muscle arises as two heads, one from the medial epicondyle of the humerus and the other from the inner margin of the olecranon and upper two-third of the posterior border of ulna. It inserts into the pisiform and functions to flex and ulnar deviate the wrist. It, however, continues to function as a flexor of the elbow. The two heads form a long tunnel in the medial elbow through which the ulnar nerve passes called the *Cubital Tunnel*.

Extensor Carpi Radialis Longus

The extensor carpi radialis longus (ECRL) arises from the lower third of the external supracondylar ridge, external intermuscular septum and common extensor origin. It inserts into the base of the metacarpal bone of the index finger and functions to extend and radially deviate the wrist.

Extensor Carpi Radialis Brevis

The extensor carpi radialis brevis (ECRB) arises from the lateral epicondyle of the humerus, the lateral ligament of the elbow and from the external intermuscular septum. It inserts into the base of the metacarpal bone of the middle finger and functions to extend and radially deviate the wrist.

MECHANICS (NORMAL ROLL AND GLIDING)

The movements possible in the elbow and radioulnar joints are flexion, extension, pronation and supination. Wrist movements have a profound influence on the elbow and will be dealt in the next chapter. Flexion and extension at the elbow are characterized by the lateral gliding occurring in the olecranon fossa and the inferior and superior movement occurring at the radial head. In extension, the ulna glides medially in the olecranon fossa, the radius moves distal and caudal on the ulna and the radial head glides posteriorly on humerus. A valgus angulation occurs at the elbow joint and delays contact between the ulna and the humerus. This is to accommodate the soft tissue structures. During flexion, the reverse occurs. The radial head glides more proximal and cephalic on the ulna, with the ulna gliding laterally in the olecranon fossa. The radial head glides anteriorly on the humerus. Typically, the caudal or inferior movement with restriction of medial and lateral glide of the olecranon at the olecranon fossa are the common restriction patterns.

Pronation and supination are a little more complex as this not only involves the superior and inferior radioulnar joints but also the ulnohumeral, radiohumeral and radiocarpal joints.

During pronation, the radial head twists on the capitulum, swings on the ulna and moves laterally. At the inferior radioulnar joint, the ulna moves into slight extension and abduction and hence glides posteriorly and the radius swings medially over the ulnar styloid.

During supination, the radial head reverses the movements and moves medially. At the inferior radioulnar joint the ulna moves into slight flexion and adduction and hence glides anteriorly and the radius swings laterally over the ulnar styloid.[2]

This probably explains the fact that trauma to the wrist can significantly affect the elbow joint and vice versa. The clinician must also understand that this is not just by the joint mechanics but also by the muscular influences over both joints.[3,4]

MECHANISM OF DYSFUNCTION

Symptoms of elbow dysfunction are described as lateral, medial and posterior. The lateral component has received more attention, however, is often prone to dysfunction. The medial and posterior components warrant attention.

Medial and Anterior Elbow Dysfunction

The medial component of the elbow is often strained during activities that involve excessive wrist flexion and throwing. Both activities are described.

Throwing

Throwing[5] involves a starting position of shoulder extension with abduction and external rotation, while the elbow is flexed. Then the motion consists of the trunk and shoulder moving rapidly forward while leaving the arm behind. This causes an extension moment at the elbow which is rapid and jerky. This will cause the radius to glide inferiorly with the radial head gliding posterior. This causes a valgus stress at the medial aspect of the elbow and increased tensile forces. However, if the arthrokinematic radial inferior glide is restricted it increases compressive forces on the lateral side which further increases the tensile forces on the medial side of the elbow. The medial collateral ligament is most vulnerable. In addition it causes overuse injury of the musculature, capsular injury, ulnar traction spurs and medial epicondylitis.

Wrist Flexion

Wrist flexion has a significant influence over the medial aspect of the elbow. At the distal radioulnar joint, wrist flexion causes an inferior radial glide. The hamate, capitate, trapezoid and scaphoid are loose packed and ulnar deviation occurs. Restriction of joint play followed by impact/cumulative stress on a flexed wrist (golf, cricket batsman, occupational) causes a more medially directed force over the common flexor origin. This is also called a golfers elbow. The pronator teres, flexor carpi radialis and ulnaris are involved. Prolonged irritability of the soft tissue can throw off an effusion or cause a fibrous entrapment of the ulnar nerve causing an ulnar nerve involvement. The two heads of the flexor carpi ulnaris forms the 'cubital tunnel' through which the ulnar nerve passes.[6] Hypertrophy or repeated microtrauma can irritate the ulnar nerve causing a cubital tunnel syndrome.

The median nerve or its anterior interosseous branch can similarly be pinched as it passes through the two heads of the pronator teres causing a pronator or anterior interosseous syndrome.[6] Thus the common pathologies occurring secondary to a medial and anterior elbow dysfunction are:
- Medial epicondylitis, golfers elbow.
- Medial collateral ligament strain.
- Ulnar traction spur.
- Pronator syndrome.
- Anterior interosseous syndrome.
- Cubital tunnel syndrome.

Posterior Elbow Dysfunction

Posterior elbow pain is also described as an overuse and the mechanics requires consideration. Direct pressure or trauma is an obvious causative factor, however, both mechanisms described in medial elbow pain (throwing/wrist flexion) are additional causative factors. Interestingly, it is a combination of both.

Throwing comprises a violent elbow extension with wrist flexion and ulnar deviation. Hence, faulty mechanics of these component motions can irritate triceps and its underlying bursa causing triceps strain and olecranon bursitis. This is particularly seen with faulty mechanics of ulnar glide in the olecranon fossa. If prolonged, the 'snap back' that occurs secondary to the open chain motion (including punching in the air like martial artists would do) could cause a posterior impingement. The posteromedial aspect of the olecranon offers attachment to the flexor carpi ulnaris and can cause posterior elbow pain due to dysfunction of this muscle. In addition, inadequate medial and lateral glide of the olecranon at the posterior elbow may irritate the soft tissue with prolonged activity and cause posterior elbow pain and impingement. Thus the common pathologies occurring in a posterior elbow dysfunction are:

- Triceps strain.
- Olecranon bursitis.
- Flexor carpiulnaris (FCU) strain.
- Posterior impingement.

Lateral Elbow Dysfunction

This entity has long been described and for most clinicians the first thought process is a 'tennis elbow'. Although this is the most common lesion that occurs in the lateral elbow complex, other causative factors are also described.

The two functional factors are considered again, throwing and, but however, wrist extension. It is commonly seen in racquet sports, but also in occupational situations as in hammering, typing, etc. Excessive supination as in the constant use of a screwdriver as an electrician or a carpenter would do, predisposes to a dysfunction.

Throwing, as described earlier, causes compressive forces over the radial head. However, faulty arthrokinematics can cause an increase in these compressive forces predisposing to dysfunction including a radial head compression and fibrillation.

Wrist extension should be considered in detail due to its intricate mechanics and vulnerability. The mechanics has been described in the chapter on 'principles of diagnosis'. To review, during wrist extension.[2]

- The distal row moves dorsal and the proximal row moves volar.
- The predominant movement happens in the radially placed radiocarpal joint.
- The scaphoid and lunate glides anterior on the radius.
- This accompanied by the action of the ECRL, ECRB that are powerful wrist extensors and radial deviators causes the wrist to deviate radially.
- The radius glides cephalad on ulna.

Thus when a blow is received on an extended hand, the force is taken via the 3rd metacarpal to the capitate, lunate, scaphoid and then to the radius and common wrist extensors.

Cumulative stress can involve the tenoperiosteal junction of the common extensors, most commonly ECRB, and less commonly ECRL and extensor digitorum. However, any faulty alteration of the arthrokinematics described above or excessive cephalad movement of the radius can cause compressive forces at the radial head and increase contraction stresses of the common extensor origin.

Soft tissue dysfunction can cause pain and nerve entrapment in the lateral elbow area. The major branch of the radial nerve in the forearm is the posterior interosseous nerve. This nerve can be compressed near the lateral epicondyle as it passes through the two heads of supinator in the 'arcade of Frohse'. Fibrous compression can occur during hypertrophic states of the supinator and forearm extensors causing a 'radial tunnel syndrome'.[7] There is no sensory deficit and may mimic a lateral epicondylalgia. Thus collectively the common pathologies occurring in a lateral elbow dysfunction are:

- Lateral epicondylalgia, 'tennis elbow'.
- Radial tunnel syndrome.
- Ligamentous strain, (lateral collateral, annular).
- Radial head compression/fibrillation.

ELBOW JOINT SOMATIC DIAGNOSIS

Ulna Medial/Lateral

The patient is seated and the clinician is seated by the side of the elbow to be examined. The clinician then grasps the proximal radioulnar joint circumferentially and stabilizes the arm between the trunk and elbow. The clinician then glides the elbow medially and laterally in Figure 16.1 and senses for restriction.[8] Then with the patient seated, the clinician places the thumb and index finger on either side of the olecranon in the olecranon fossa (Fig. 16.2). Now the elbow is flexed and extended and the clinician feels for medial and lateral movement of the olecranon in the olecranon fossa. During extension the medial space increases and during flexion it decreases. Altered states with pain and local tenderness indicate dysfunction.

A restriction in medial glide is more frequently seen and is sensed as an adduction restriction during examination. This would mechanically interfere with normal extension.

Hence during activities that incorporate violent or repetitive extension, a restricted glide of the ulna can irritate the posterior structures mainly the olecranon bursa, predisposing to a bursitis. The flexor carpi ulnaris is yet another structure that is predisposed to dysfunction owing to one of its attachments to the olecranon.

Radial Head Superior/Inferior

The patient is seated and the clinician faces the patient. The head of the radius is palpated with the index finger and moved slightly proximally to palpate the hollow dip between the radial head and the capitulum of the humerus. The patients' elbow is now flexed and extended while this hollow space is palpated. During this process the clinician can actually feel the space decrease during flexion and increase during extension (Fig. 16.3). The clinician senses for the movement and palpates the space in terminal extension. The two side are compared. A decrease in the space will denote a superior radial head dysfunction and vice versa.

A restriction in inferior glide is most common on extension/throwing. This increases compressive forces on the lateral aspect and tensile forces on the medial aspect.

Radial head dysfunctions can affect mechanics at the wrist and increase stresses on the radial head especially during wrist extension and predispose to lateral epicondylitis.

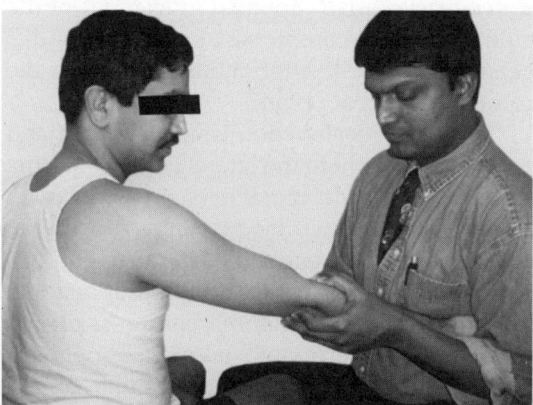

Fig. 16.1: Assessing medial and lateral ulna.

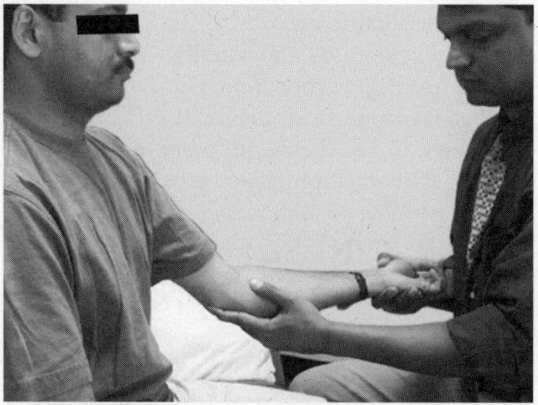

Fig. 16.2: Assessing medial and lateral ulna.

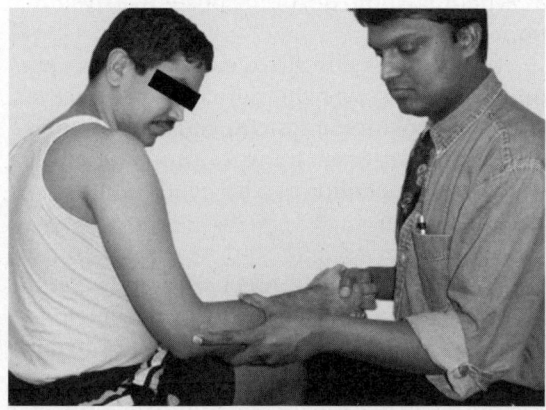

Fig. 16.3: Assessing superior radius.

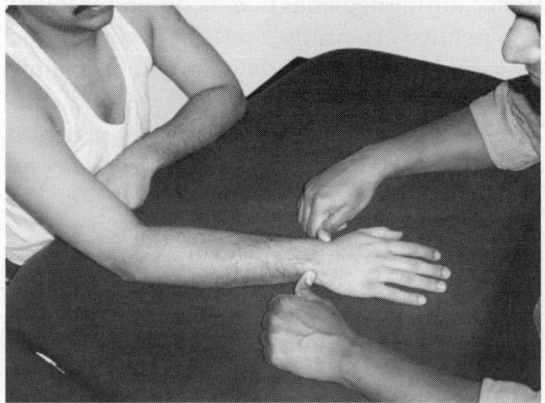

Fig. 16.4: Assessing ulnar variance.

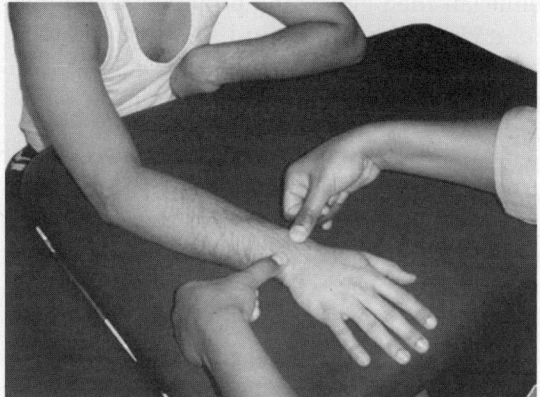

Fig. 16.5: Assessing posterior ulna styloid.

Ulnar Variance

The patient is seated with the forearm resting on the table and the clinician faces the forearm to be treated. The thumbs of the clinician palpate both styloid processes and move slightly inferior to the tips of the styloid processes. Normally, the radial styloid extends more inferiorly and both sides are compared (Fig. 16.4). If the radial styloid appears higher in comparison to the opposite side it is considered a positive ulnar variance and can also indicate a superior radial head dysfunction.

This has an implication both at the elbow and wrist. The implication in the elbow is as described for a superior radial head dysfunction. Those at the wrist will be described in the next chapter on the wrist and hand.

Ulnar Styloid Posterior

The patient is seated with the forearm resting on the table and the clinician facing the forearm. The thumbs of the clinician are placed on both the styloid processes and the clinician observes for asymmetry (Fig. 16.5). The ulnar styloid is normally slightly posterior in comparison to the radial styloid, but increased posteriority in comparison to the opposite side suggests a posterior ulna styloid dysfunction.

A posterior distal ulna can restrict/affect mechanics of supination and prolonged overuse in the presence of this dysfunction can cause hyperactivity and irritability of the supinator predisposing to a radial tunnel syndrome.

TREATMENT FOR SPECIFIC SOMATIC DYSFUNCTION

Ulna Medial/Lateral

The patient is lying prone and the clinician faces the patient from the side of the elbow to be treated. The patients' arm is flexed to about 70 to 90° and is hanging by the side of the table. The clinician stabilizes the condyles of the humerus and grips the olecranon with the thumb, index, and middle fingers. The olecranon is mobilized in a medial and lateral direction (Figs 16.6 and 16.7). An alternative position in supine lying is also illustrated.

Radial Head Superior/Inferior

For a superior dysfunction, the patient is in a side lying position and the clinician faces the patient from the side to be treated with the patient's elbow flexed to 45°. One hand of the clinician grasps the lower end of the radius just above the wrist (Figs. 16.7 to 16.9). The other hand stabilizes the upper arm at the midshaft of the humerus. A gentle distraction is applied at the lower end of the radius, while the other hand stabilizes and offers counter pressure for the distraction. Alternately a towel/strap or sheet is placed under the shaft of the humerus and hooked under the trunk of the patient. A mobilization strap if available can be incorporated. Now the clinician offers a distraction at the lower end of the radius,

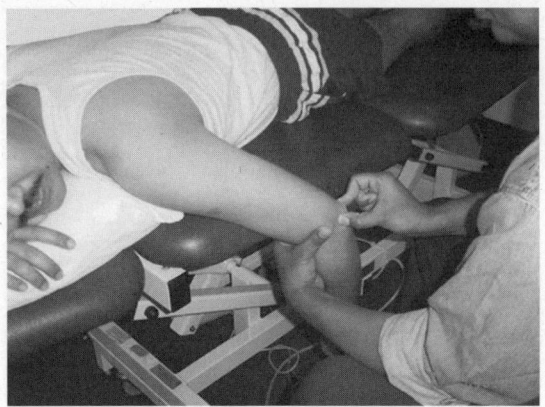

Fig. 16.6A: Olecranon medial and lateral glide.

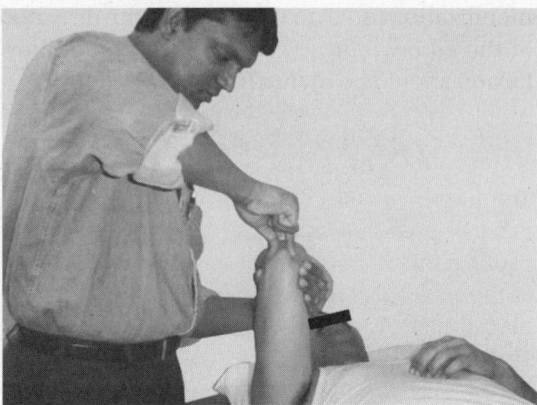

Fig. 16.6B: Olecranon medial and lateral glide.

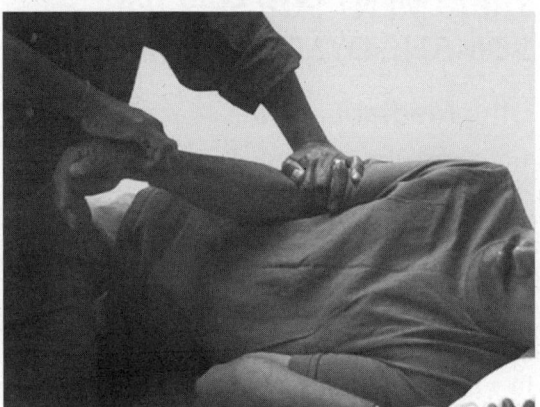

Fig. 16.7: Radius inferior glide

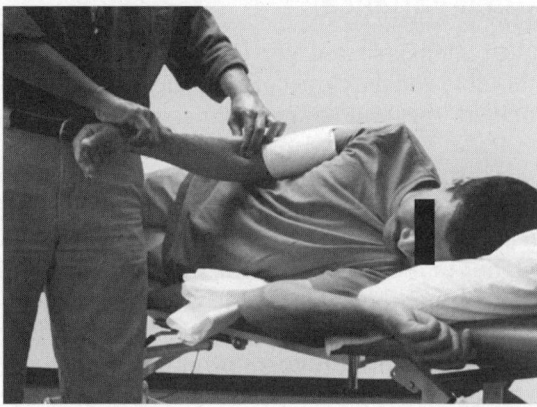

Fig. 16.8: Radial head superior/inferior glide.

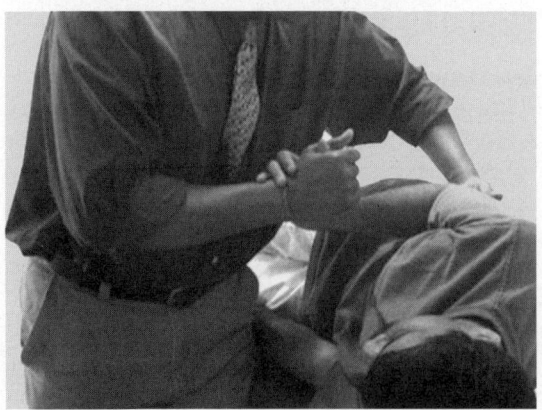

Fig. 16.9: Radius superior glide.

while the other hand glides the radial head in an anterior or posterior direction. This further mobilizes the radial head for ease of superior and inferior movement.

For an inferior dysfunction, the patient and the clinician position are as above. The elbow of the patient is in 90 to 100° of flexion. The thenar eminence of the clinicians' hand contacts the thenar eminence of the patient (right thenar eminence contacts the right thenar eminence of the patient and vice versa). The clinicians' thumb is hooked around the thumb of the patient. The clinician then stabilizes the condyles of the humerus with the other hand and exerts a mobilization force on the radius in the direction of the elbow joint. Wrist extension and elbow flexion should be maintained.

Ulnar Styloid Posterior

The patient is lying supine with the elbow in extension and pronation. The thenar eminence of one hand of the clinician stabilizes the dorsum of the lower end of the radius, while the ulna is placed just a little outside the edge of the table. The thenar eminence of the other hand is placed on the dorsum of the lower end of the ulna. An inferiorly directed mobilization force is imparted on the ulna to glide it anteriorly (Fig. 16.10).

Ulnar Variance

The treatment technique is as described for a superior dysfunction of the radius.

TREATMENT FOR OVERALL IMPROVEMENT IN RANGE OF MOTION (TJP: TRACTION AND PASSIVE GLIDING)[2,9]

Joint Basics: Humeroulnar-radial

Type of joint	Diarthrodial hinge
Degrees of freedom	Flexion, extension, abduction, adduction
Range of motion	Flexion: 0–150°, extension: 0–10° hyperextension
Capsular pattern	Flexion more than extension
Loose packed position	70–90° of flexion and 10–35° of supination

Joint Basics: Superior radioulnar

Type of joint	Diarthrodial pivot
Degrees of freedom	Pronation, supination
Range of motion	Pronation and supination: 0–80°
Capsular pattern	Equal pronation and supination
Loose packed position	70° flexion and 30° supination

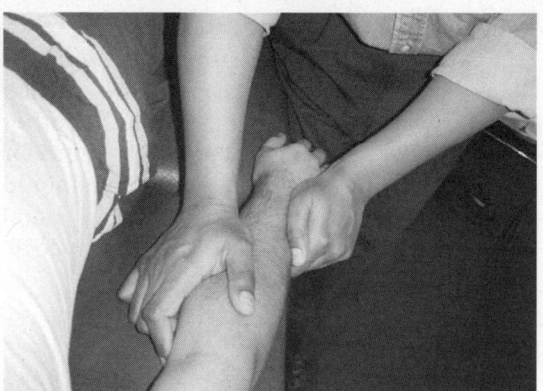

Fig. 16.10: Ulna anterior glide

To Improve Flexion

- Ulna distraction
- Superior glide of the radius
- Anterior glide of radial head
- Radioulnar retraction..

To Improve Extension

- Caution is exercised to avoid myositis ossificans of the brachialis
- Ulna distraction
- Inferior glide of the radius
- Posterior glide of radial head.

Medial and lateral glide of ulna styloid as in treatment for specific somatic diagnosis section.

To Improve Pronation

- Posterior glide of radial head
- Posterior glide of ulnar styloid
- Radioulnar retraction.

To Improve Supination

- Anterior glide of radial head
- Anterior glide of ulnar styloid
- Radioulnar retraction.

Ulna Distraction (Fig. 16.11)

The patient is lying supine and the clinician, seated, faces the patient from the side to be treated, with the patient's elbow flexed to 90°. One hand of the clinician grasps the upper shaft of the ulna just below the joint level and the arm rests on the clinician's shoulder. The other hand stabilizes the upper arm at the midshaft of the humerus. A gentle distraction is applied at the upper end of the ulna, while the other hand stabilizes and offers counter pressure for the distraction. *Note:* Ulna distraction should be a preceding maneuver for medial and lateral glide of the olecranon in th treatment for specific somatic diagnosis section.

Superior Glide of the Radius (Fig. 16.12)

The patient is in a side lying position and the clinician faces the patient from the side to be treated with the patient's elbow flexed to 90 to 100°. The thenar eminence of the clinicians' hand contacts the thenar eminence of the patient (right thenar eminence contacts the right thenar eminence of the patient and vice versa). The clinicians' thumb is hooked around the thumb of the patient. The clinician then stabilizes the condyles of the humerus with the other hand and exerts a downward mobilization force on the radius as the radius terminates at the thenar eminence. Wrist extension and elbow flexion should be maintained.

Inferior Glide of the Radius (Fig. 16.13)

The patient is in a side lying position and the clinician faces the patient from the side to be treated with the patient's elbow flexed to 45°. One hand of the clinician grasps the lower end of the radius just above the wrist. The other hand stabilizes the upper arm at the midshaft of the humerus. A gentle distraction is applied at the lower end of the radius, while the other hand stabilizes and offers counter pressure for the distraction. Elbow extension and wrist flexion is maintained.

Anterior/posterior Glide of Radial Head

The patient is in a side lying position and the clinician faces the patient from the side to be treated with the patient's elbow flexed to 90°. One hand of the clinician grasps the lower end of the radius just above the wrist. The other hand stabilizes the upper arm at the midshaft of the humerus. A gentle distraction is applied at the lower end of the radius, while the other hand stabilizes and offers counter pressure for the distraction. Alternately a towel or sheet is placed under the shaft of the humerus and hooked

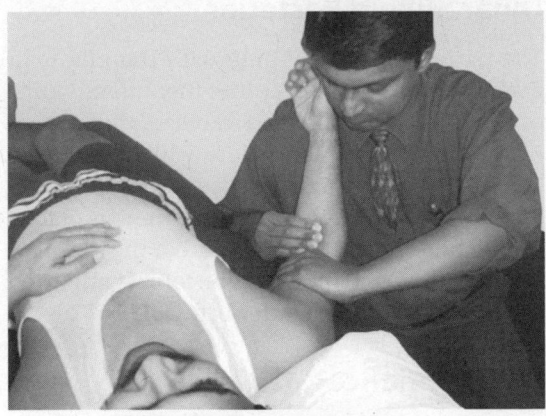

Fig. 16.11: Ulna distraction.

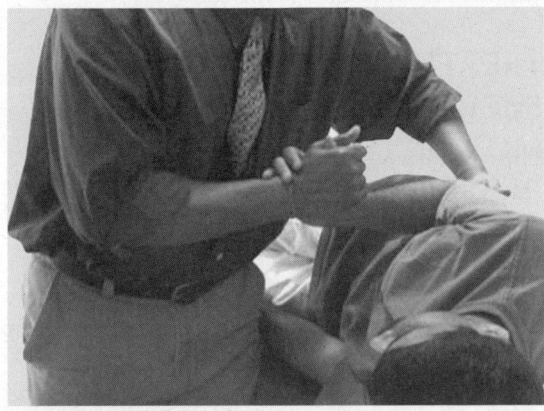

Fig. 16.12: Superior glide radius.

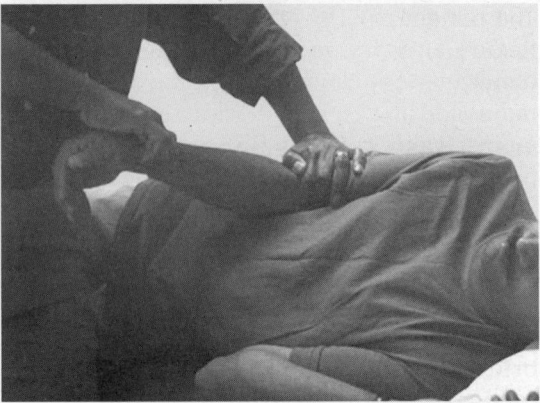

Fig. 16.13: Radius inferior glide.

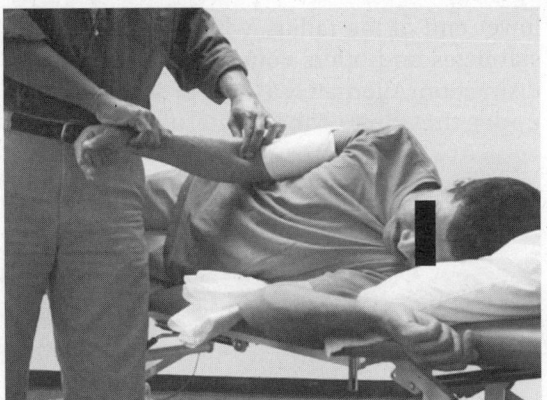

Fig. 16.14: Radius anterior posterior glide.

under the trunk of the patient. A mobilization strap if available can be incorporated. Now the clinician offers a distraction at the lower end of the radius, while the other hand glides the radial head in an anterior direction to improve flexion or posterior direction to improve extension.

Radioulnar Retraction (Figs. 16.14 and 16.15)

The patient is lying supine with the elbow extended and supinated. The clinician faces the patient from the side of the elbow to be treated. Both thenar eminences are placed on either sides of the forearm on the radius and ulna, respectively. A posteriorly directed pressure is applied via both thenar eminences so as to retract the radius and ulna.

Anterior/posterior Glide of Ulna Styloid

The patient is lying supine with the elbow in flexion and supination. The thumbs of both hands of the clinician hold the lower end of the radius and ulna (styloids). With a firm grip on the radial styloid, the ulna is glided in an anterior/posterior direction (Fig. 16.16).

MYOFASCIAL TENDER POINTS

The concept of addressing myofascial tender points is to decrease actin and myosin cross-bridging and myofibrillar restriction. Their

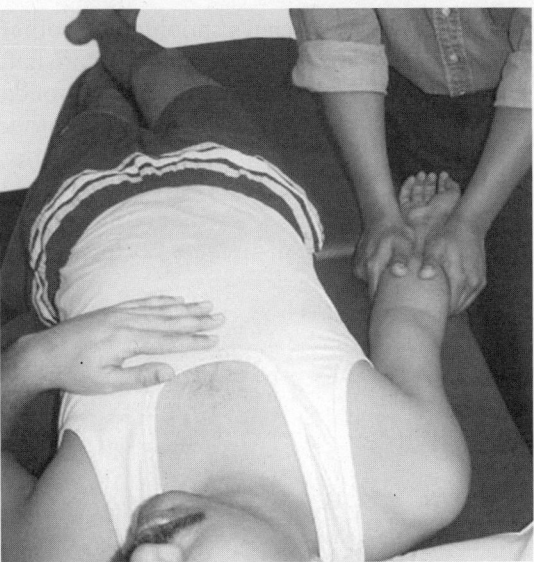

Fig. 16.15: Radioulnar retraction.

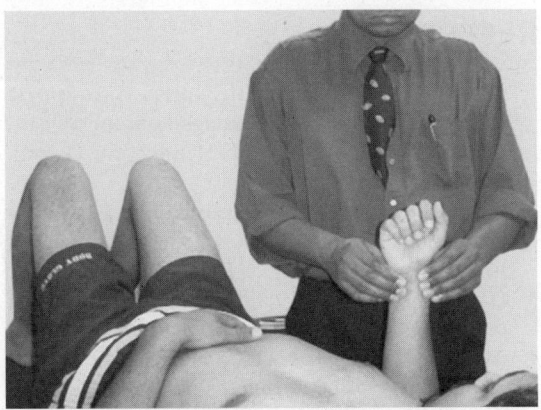

Fig. 16.16: Ulna styloid anterior/posterior glide.

continual presence may encourage chemical accumulation, early fatigue and decreased muscle performance with accompanying pain and dysfunction. They may be best treated with frictions and electrotherapy. Tender points secondary to aberrant gamma efferents may require an alternate positional release approach and the reader is encouraged further reading in the area of 'strain counterstrain' methods. The following are some common dysfunctional points of the elbow (Figs. 16.17 and 16.18).

1. Extensor carpi ulnaris
2. Extensor carpi radialis brevis
3. Extensor carpi radialis longus
4. Brachioradialis

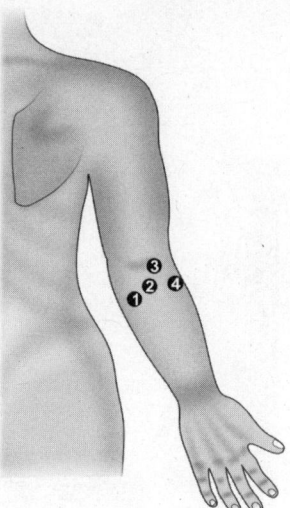

1. Supinator
2. Pronator teres
3. Flexor carpi radialis
4. Flexor carpi ulnaris
5. Flexor digitorum superficialis/ profundus

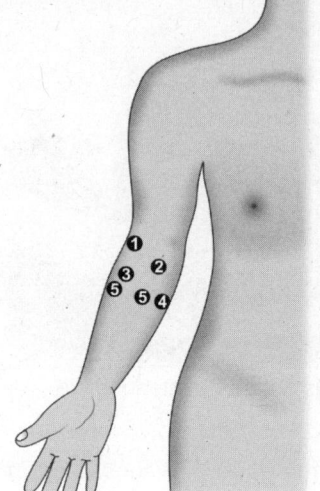

Fig. 16.17: Myofascial tender points: Elbow (posterior).

Fig. 16.18: Myofascial tender points: Elbow (anterior).

REFERENCES

1. Norris CM. The Knee. In: Norris CM. Sports Injuries: Diagnosis and management for physiotherapists 1993. Butterworth-Heinemann, Oxford, pp:169-192.
2. Patla CE, Paris SV. EI Course Notes: Extremity Evaluation and manipulation, 1996. St. Auguatine, Institute press.
3. Davies C. The trigger point therapy workbook, 1st edn, 2001, New Harbinger Publication, Oakland.
4. Cyriax J. Textbook of orthopaedic medicine, vol 1: Diagnosis of soft tissue lesions, 1982, Bailliere Tindall, Philadelphia.
5. Andrews JR, et al. Physical examination of the thrower's elbow. J Orthop Sports Phys Ther. 1993;17:296-304.
6. Chabon SJ. Uncommon compression neuropathies of the forearm. Physician Assistant. 1990; 14(9):65.
7. Moss SH, Switzer HE. Radial tunnel syndrome: a spectrum of clinical presentations. J Hand Surg Am. 1983;8:414-20.
8. Greenman PE. Principles of Manual Medicine, 1996, Williams and Wilkins, Baltimore.
9. Kaltenborn F. Mobilization of the extremity joints: Examination and basic treatment techniques, 3rd edn, 1980, Olaf Norlis Bokhandel Universitetsgaten, Oslo, Norway.

CHAPTER 17

Wrist and Hand

The hand is the most sensitive and prehensile organ of the body. 25% of the pacinian corpuscles of the body are situated in the hand. It is not only an essential organ to perform functional activity, but it is also the primary organ for tactile perception. If one tends to feel in the absence of visual feedback, the only structure in the body that is primarily incorporated is the hand. Hence, functional motor and sensory integrity of the hand is essential.

The hand is essentially considered with the wrist, and forearm is also an important component of the structural complex. Lesions of the elbow are strongly influenced by the movements of the wrist and their two joint musculature. As many of the muscles that are rendered pathological arise from the elbow and forearm, a detailed examination of the elbow is recommended when treating mechanical dysfunctions of the wrist and hand.

OSSEOUS ANATOMY

Distal Radioulnar Joint

This joint is formed by the head of the ulna received into the sigmoid cavity at the inner side of the lower end of the radius. The ulna and radial movement are equally significant.

Radiocarpal

The radius articulates with the scaphoid and lunate to form the radiocarpal (wrist) joint. Stability of the wrist is enhanced by a fibrocartilaginous disk that runs from the ulnar side of the radius to the ulnar styloid. This is called the triangular fibrocartilaginous complex (TFCC) and the lunate and triquetrum also articulate with it. This structure is clinically significant and can be damaged by the forced extension and pronation.[1]

Intercarpal

This is formed by joints between the individual bones of the carpals. They are held together by the intercarpal ligaments.

Midcarpal

This joint is formed by the articulation of the proximal and distal row of carpal bones. Their ligamentous integrity is not as much as the intercapal joints and hence favors greater mobility than the intercarpal joints.

Carpometacarpal

This is formed by the articulation of the distal rows of the carpal bones and the 1st to 5th metacarpal bones.

Intermetacarpal

The four inner metacarpal bones articulate with one another on each side by small surfaces covered with cartilage. These are the intermetacarpal joints and are strengthened by the dorsal, palmar and interosseous ligaments.

Metacarpophalangeal

This is a condyloid joint formed by the rounded head of the metacarpal bone articulating into a shallow cavity in the extremity of the phalanx. They are strengthened by the collateral, palmar, and deep transverse metacarpal ligaments.

Interphalangeal

These are hinge joints and are formed by the articulation of the condyles of the phalanges. They are held together by a fibrous capsule and the palmar and collateral ligaments. An interesting feature is that a certain amount of rotation occurs in these joints on flexion, so that the pulp of the tip of the fingers face the pulp of the thumb.

LIGAMENTOUS ANATOMY

There are several ligaments in the wrist and hand and some are more vulnerable to injury than others.[2] The following ligaments of the wrist and hand are described for the fact that they are more susceptible to injury and hence clinically relevant.

Scapholunate/Lunate, Capitate

A wrist sprain is a common diagnosis and are often involving the intercarpal ligaments of the wrist. The scapholunate and lunate, capitate ligaments are the most commonly involved and as their names suggests, their attachments are self explanatory.

Transverse Carpal

The transverse carpal ligament runs from the scaphoid tubercle to the hamate and hence lateral to medial. It is otherwise known as the flexor retinaculum. It forms the roof of the carpal tunnel and offers attachment to the thenar and hypothenar muscles. It also maintains the transverse carpal arch and prevents bow stringing of the flexor tendons. The other important function of this structure is to offer protection for the median nerve.

Ulnar Collateral Ligament of Thumb

The ulnar collateral ligament of the thumb is the primary stabilizer of the MCP of the thumb. It runs from the metacarpal bone of the thumb to the base of the proximal phalanx of the thumb. It prevents and stabilizes the thumb from an abduction strain. It is commonly injured in sport and in occupational situations.

Collateral Ligament

The metacarpophalangeal (MCP) and interphalangeal (IP) joints have obliquely placed ligaments that are lax in extension and become increasingly taut in flexion. These ligaments prevent abduction and adduction strains to the joint and are hence vulnerable during such forceful movements. They are also contracted in length by faulty immobilization resulting in stiffness and impairment.

Pisohamate Ligament

These are essentially two fibrous bands, pisohamate and pisometacarpal ligaments that run from the pisiform and hamate and the pisiform and fifth metacarpal. These are in reality extensions of the flexor carpi ulnaris muscle and are susceptible to dysfunction (see elbow joint).

MUSCULAR ANATOMY

The muscles of the hand and fingers are elaborate and intricate and hence only the muscles that are clinically relevant are mentioned. Injuries to the muscles of the hand are often occupational or sport related. As mentioned earlier, the injury could primarily occur as a result of faulty muscle mechanics rather than faulty joint arthrokinematics. The common muscles that are susceptible to injury are:

Interossei

These muscles are elaborate and originate from the metacarpal bones and insert into the extensor expansion and the base of the proximal phalanx. They are commonly strained in overuse sydromes and are a source of pain in the hand.

Extensor Digitorum Communis

This muscle originates from the common extensor origin on the lateral epicondyle of humerus and the deep antebrachial fascia. It inserts as medial and lateral bands into the bases of the middle and distal phalanx, respectively. This muscle is commonly involved as an occupational injury due to periodic overuse[3] as in repetitive movements, (keyboard operators). The tendon or the sheath covering the tendon can be inflamed and is a source of hand and elbow pain. This muscle is also strained with excessive gripping motion.

Flexor Digitorum Profundus/Superficialis

The former muscle originates from the common flexor origin at the medial epicondyle of humerus, ulnar collateral ligament of the elbow and deep antebrachial fascia with two other heads from the ulna and radius. It inserts into the sides of the middle phalanges excluding the thumb. The latter muscle arises from the proximal part of the ulna, and interosseous membrane and deep antebrachial fascia. They insert into the bases of the distal phalanx, excluding the thumb. They work to flex the digits and assist in flexing the wrist.

These muscles are commonly strained with prolonged gripping motion and are seen in occupational situations. They are also seen as sport injuries and the former muscle can also be a source of medial elbow pain. The flexor sheath is also described to be inflamed secondary to overuse.

Abductor Pollicis Longus/Extensor Pollicis Brevis

The former muscle arises from the posterior surface of the middle one-third of ulna and radius and inserts into the base of first metacarpal bone on the radial side. It abducts the carpometacarpal (CMC) joint and wrist and extends the CMC joint of the thumb.

The latter muscle arises from the posterior surface of the body of radius, distal one-third, and inserts into the base of proximal phalanx of thumb. It extends the MCP joint of the thumb and extends and abducts the CMC joint. They form the radial border of the anatomical snuff box. These two tendons pass together on the lateral side of the radial styloid into a fibro-osseous tunnel. These two tendons with the tunnel are prone to overuse injuries at this location.

MECHANICS (NORMAL ROLLING AND GLIDING)

The mechanics at the wrist are complicated as for the fact that there are several articulations involved.[4,5] The four motions that occur in the wrist, however, occur as coupled motions. In that, flexion always occurs with ulnar deviation and extension occurs with radial deviation. The clinician must remember that wrist motion is not complete without adequate gliding motion of the radius or adequate mobility between the distal radius and ulna.

WRIST EXTENSION WITH RADIAL DEVIATION

The distal row moves dorsal and the proximal row moves volar.

The predominant movement happens in the radially placed radiocarpal joint.

The scaphoid and lunate glides anterior on the radius.

This accompanied by the action of the extensor carpi radialis longus (ECRL), extensor carpi radialis brevis (ECRB) that are powerful wrist extensors and radial deviators causes the wrist to deviate radially.

The radius glides cephalad on ulna.

WRIST FLEXION WITH ULNAR DEVIATION

The distal row moves volar and the proximal row moves dorsal.

The predominant movement happens in the radiocarpal joint.

The scaphoid and lunate glides posterior on the radius.

This accompanied by the action of the flexor carpi ulnaris (FCU) which is the most powerful wrist flexor and ulnar deviator, which causes the wrist to deviate ulnar.

The radius glides caudal on ulna.

In a pure radial deviation there is an ulnar glide of the proximal row of bones.

In a pure ulnar deviation there is a radial glide of the proximal row of bones.

MECHANISM OF DYSFUNCTION

As previously mentioned, mechanical injury to the wrist and hand occurs as overuse syndromes with primarily, lesions of the soft tissue responsible for the activity.[3,6] Although much of the motion in the wrist and hand occur as open chain activity, a significant proportion of activity occurs in a closed chain fashion (push ups, falling on the hand, etc.). Hence, joint arthrokinematics is still an integral portion of the evaluation. The soft tissue lesion in many instances may be secondary to restricted or faulty arthrokinematics.

Common Pathologies Secondary to Mechanical Dysfunction

Triangular Fibrocartilage Complex

This is a triangular structure that arises from the ulnar margin of the radius and extends to insert into the base of the ulnar styloid. Distally, it attaches to the lunate, triquetrum, hamate and base of the fifth metacarpal. This area is often described as the ulna-meniscal-triquetral joint. The triangular fibrocartilage complex is synonymously described as a disk or meniscus.

It normally helps to absorb shock and when intact, the radius takes 60% of the axial loading. In its absence, the axial loading can increase up to 95%.

The length of the ulna with respect to the radius is also a concern. Normally the radius is longer than the ulna at the level of the wrist. This is called a negative ulna variance. If the ulna increases in relative length, as with growth plate deficiencies or restriction in caudal glide of the radius, the ulna can be apparently longer increasing compressive forces on the triangular fibrocartilage complex (TFCC) and predisposing to wrist pain and dysfunction.

The TFCC hence functions to provide a continuous gliding surface for its relevant articulation, and provides a flexible mechanism for stable rotational movements of the radiocarpal unit along the ulnar axis.

De Quervain's Disease

The abductor pollicis longus and extensor pollicis brevis form the radial border of the anatomical snuff box. These two tendons pass together on the lateral side of the radial styloid into a fibro-osseous tunnel. These two tendons with the tunnel are prone to overuse injuries at this location.[7] Activities involving repetitive flexion and ulnar deviation from and extended, radial deviation position of the wrist can cause friction between the tendons, between the tendon and the sheath and between the tendon and the bony structures in close proximity to them. Inflammation is caused leading to thickening and stenosis of the tunnel. Faulty arthrokinematics of flexion and unlar deviation can further increase stress on the tendons.

Muscles and Tendons

Overuse strains are seen in several of the small muscles of the hand and forearm[8,9] the most commonly involved are interossei, flexor digitorum profundus and superficialis. As mentioned earlier these may occur secondary to faulty arthrokinematics as well. Similarly the extensor tendons and tendon sheaths are also prone to injury secondary to overuse. It is also important to address the normal arthrokinematics of extension and radial deviation.

Ligament Strains

The scapholunate and lunate, capitate ligaments are susceptible to strains and is commonly seen secondary to overuse and extension strains at the wrist. This could be a fall on an extended hand, push up exercises, gymnastics, or a disabled patient that pushes his/her body up during transfers and during crutch walking. The lunate also has a tendency to sublux anteriorly causing ligamentous stress. Improperly diagnosed wrist sprains may involve these ligaments that are subjected to chronic irritation. Pain is usually elicitable on the dorsum of the flexed wrist.

Transverse Carpal

The transverse carpal ligament runs from the scaphoid tubercle to the hamate and forms the roof of the carpal tunnel. Of the many factors that compromise the tunnel, a contracture of this structure can also be a predisposing factor to median nerve irritation at the carpal tunnel.

Ulnar Collateral Ligament of Thumb (Gamekeepers Thumb)

The ulnar collateral ligament of the thumb is the primary stabilizer of the MCP of the thumb. It runs from the metacarpal bone of the thumb to the base of the proximal phalanx of the thumb. It prevents and stabilizes the thumb from an abduction strain. Hence, typically stressed during skiing or when the thumb gets stuck in a sweater and is pulled laterally. It is also stressed with chronic overuse and occupational situations.

Collateral Ligament

The MCP and IP joints have obliquely placed ligaments that are lax in extension and become increasingly taut in flexion. These ligaments prevent abduction and adduction strains to the joint and are hence vulnerable during such forceful movements. They are also contracted in length by faulty immobilization resulting in stiffness and impairment.

Pisohamate Ligament

These are essentially two fibrous bands, the pisohamate and the pisometacarpal ligaments that run from the pisiform and hamate and the pisiform and fifth metacarpal. These are in reality extensions of the flexor carpi ulnaris muscle and are susceptible to dysfunction with prolonged and repetitive flexion movements of the wrist. This is seen in occupational situations and in sport as in volleyball, cricket and golf. Hence, faulty arthrokinematics of wrist flexion and ulnar deviation is a causative factor as well. There is also evidence of susceptibility of the ulnar nerve.

Carpometacarpal Arthrosis

This is an obvious arthrokinematic restriction that occurs in the CMC joint of thumb as it is most vulnerable for osteoarthritis. It is seen during chronic overuse involving gripping or racquet sports. The restriction is usually in the direction of abduction. Since it restricts thumb mobility, it can significantly affect function including the sharp pain that it is associated with.

Intersection Syndrome

Intersection syndrome is tenosynovitis of the radial wrist extensors, extensor carpi radialis longus, and extensor carpi radialis brevis. The condition also affects the extensor pollicis brevis (EPB) and abductor pollicis longus (APL) causing pain and swelling of these muscle bellies. It is characterized by pain and swelling in the distal dorsoradial forearm. It can be caused by direct trauma to the second extensor compartment. It is more commonly brought on by activities that require repetitive wrist flexion and extension. Weightlifters, rowers, and other athletes are particularly prone to this condition. While this condition occurs at the intersection of the first and second extensor compartments, many contend that the condition is a tenosynovitis of the ECRL and ECRB tendons. However, the condition has long been held to be caused by friction from the overlying EPB and APL tendons. Tensile and shearing stresses in the tendons and peritendinous tissues may lead to thickening, adhesions, and cellular proliferation. Subsequent swelling and proliferation of tenosynovium may cause pain as these tissues are compressed within the unyielding second extensor compartment. Patients with intersection syndrome complain of radial wrist or forearm pain. Symptoms may be exacerbated by repetitive wrist flexion and extension.

Nerve Entrapments

Carpal tunnel syndrome: This is a commonly described condition involving compression of the median nerve at the wrist and has several causative factors. The ones that are relevant to the manual therapist are:
- Fibrosis or contracture of the transverse carpal ligament
- Alteration of the bony margins of the tunnel secondary to injury, arthrokinematic restriction and faulty alignment secondary to fractures (Colles'). The carpals that are of concern are hamate/pisiform and trapezium/scaphoid. A tight ligament or faulty arthrokinematics can alter the patency of the tunnel resulting in symptoms. An anterior subluxation of the lunate can also predispose to a medial nerve compression.

The size of the structures within the canal may be increased if they are inflamed secondary to overuse. The structures are the flexor tendons and hence the cause for flexor tendon irritation should be addressed.[10,11]

Guyons canal syndrome: This condition describes an ulnar nerve irritation that is characterized by a stretching of the nerve by a faulty combination of hyperextension and ulnar deviation of the wrist.[10,11] It is commonly seen in cyclists. The nerve then gets irritated between the pisiform and hook of the hamate. Faulty arthrokinematics during extension of wrist may also be a causative factor.

Radial nerve neuritis: The superficial radial nerve can be compressed at the level of the distal third of the forearm between the tendons of ECRL and brachioradialis.[10,11] This occurs secondary to prolonged and repetitive ulnar deviation and pronation and the nerve is irritated due to a scissor like action of these two tendons. It is hence seen in occupational situations like unscrewing a screwdriver or wringing clothes before drying.

WRIST AND HAND SOMATIC DIAGNOSIS

Ulnar Variance

The patient is seated with the forearm resting on the table and the clinician facing the forearm. The thumbs of the clinician palpate both styloid processes and move slightly inferior to the tips of the styloid processes. Normally, the radial styloid extends more inferiorly and both sides are compared (Fig. 17.1). If the radial styloid appears higher in comparison to the opposite side it is considered a positive ulnar variance and can also indicate a superior radial head dysfunction.

Radial Head Superior/Inferior

The patient is seated and the clinician faces the patient. The head of the radius is palpated with the index finger and moved slightly proximally to palpate the hollow dip between the radial head and capitulum of the humerus. The patients' elbow is now flexed and extended, while this hollow space is palpated. During this process the clinician can actually feel the space decrease during flexion and increase during extension. The clinician senses for the movement and palpates the space in terminal extension. The two sides are compared. A decrease in the space will denote a superior radial head dysfunction and vice versa (Fig. 17.2).

Ulna Posterior

The patient is seated with the forearm resting on the table and the clinician facing the forearm. The thumbs of the clinician are placed on both

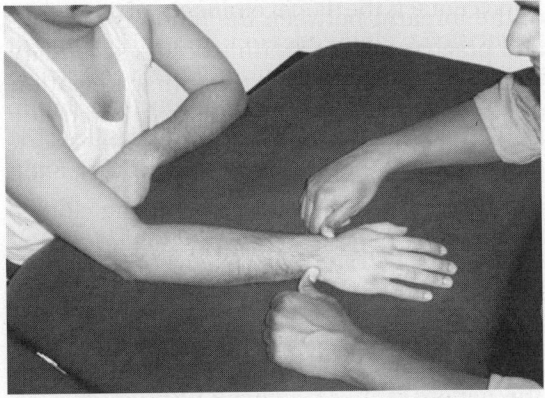

Fig. 17.1: Assesing ulnar variance.

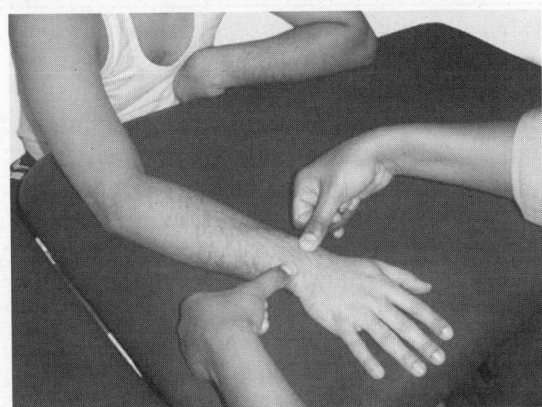

Fig. 17.3: Assessing posterior ulna styloid.

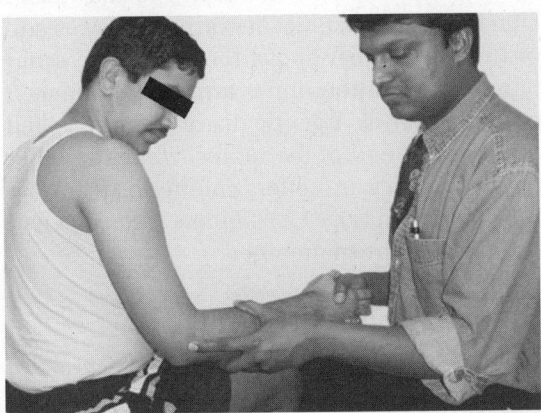

Fig. 17.2: Assessing radial head superior inferior.

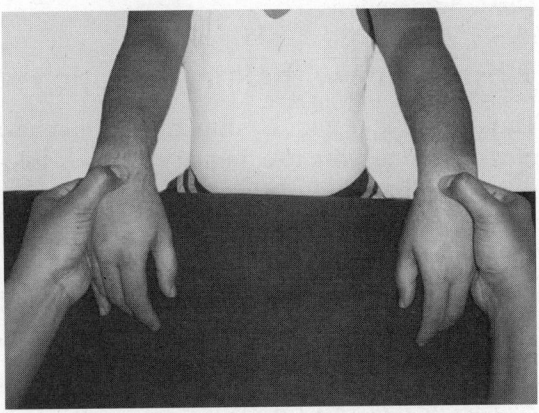

Fig. 17.4: Assessing anterior lunate.

styloid processes and the clinician observes for asymmetry. The ulnar styloid is normally slightly posterior in comparison to the radial styloid, but increased posteriority in comparison to the opposite side suggests a posterior ulna styloid dysfunction (Fig. 17.3).

Lunate Anterior

The patient is seated and the clinician faces the patient. The patients' wrist is in neutral and the clinician first palpates the scaphoid just at the base of the thumb. As the clinicians palpating finger moves medially a hollow dip is palpated just next to the scaphoid which is the lunate. Both sides are palpated and the clinician flexes both wrists of the patient in figure 17.4. The lunate becomes more prominent as the wrist is flexed. The side that shows less prominence on full wrist flexion is an anteriorly restricted lunate. An anterior dysfunction of the lunate can cause a stress on the scapholunate and lunate-capitate ligaments predisposing to a strain

ASSESSMENT OF RESTRICTION OF JOINT PLAY

Wrist Extension with Radial Deviation

The patient is seated and the clinician faces the hand to be examined. The patient pronates the forearm and extends the wrist. At about 60° of extension, the clinician observes for a radial deviation occurring at the wrist. Then the wrist is taken to neutral and the clinician grasps the triquetrum (with the pisiform) and the lunate, and glides it volarly and observes for restriction. Lastly, the wrist is in neutral and the radial and ulnar styloids are palpated. Now, the patient is asked to extend the wrist, and on terminal extension, the radius is felt to glide superiorly or in a cephalad direction (Fig. 17.5). Comparison is made with the other side to sense a dysfunction. Lack of radial deviation on extension, restriction of a volar glide of triquetrum and lunate and inadequate cephalad glide of radius indicates a dysfunction. This can predispose to a lateral elbow dysfunction.

Wrist Flexion with Ulnar Deviation

The reverse is tested. Dysfunction in mechanics may predispose to a medial and a possible posterior elbow dysfunction.

TREATMENT FOR SPECIFIC SOMATIC DYSFUNCTION

Radial Head Superior/Inferior

Superior Glide of the Radius

The patient is in a side lying position and the clinician faces the patient from the side to be treated with the patient's elbow flexed to 90 to 100°. The thenar eminence of the clinicians' hand contacts the thenar eminence of the patient (right thenar eminence contacts the right thenar eminence of the patient and vice versa). The clinicians' thumb is hooked around the thumb of the patient. The clinician then stabilizes the condyles of the humerus with the other hand and exerts an upward mobilization force on the radius as the radius terminates at the thenar eminence (Fig. 17.6). Wrist extension and elbow flexion should be maintained.

Inferior Glide of the Radius

The patient is in a side lying position and the clinician faces the patient from the side to be treated with the patient's elbow flexed to 45°. One hand of the clinician grasps the lower end of the radius, just above the wrist. The other hand stabilizes the upper arm at the midshaft of the humerus. A gentle distraction is applied at the lower end of the radius, while the other hand stabilizes and offers counter pressure for the distraction (Fig. 17.7). Elbow extension and wrist flexion are maintained.

Ulnar Styloid Posterior

The patient is lying supine with the elbow in extension and pronation. The thenar eminence of one hand of the clinician stabilizes the dorsum of the lower end of the radius, while the ulna is placed just a little outside the edge of the table. The thenar eminence of the other hand is placed on the dorsum of the lower end of the ulna. An

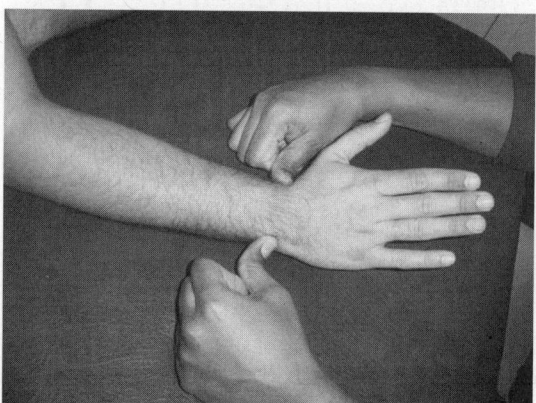

Fig. 17.5: Assessing restriction of joint play.

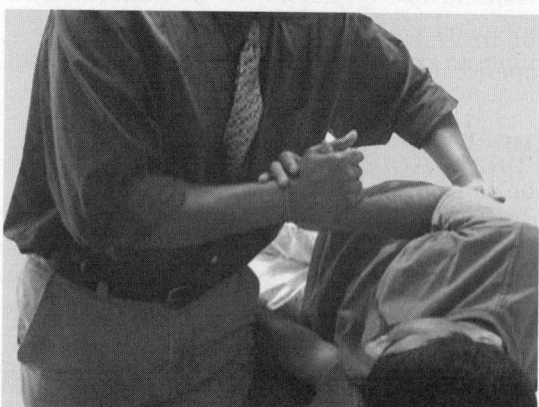

Fig. 17.6: Radius superior glide.

Wrist and Hand

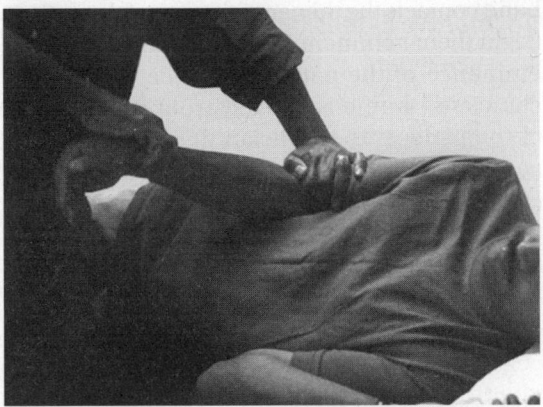

Fig. 17.7: Radius inferior glide.

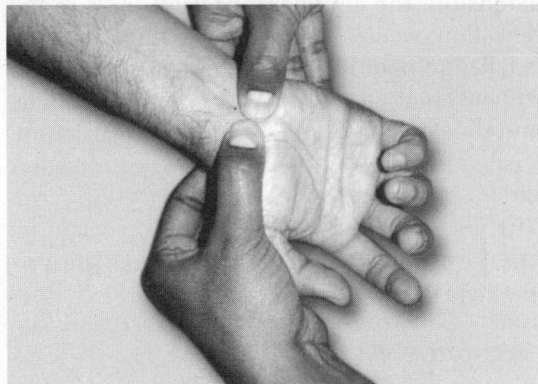

Fig. 17.9: Lunate posterior glide.

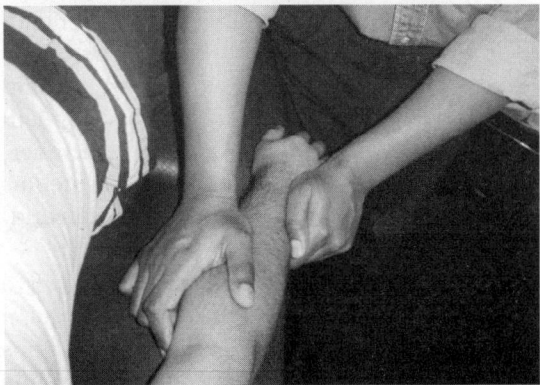

Fig. 17.8: Ulna styloid anterior glide.

inferiorly directed mobilization force is imparted on the ulna to glide it anteriorly (Fig. 17.8).

Positive Ulnar Variance

The treatment technique is as described for a superior dysfunction of the radius.

Lunate Anterior

The patient is seated and the clinician faces the patient's hand to be treated. The patients hand is in supination and the clinician palpates the pisiform on the ulnar border of the wrist. Moving laterally, the lunate is palpated and held by the thumb ventrally and the index/middle finger dorsally. A glide is imparted in a dorsal direction to glide the lunate posteriorly (Fig. 17.9).

Wrist Extension with Radial Deviation

This is done as a combination of a cephalic motion of the radius as described for an inferior radial dysfunction. This is followed by a technique similar to an anterior lunate dysfunction, except that the lunate is glided in a volar direction. A similar procedure is applied to the triquetrum, just medial to the lunate.

In addition, the radiocarpal joint is distracted and the distal row of carpal bones are glided in a dorsal direction. The proximal row of carpal bones are glided in a volar and ulnar direction.

Wrist Flexion with Ulnar Deviation

The exact reverse of the above is done to improve wrist flexion with ulnar deviation.

TREATMENT FOR OVERALL IMPROVEMENT IN RANGE OF MOTION[4,12] (TJP: TRACTION AND PASSIVE GLIDING)

Radiocarpal Joint

To Improve Wrist Flexion

- Radiocarpal distraction
- Radiocarpal dorsal glide
- Midcarpal volar glide
- Caudal movement of radius.

To Improve Wrist Extension

- Radiocarpal distraction
- Radiocarpal volar glide
- Midcarpal dorsal glide
- Cephalad movement of radius.

To Improve Radial Deviation

Radiocarpal distraction with ulnar glide of proximal row.

To Improve Ulnar Deviation

Radiocarpal distraction with radial glide of proximal row (Fig. 17.10).

Metacarpophalangeal Joints

To Improve Flexion

- Distraction rotation
- Volar glide
- Medial/lateral glides.

To Improve Extension

- Distraction rotation
- Dorsal glide
- Medial/lateral glides

PIP/DIP Joints

To improve flexion
- Distraction
- Volar glide
- Medial/lateral glide.

To Improve Extension

- Distraction
- Dorsal glide
- Medial/lateral glide.

TECHNIQUE

Radiocarpal Joint

Radiocarpal Distraction

The patient is seated with the hand resting on the treatment table or wedge and the clinician is facing the arm to be treated. One arm of the clinician grips and stabilizes the distal radius and ulna, while the other hand grips the proximal row of carpal bones. While stabilizing the radius and ulna, the other hand exerts a long axis distraction (Fig. 17.11).

Radiocarpal dorsal glide (pisiform, triquetrum, lunate, scaphoid/lunate and scaphoid mainly): The patient is seated with the forearm supinated and the hand resting on the treatment table or on a wedge and the clinician is facing the arm to be treated. The wedge is at the level of the radial and ulnar styloid. One arm of the clinician grips and stabilizes the distal radius and ulna, while the other hand grips the proximal row of carpal bones. While stabilizing the radius and ulna, the other hand exerts a dorsal glide in the inferior direction (Fig. 17.12).

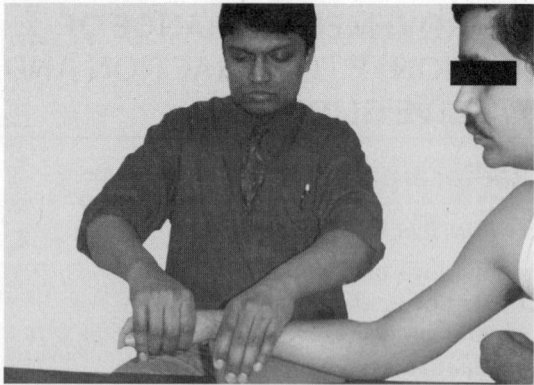

Fig. 17.10: Radiocarpal ulnar and radial glide.

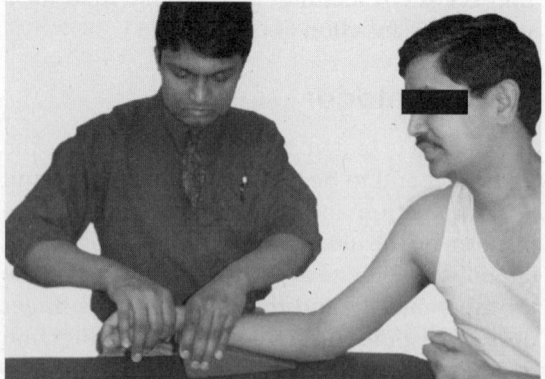

Fig. 17.11: Radiocarpal distraction.

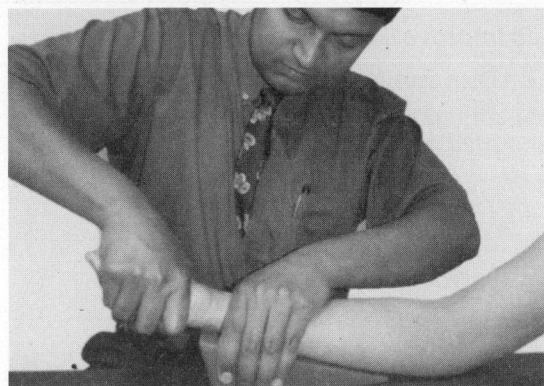

Fig. 17.12: Radiocarpal dorsal glide.

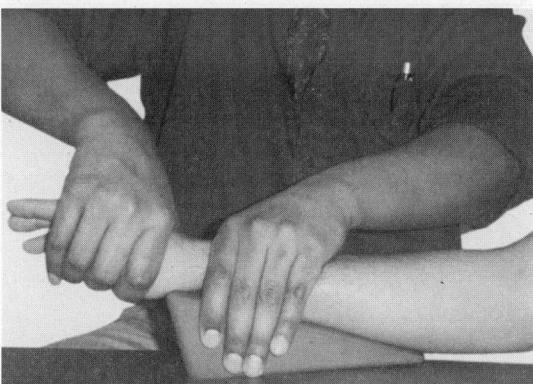

Fig. 17.13: Midcarpal volar glide.

Midcarpal volar glide (trapezium, trapezoid, capitate, hamate): The patient is seated with the forearm pronated and resting on the treatment table or on a wedge. The proximal row of carpal bones are resting on the edge of the table or on a wedge. The distal row (midcarpal) consists of the trapezium, trapezoid placed laterally and capitate, hamate are placed medially. One arm of the clinician grips and stabilizes the distal radius and ulna, while the other hand grips the distal row of carpal bones. While stabilizing the radius and ulna, the other hand exerts a volar glide in the inferior direction (Fig. 17.13).

Caudal/Cephalad Movement of Radius

Refer Chapter 16 for details on this technique.

Radiocarpal volar glide (pisiform, triquetrum, lunate, scaphoid/lunate and scaphoid mainly): The patient is seated with the forearm pronated and the hand resting on the treatment table or wedge and the clinician is facing the arm to be treated. The wedge is at the level of the radial and ulnar styloid. One arm of the clinician grips and stabilizes the distal radius and ulna, while the other hand grips the proximal row of carpal bones. While stabilizing the radius and ulna, the other hand exerts a volar glide in the inferior direction (Fig. 17.14).

Midcarpal dorsal glide (trapezium, trapezoid, capitate, hamate): The patient is seated with the forearm supinated and resting on the treatment

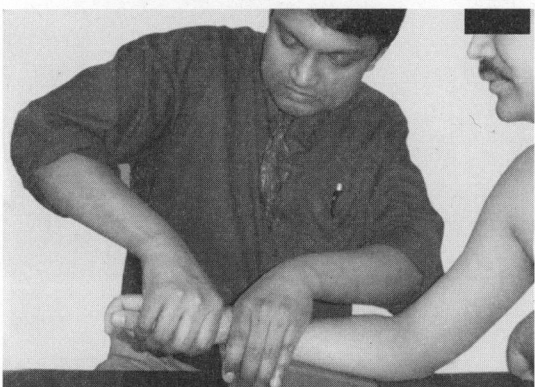

Fig. 17.14: Radiocarpal volar glide.

table or on a wedge. The proximal row of carpal bones are resting on the edge of the table or on a wedge. The distal row (midcarpal) consists of the trapezium, trapezoid placed laterally and the capitate, hamate are placed medially. One arm of the clinician grips and stabilizes the distal radius and ulna, while the other hand grips the distal row of carpal bones. While stabilizing the radius and ulna, the other hand exerts a dorsal glide in the inferior direction (Fig. 17.15).

Ulnar and Radial Glide of Proximal Row

The patient/clinician and hand position are the same as for distraction. Stabilizing the distal radius and ulna, the other hand grips the proximal row of carpal bones and applies a long axis distraction. It then glides it in an ulnar and radial direction, in the direction of the little finger.

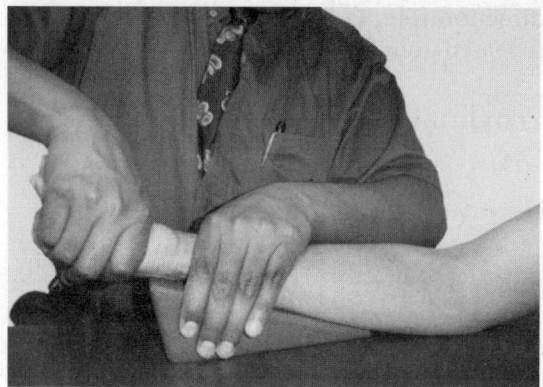

Fig. 17.15: Midcarpal dorsal glide.

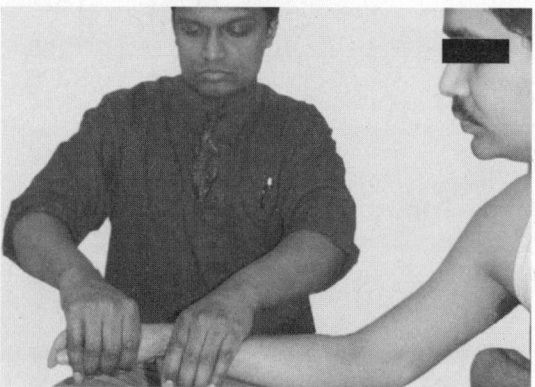

Fig. 17.16: Proximal row ulnar and radial glide.

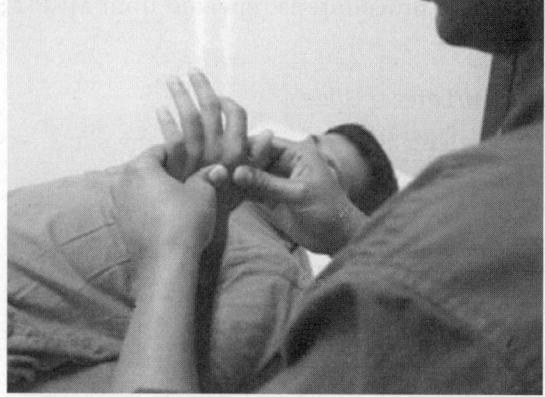

Fig. 17.17: Intermetacarpal and intercarpal joints.

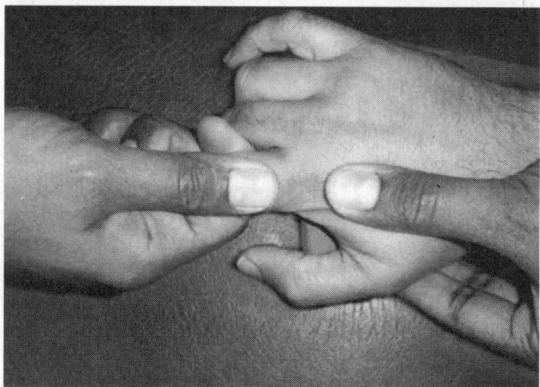

Fig. 17.18: Metacarpophalangeal distraction and rotation.

Note that the movement is in a semicircular arc and not in a straight plane (Fig. 17.16).

Intermetacarpal and Intercarpal Joints

The patient is in supine lying or sitting and the clinician faces the patient. The clinician grips either metatarsal heads and glides them in an anterior/posterior direction to mobilize the intermetacarpal joints. Gliding the intercarpal joints is similar to gliding the lunate in the section 'lunate anterior'. However, the clinician takes time to glide all the carpal bones individually. Joint play of the intermetacarpal and intercarpal joints which are essential for overall improvement of wrist mobility (Fig. 17.17).

Metacarpophalangeal Joints

Distraction and Rotation

The patient is seated with the arm resting on the treatment table. On hand of the clinician grips and stabilizes the metacarpal, while the other hand grips the proximal phalanx. While the metacarpal is stabilized, the other hand exerts a long axis distraction through the proximal phalanx. Then it is gently rotated in and out as in a wringing motion (Fig. 17.18).

Volar Glide

The patient/clinician and hand positions are the same as for a distraction. Stabilizing the metacarpal bone, the proximal phalanx is distracted and glided in an inferior direction (Fig. 17.19).

The same procedure is repeated from MCP 1 through 5.

Medial/Lateral Glides

The patient/clinician position is the same as for distraction but the hand position is moved to the medial and lateral aspect of the proximal phalanx. Stabilizing the metacarpal bone, proximal phalanx is distracted and glided in a medial and lateral direction (Fig. 17.20).

Dorsal Glide

The patient/clinician and hand positions are the same as for a distraction excepting that the palmar surface of the hand is facing up. Stabilizing the metacarpal bone, the proximal phalanx is distracted and glided in an inferior direction (Fig. 17.21). The same procedure is repeated from MCP 1 through 5.

Proximal Interphalangeal Joint/ Distal Interphalangeal Joint

Distraction and Rotation

The procedure is the same as for an MCP distraction except that the proximal phalanx is stabilized, while the distal phalanx is distracted (Fig. 17.22).

Volar glide: The procedure is the same as for a volar glide of the MCP except that the proximal phalanx is stabilized, while the distal phalanx is distracted and glided inferior (Fig. 17.23).

Medial/lateral glides: The procedure is the same as for a medial/lateral glide of the MCP except

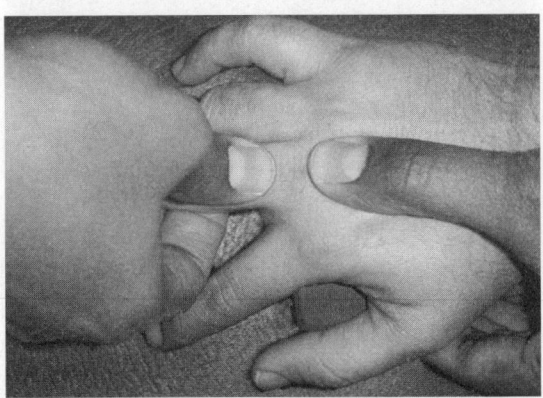

Fig. 17.19: Metacarpophalangeal volar glide.

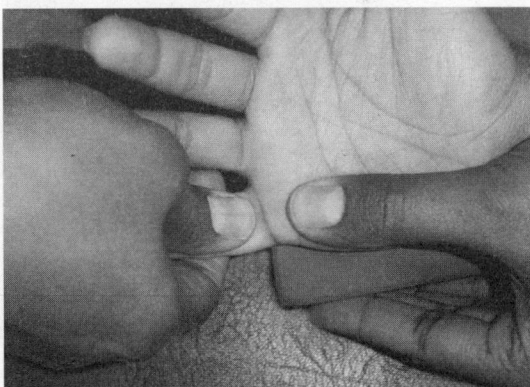

Fig. 17.21: Metacarpophalangeal dorsal glide.

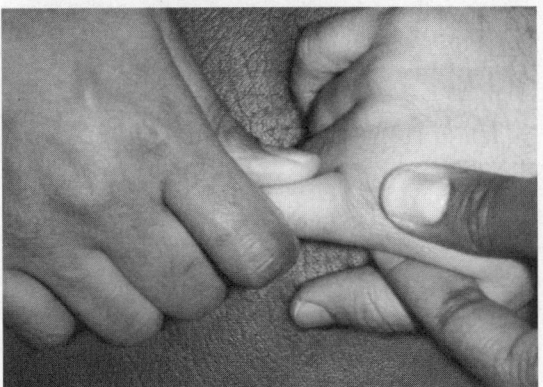

Fig. 17.20: Metacarpophalangeal medial/lateral glide.

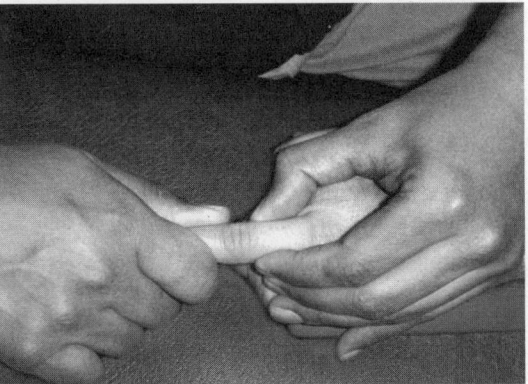

Fig. 17.22: PIP/DIP distraction and rotation lateral hold.

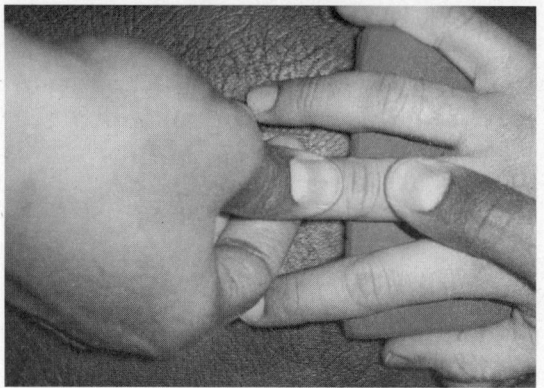

Fig. 17.23: PIP/DIP volar glide.

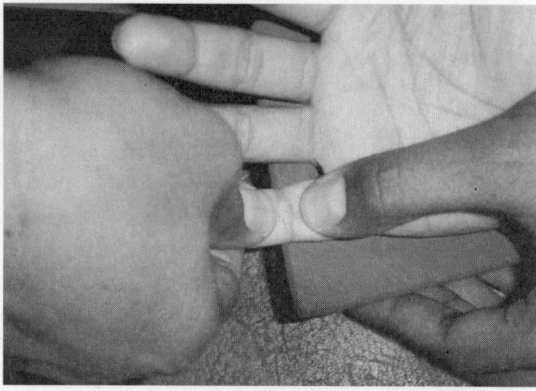

Fig. 17.25: PIP/DIP dorsal glide.

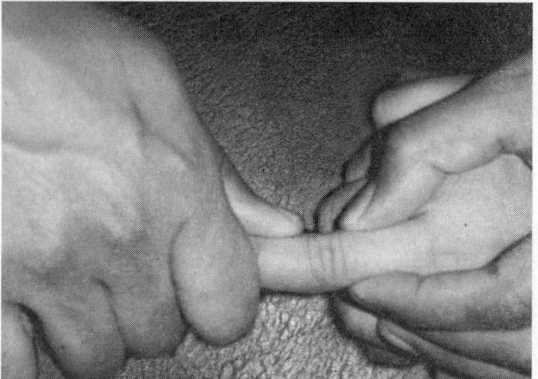

Fig. 17.24: PIP/DIP medial/lateral glide.

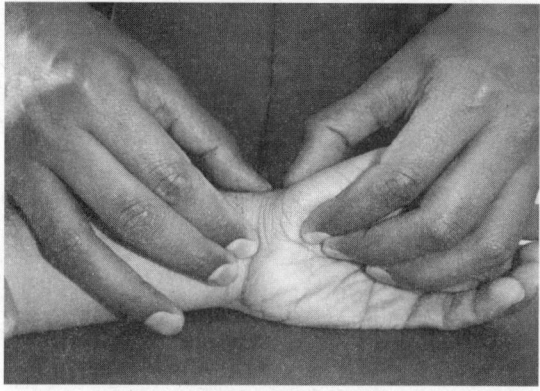

Fig. 17.26: CMC palmar glide.

that the proximal phalanx is stabilized and the distal phalanx is distracted and glided medial/lateral (Fig. 17.24).

Dorsal glide: The procedure is the same as for a volar glide of the MCP except that with the palmar surface facing up the proximal phalanx is stabilized, while the distal phalanx is distracted and glided inferior (Fig. 17.25).

Carpometacarpal Joints

Palmar Glide Parallel to Palm

The patient is seated with the hand to be treated in the midprone position. The thumb and index finger of the clinician grips the trapezium. The thumb and index finger of the other hand grips the first metacarpal. The first metacarpal is then glided across the palm for flexion and away from the palm for extension (Fig. 17.26).

Palmar Glide at Right Angles to the Palm

The patient is seated with the hand to be treated in a semisupinated position. The thumb and index finger of the clinician grips the trapezium. The thumb and index finger of the other hand grips the first metacarpal. The first metacarpal is then glided into the palm for abduction and at right angles away from the palm for adduction (Fig. 17.27). The thumb position should be more proximal and is shown more distal for ease of illustration.

PROPHYLAXIS

Exercise prescription for the elbow, forearm, wrist and hand is more pathology specific rather than mechanical dysfunction specific. At the elbow and forearm the muscles that require attention are:

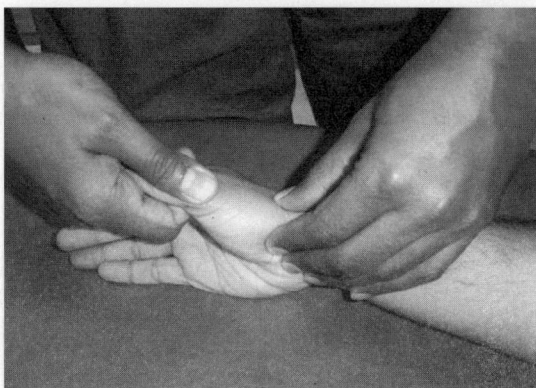

Fig. 17.27: CMC palmar glide (metacarpal hold should be more proximal).

- Triceps brachii
- Biceps brachii
- Supinator
- Flexor carpi ulnaris
- Pronator teres.

These muscles are commonly dysfunctional and should be addressed according to the pathology. Hence as being pathology specific, they may require stretching, strengthening or myofibrillar mobilization as appropriate.

The interosseous membrane is yet another structure that requires attention. The radius and ulna have the capability of rolling inwards and outwards and the interosseous membrane has a tendency to tighten and prevent this motion.

At the level of the elbow are the muscles that act on the wrist, which includes the common flexor and extensor origin. At the common extensor origin, the muscles that require attention are:

- Extensor carpi radialis brevis
- Extensor carpi radialis longus
- Extensor digitorum.

The flexor carpi ulnaris at the common flexor origin requires attention in a medial elbow dysfunction. Again, exercise management is pathology specific and the muscles may be stretched or strengthened as appropriate including myofibrillar mobilization of the MTPs.

The wrist and hand are obviously more complex in their musculature. As in the elbow, management is more pathology specific rather than mechanical dysfunction specific. The structures that require attention are:

- Flexor digitorum superficialis
- Flexor digitorum profundus
- Flexor digiti minimi
- Lumbricals
- Interossei
- Abductor pollicis longus
- Extensor pollicis brevis
- Extensor pollicis longus.

Overall, the muscles of the forearm, wrist and hand are more susceptible to neural, avulsion and anatomical disruption type of injuries. From a somatic dysfunction perspective, their vulnerability is relatively lesser. Hence the reason for exercise prescription being more pathology oriented rather than from a mechanical dysfunction perspective.

The other area to be considered in management, as in the ankle and foot are corrective orthotics. Appropriate splinting should be advocated be it static or dynamic to address dysfunction. This being a very elaborate topic warrants further reading but definitely a strategy worth considering.

MYOFASCIAL TENDER POINTS

The concept of addressing myofascial tender points is to decrease actin and myosin crossbridging and myofibrillar restriction. Their continual presence may encourage chemical accumulation, early fatigue and decreased muscle performance with accompanying pain and dysfunction. They may be best treated with frictions and electrotherapy. Tender points secondary to aberrant gamma efferents may require an alternate positional release approach and the reader is encouraged further reading in the area of 'strain counterstrain' methods. The figure illustrate some common dysfunctional points of the wrist and hand (Fig. 17.28).

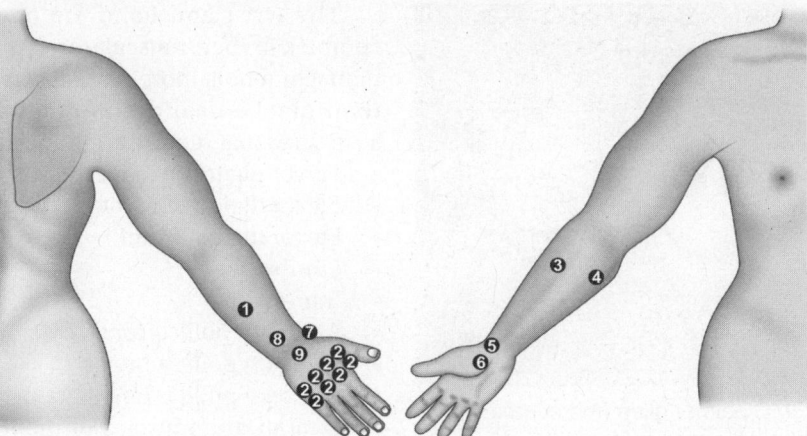

Fig. 17.28: Myofascial tender points: Wrist and hand (posterior) 1. Extensor digitorum; 2. Dorsal interrossei; 3. Brachioradialis; 4. Flexor carpi ulnaris; 5. Abductor pollicis brevis; 6. Adductor pollicis; 7. Abductor pollicis longus\extensor pollicis brevis, extensor pollicis longus (dequervain's); 8. Abductor pollicis longus, extensor carpi radialis longus and brevis (intersection syndrome); 9. Scapholunate ligament.

REFERENCES

1. Magee DJ. Orthopedic Physical Assessment, 4th edn, 2002. WB Saunders, Philadelphia.
2. Norris CM. The Knee. In: Norris CM. Sports Injuries: Diagnosis and management for physiotherapists 1993. Butterworth-Heinemann, Oxford, pp:169-192.
3. Poole BC. Cumulative trauma disorder of the upper extremity from occupational stress. J Hand Ther. 1988;1:172-80.
4. Patla CE, Paris SV. EI Course Notes: Extremity Evaluation and manipulation. 1996. St. Auguatine, Institute press.
5. Zong-Ming Lia, Laurel Kuxhausa, Jesse A. Fiskb, et al. Coupling between wrist flexion-extension and radial–ulnar deviation. Clinical Biomech (Bristol Avon). 2205;20:177-83.
6. Conwell HE. Injuries to the wrist. Clin Symp. 1982;22(1):14.
7. Viegas SF. Trigger thumb of de Quervain's disease. J Hand Surg Am. 1986;11:235-7.
8. Nakano KK, et al. Anterior interosseous nerve syndrome. Arch Neurol. 1977;34:477.
9. Werner CO, et al. Clinical and neurophysiological characteristics of the pronator syndrome. Clin Orthop. 1985;197:231-36.
10. Wadsworth C. Peripheral nerve compression neuropathies. Home study course 97-2. Orthopedic Section, American Physical Therapy Association.
11. Nugent K. Nerve injuries of the upper extremity. Orth Phys Ther Clinics of North Am. 2001;10:635-48.
12. Kaltenborn F. Mobilization of the extremity joints: Examination and basic treatment techniques, 3rd edn, 1980, Olaf Norlis Bokhandel Universitetsgaten, Oslo, Norway.

PART 2

A Manual Therapy Approach to Mechanical Peripheral Nerve Entrapment Dysfunction

Chapter 18: Introduction
Chapter 19: Relevant Anatomy
Chapter 20: Understanding Mechanical Nerve Dysfunction
Chapter 21: Examination
Chapter 22: Treatment

CHAPTER 18

Introduction

Peripheral nerve injury is an entity that is commonly encountered by physical therapists in their day-to-day practice. The scope of management would be to rely on the medical model to determine the type and status of the injury depending on the extent of disruption of nerve tissue and the resultant sequelae from a motor and functional perspective. Essentially then diagnostic determinants are based on the classification by Seddon[1] and are as follows:
- Neurapraxia
- Axonotmesis
- Neurotmesis

The first category is referred to the physical therapist for the most part and of a lesser prevalence category two. Category three is invariably a surgical referral. In any given situation there is an obvious functional loss by the time the patient is on your treatment table, say a 'foot drop' or a 'wrist drop'. Pain as the main entity, without obvious functional loss may not be considered from a neural perspective. It is usually seen as a global neuro-orthopedic entity as in 'cervical spondylosis with radiculopathy' or 'sciatica'.

The bigger focus in this literature review is 'pain' and the neural determinants of pain, hence the diagnostic criteria may not follow the Seddon classification. Rather the pathologies of reference are *preneuropraxic* and 'pain' invariably being a bigger factor than 'motor loss'.

As physical therapists, we are most concerned about movement and we aim to treat pathologic motion. We apply this sound conceptual basis to the musculoskeletal system and call it biomechanics for normal movement and pathomechanics for abnormal motion. Can the peripheral neural system be considered a movable system and can the above concepts be applied to it? Most certainly and the concept long described. The pioneers in this field call it neurodynamics and are principally concerned about the movement of peripheral neural tissue.[2]

As our body moves, and along with it the extremities, the soft tissue including muscle fascia and ligaments modify their length to adapt for the movement changes. The peripheral nerves that traverse the extremities will hence also have to modify their length to adapt for the length changes with movement. It is obvious then that a certain amount of gliding occurs in these nerves and this helps to adapt for the changes in length. Hence, the postulation is from the origin of the nerve in the spinal cord to its termination, it has to traverse through connective tissue, bone, muscle and fascia which may be in the form of fibro-osseous tunnels, and these are the milieu through which they glide. They may hence, due to faulty mechanics and dysfunctional states, be entrapped in these areas that they traverse through and result in pathology. The chemical effusion that results from dysfunctional states of the mileu has also been considered as added predisposition to dysfunction and pain.[3] We call this an external entrapment. In addition the nerve can experience entrapment in the individual nerve fascicles which would also result in dysfunction. This would constitute an internal entrapment.

Mechanical extremity nerve pain has been traditionally viewed as originating from abnormal changes in the spinal canal. The most common described causes are herniations of the nucleus pulposis, degenerative spinal and foraminal stenosis, fractures and spondylolisthesis. The term mechanical implies pathology of a neuromusculoskeletal origin rather than a disease process as in neurilemomas, anerysms, tumors, hematomas, diabetes, etc. However, contemporary research has shown that radicular pain may not necessarily occur secondary to changes within the spine.[4] Nerve irritation that occur outside the spine are called extraspinal lesions. When a detail clinical and radiological investigation rules out the possible existence of a nonmechanical cause (tumors, abscesses, nerve disease, etc.) for nerve pain, the situation may leave the clinician to investigate the possible mechanical origin of the pain. Standard examination procedures however, aim at identifying a spinal origin for the symptoms, unfortunately though, a variety of possible extraspinal causes may exist. These extraspinal sites of nerve irritation may be bone, muscle, fascia, and ligaments that the nerve glides through following its exit at the vertebral foramen. Awareness of this fact is mandatory as mechanical radicular pain in the extremities, by default, are assumed to be of a spinal origin. Indeed, most often it is the case, but what if not. Newer research has made it easier by the application of clinical prediction rules, as in a cluster of tests to identify the presence of pain of a spinal origin.[5] If symptoms are not modified or altered by the application of this cluster of tests, then the assumption is made that the pain is not of a spinal origin. However, it is considered astute to prioritize the possibility of a spinal origin of symptoms and hence careful examination is warranted.

A collective description of spinal and extraspinal mechanical causes of radicular pain in the spine and extremity may enable the clinician to make a differential diagnosis and arrive at a more specific conclusion as to the site of irritation. This literature review aims to collectively describe the possible spinal and extraspinal causes of radicular pain which are of a mechanical origin to enable the clinician to make a more accurate diagnosis and help avoid unnecessary and expensive diagnostic and surgical procedures.

REFERENCES

1. Kaye Andrew H. Essential Neurosurgery, 1991, Churchill Livingstone. pp. 333-4.
2. Nee RJ, Butler D. Management of peripheral neuropathic pain: integrating neurobiology, neurodynamics, and clinical evidence: Physical Therapy in Sport. 2006;2:36-49.
3. Takahashi N, Yabuki S, Aoki Y, et al. Pathomechanisms of nerve root injury caused by disk herniation: an experimental study of mechanical compression and chemical irritation. Spine. 2003;28:435-41.
4. Lewis AM, Layzer R, Engstrom JW, et al. Magnetic resonance neurography in extraspinal sciatica. Arch Neurol. 2006;63:1469-72.
5. Wainner RS, Fritz JM, Irrgang JJ, et al. Reliability and diagnostic accuracy of the clinical examination and patient self-report measures for cervical radiculopathy. Spine. 2003;28:52-62.

CHAPTER
19

Relevant Anatomy

INTRODUCTION

The nervous system is broadly divided into three parts, central, peripheral (which consists of the 31 pairs of spinal nerves, and the 12 pairs of cranial nerves) and autonomic. The description herein is mainly the peripheral nervous system comprising the spinal nerves which originate from the spinal cord.

The spinal nerves originate from the spinal cord as two roots, anterior (ventral) root and posterior (dorsal) root. The ventral root carries motor impulses and dorsal root carries sensory impulses. These two nerve roots joint to form the mixed spinal nerve. Just short of joining together is a small bulbous structure in the sensory posterior dorsal root called the dorsal root ganglion (DRG). The cell bodies of sensory nerves that convey somatosensory information to the brain are found in the dorsal root ganglion. These somatosensory neurons are unipolar, where the axon splits in two and sends one branch to the sensory receptor and the other to the brain for processing. The cell bodies found in the dorsal root ganglia are mostly somatosensory, but other sensory representations also occur. This part of the peripheral nervous system is encased in the spinal canal of the vertebral bodies. The mixed spinal nerve exits from the bony spinal canal through the intervertebral foramen. The nerve at this time is divided into two parts:
1. Anterior (ventral) primary ramus.
2. Posterior (dorsal) primary ramus.

It is the anterior primary ramus that has received most of the attention as these are the structures that form the peripheral nerves. However, the posterior primary ramus which is the beginning to receive attention has a complex innervation and knowledge of its anatomy is required to understand the complexity of pain patterns arising from nerve irritation at the intervertebral foramen.[1] The anterior primary ramus being the actual peripheral nerve is what is being described first, upon exit from the intervertebral foramen (Fig. 19.1).

Upon thus exiting from the spine (intervertebral foramen), the nerve root forms the nerve plexus and nerve trunk. In the nerve plexus, these nerves decide on their respective destinations and emerge as single nerves to run towards their single area of supply. These single isolated nerves are the peripheral nerves whose disturbance in conduction and function are seen as nerve pathologies in our day-to-day practice.

The posterior primary ramus as it travels out of the spine first sends a supply to the facet joint above the level it emerges from. It then supplies the multifidus muscle and later its medial branch supplies the facet capsule and then the facet joint below the level it emerges from. In communication with the gray ramus communicans, it forms the sinuvertebral nerve and supplies the posterior longitudinal ligament, posterolateral disk, ligamentum flavum and the facet joint at the same level. Hence, it should be understood that although we are concerned

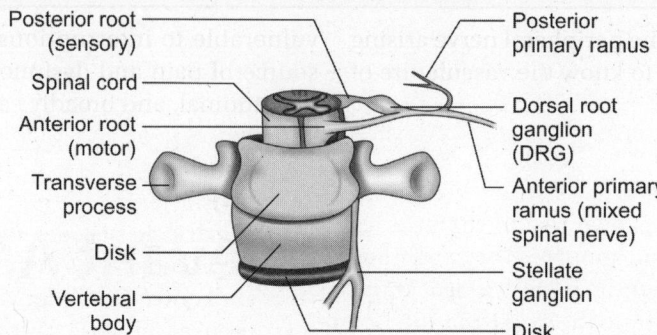

Fig. 19.1: Illustration of vertebral body, spinal cord and spinal nerve (anterior view).

about the anterior primary ramus and the peripheral nerve arising from it, the complex innervation of the other structures including posterior primary ramus (which together supply three levels of the facet same above and below) can make pain presentation appear more complex.[1]

STRUCTURE OF A PERIPHERAL NERVE[2]

The nerve cell and its process is the basic structural and functional unit of the nervous system and is called the neurone with the axon. It is embedded in the axoplasm. An axon is the peripheral extension from the nerve cell. They are surrounded by individual Schwann cells arranged in a longitudinal continuous chain forming myelinated nerve fibers. Lying next to the myelinated nerve are many nonmyelinated fibers associated with one Schwann cell. These myelinated and nonmyelinated nerve fibers are organized into bundles called fascicles and are surrounded by a strong membrane called *perineurium*. They consist of laminae of flattened cells. The fascicles are organized in groups held together by a loose connective tissue called *epineurium*. Surrounding the Schwann cells is a collagenous basement membrane which is surrounded by the innermost connective tissue layer called *endoneurium*.

The epineurium is the outermost layer of the nerve and consists of connective tissue to offer cushioning. Apparently, the quantity of connective tissue components may vary depending on their location (superficial or deep), probably as a response to loading. For example, nerves located superficially or close to a joint may contain a greater quantity of connective tissue possibly as a response to repeated loading. The other important aspect of the epineurium is the presence of a highly structured vascular system which is important for the well-being of the nerve.

The perineurium is the next layer and are seen as coverings for the fascicles seen within the epineurium. The perineurium provides protection to the endoneurial contents and has an important role in maintaining the osmotic milieu. It also helps to protect the contents of the nerve from chemical and bacterial invasion.

The endoneurium are the contents of the fascicles that the perineurium surrounds. It helps in the maintenance of endoneurial space and fluid pressure. The cellular components are of the endoneurium are bathed in the endoneurial fluid.

NERVE VASCULARITY

The knowledge of the vascular system is important to know the basis of symptoms as most nerve pain is secondary to the interruption of the flow of blood resulting in nerve ischemia. Normal blood flow is also essential for energy supply for nerve conduction and for the intracellular movement of the cytoplasm of the neurone. Since the peripheral nervous system concerns the spinal cord and the peripheral nerve arising from it, it is of value to know the vasculature of the spinal cord first.

Spinal Cord

The vertebral arteries give rise to the arteries important to the blood supply of the cord. They are anterior and posterior spinal arteries. About 75% of the blood supply to the cord is via anterior spinal artery. These arteries however supply the superior portion of the cord. The rest of the cord is dependent on the supply from the segmental medullary and radicular arteries.

The segmental medullary (anterior and posterior) and radicular (dorsal and ventral) are derived from the ascending cervical, deep cervical, posterior intercostals and lumbar arteries. The medullary arteries reinforce the anterior and posterior spinal arteries. They primarily provide additional vascularization to the cord. The radicular arteries, hence, are the most relevant as far as the blood supply to the nerve root and subsequently nerve.

Nerve Root

The blood supply to the nerve root is by the 'radicular arteries' that supply the major longitudinal vessels of the cord. The nerve roots contain fascicles within them which slide on each other during movement and hence a compensatory adaptation may be required. Alongside the fascicles, a major longitudinal radicular artery is accompanied by the several collateral radicular arteries which give rise to interfascicular branches. These interfascicular branches may be stretched due to gliding fascicular motion. This increase in length is accommodated by 'compensating coils' which adapt for the change in length.

Peripheral Nerve

The vasculature of the peripheral nerve is considered to be well developed probably due to the increased mobility demands. They are vulnerable to interruptions in flow and are a source of pain and dysfunction. The supply is longitudinal, and broadly categorized into two, namely:
1. Extrinsic
2. Intrinsic

The extrinsic system run longitudinally and has several conections to the intrinsic supply by what are known as 'feeder vessels'. The extrinsic (extraneural vessel) communicates with the epineurium via the feeder vessels. They form the external part of the extrinsic vessel in the epineurium. They travel further inward to form the inner intrinsic plexus.

The epineurium is the outermost part of the nerve and hence the first to be compromised by external pressure. Thus when the nerve passes through the fibro-osseous tunnels in order to protect the nerve the epineurium is thickened.

AXONAL TRANSPORT

All cells have a cytoplasm where its constituents like mitochondria, synaptic vescicles and other cytopasmic constituents travel to and fro from the cell body. This process is known as axonal transport.

It is important to know that the axon contains 100 times the volume of the cell body but no protein synthesis takes place in them. Only the cell body and proximal dentrites contain ribosomes, the structures that manufacture proteins. These proteins that are required for neurotransmitters and membrane repair, and some lipids are routinely transported from the cell body down the length of the axon to maintain axon function. If there is deprivation of proteins due to injury, the segment distal to it will degenerate.

There are two types of axonal tansport, namely:
1. Anterograde (away from the cell body)
2. Retrograde (towards the cell body)

The speed at which anterograde transport systems function vary. Rapid transport carries neurotransmitter and transmitter/synaptic vesicles. Speeds are approximately 400 mm/day.

Slow transport carries soluble enzymes and structural proteins (microtubule, tubulin). Speed are about 1-6 mm/day.

The rate of retrograde transport is about 200 mm/day. It is important as it regulates the metabolism of the cell. In a cut axon, the signal for chromatolysis is carried by retrograde transport. Also, neurotropic viruses infect the cell body by retrograde transport (polio, herpes, rabies, etc.)

Knowledge of axonal transport is important for the physical therapist as axonal transport is dependent on vascularity and mobility. Hence, restoring nerve mobility may have an effect on the flow of blood and axoplasm which is essential for normal functioning of the nerve.

CLINICALLY RELEVANT PERIPHERAL NERVE ANATOMY

Radicular pain in the lower is defined as the pain radiating down arm or leg in a specific pattern secondary to nerve root compression. It is also defined as the pain experienced along the dermatome of a nerve due to pressure on the nerve. If a patient complains of such pain we generally think of the nerve root compression at the level of spine. However, as earlier mentioned, the nerve can be entrapped in interfaces it traverses through its course producing identical symptoms. This literature review enumerates the extra spinal causes of nerve compression in its course which produces similar pattern of pain which is often mistaken as compression of the nerve at the root level in the spine. A good understanding of the relevant anatomy may be necessary to comprehend such a speculation.

The Lower Limb[3]

Iliohypogastric Nerve

Course: The nerve arises from the ventral primary rami of L1 and occasionally from T12. It travels through the psoas major, lateral abdominal wall and penetrates the transverse abdominal muscle.

Structures supplied: The nerve supplies the lower fibers of the transverse abdominus and internal oblique. The distribution of the cutaneous sensation is a small region just superior to the pubis.

Entrapment etiopathology: The most common cause for entrapment is scar formation secondary to surgeries. Blunt trauma of the lower abdominals by contact sports, large abdomen and pregnancy are other causes. Palpation of the scar may elicit tenderness and reproduce pain in the inguinal and suprapubic area. If the cutaneous nerves are involved, radiation of symptoms into the genitalia is seen.

Ilioinguinal Nerve

Course: Arises from the T12 and L1 nerve roots and emerges from the lateral border of the psoas muscle and traverses the anterior abdominal wall to the iliac crest. This nerve passes through the internal oblique and transversus abdominus muscles.

Structures supplied: The nerve supplies the pubic symphysis, femoral triangle, penis and anterior scrotum in the male and the mons pubis and labia majora in the female.

Entrapment etiopathology: Same as the iliohypogastric nerve.

Genitofemoral Nerve

Course: It arises from the L1 and L2 ventral primary rami, passes through the psoas muscle and then splits into the genital branch and femoral branch.

Structures supplied: The genital branch supplies the cremaster muscle, spermatic cord, scrotum, and medial upper thigh in males and the labia majora and medial upper thigh in the females.

Entrapment etiopathology: Same as the iliohypogastric and ilioinguinal nerves, however, injury to this nerve is rare. Anterior thigh pain and groin pain are the symptoms mostly reported. Movements of the hip in rotation may also cause pain.

Lateral Femoral Cutaneous Nerve

Course: It arises from the L2-L3 nerve roots and divides into anterior and posterior branches. Fusion of the dorsal part forms the lateral femoral cutaneous nerve and this occurs in the region of the midpelvis. The nerve then courses over the iliacus toward the anterior superior iliac spine (ASIS), travels posterior to the inguinal ligament and superior to the sartorius muscle. The nerve then divides into anterior and posterior branches which later communicate with the patellar plexus.

Structures supplied: Lateral thigh just proximal to the patella and the skin from the greater trochanter to the midthigh.

Entrapment etiopathology: This nerve may be compressed under the inguinal ligament and sartorius muscle secondary to pressure and tight garments. Other causes for entrapment are diabetes, growths, fibroids and diverticulitis. Patients present with pain in the anterolateral thigh with burning and tingling which increases with standing and walking. Symptoms may be reproduced by pressure over the medial aspect of the ASIS and over the origin of the sartorius. This entrapment syndrome is described as 'meralgia paresthetica' (Fig. 19.2).

Femoral Nerve

Course: It arises from the posterior divisions of the ventral primary rami of L2, L3, and L4 within the psoas major muscle and passes between the psoas and iliacus muscle. It then passes under the inguinal ligament and divides into sensory branches in the proximal thigh which is the lateral femoral cutaneous nerve. It also divides into the medial femoral cutaneous nerve which ultimately communicates with the saphenous nerve.

Structures Supplied: It inervates the upper and anterior thigh and muscular branches to the quadriceps muscle. One of the major branches is the lateral femoral cutaneous nerve as discussed above. It provides sensation to the anteromedial thigh and patella area.

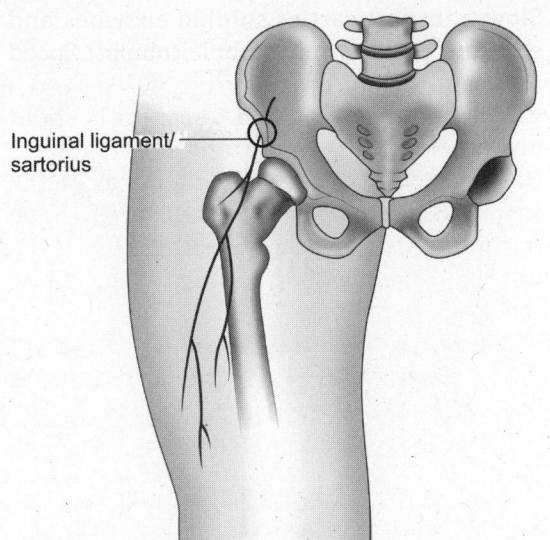

Fig. 19.2: Lateral femoral cutaneous nerve.

Entrapment etiopathology: The most common site of entrapment is below the inguinal ligament and hence dysfunctions of the innominate or prolonged flexion, abduction, external rotation may cause entrapment (Fig. 19.3). The femoral nerve lacks protection close to the femoral head, tendon insertion of the vastus intermedius, psoas muscle and hip joint capsule. Hence, dysfunctional states of these structures can cause entrapment. Other causes for entrapment are pregnancy secondary to pressure from fetus, psoas abcesses and a prominent iliopectineal eminence. Patients present with anteromedial thigh pain with numbness and inguinal pain. If the saphenous nerve is involved, anteromedial knee pain may be present. Weakness of knee extension and hip flexion may depend on the severity of injury.

Saphenous Nerve

Course: It is a pure sensory nerve that arises from the L3 and L4 spinal segments. It enters the Hunter's canal in the distal third of the thigh between the vastus medialis obliquus (VMO) and adductors. The nerve may also pass through the sartorius muscle.

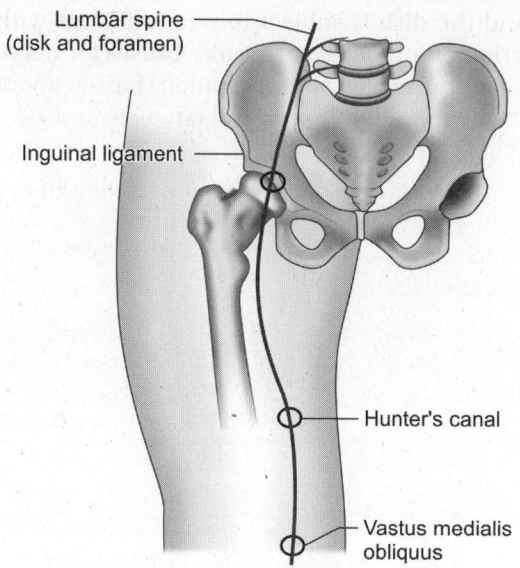

Fig. 19.3: Femoral and saphenous nerve.

Structures supplied: Offers sensory supply to the medial lower thigh and knee.

Entrapment etiopathology: This nerve can be entrapped in the Hunter's canal by dynamic muscle contractions of the VMO and adductors. Often, contusions to the medial thigh or medial knee surgeries also cause dysfunction. Patients present with pain in the thigh, knee pain about the infrapatellar region, and possibly paraesthesias in the leg and foot. Deep palpation over the medial aspect of the thigh and over the vastus medialis reproduces symptoms.

Obturator Nerve

Course: This nerve is formed by a fusion of the anterior branches of the anterior primary rami of L2, L3, and L4. It emerges from the medial border of the psoas and travels through the pelvis to enter the obturator foramen. Just prior to entering the thigh, the nerve divides into an anterior and posterior branch. The nerve passes through the pectineus, adductor longus and adductor brevis muscle. The nerve terminates at the distal aspect of the adductor longus and communicates with the anterior cutaneous branches of the femoral and saphenous nerves.

Structures supplied: It supplies the adductor brevis, adductor longus, and gracilis muscles. The skin of the medial and distal thigh region. It also supplies half of the adductor magnus.

Entrapment etiopathology: The obturator nerve can get entrapped as it passes through the adductor brevis, adductor magnus and pectineus. The obturator canal is an opening through which the obturator nerve and vessels pass from the pelvic cavity into the thigh (Fig. 19.4). Often times the nerve can get entrapped here secondary to surgery or arthroplasty. The main symptom is groin pain. Deep palpation may reveal tenderness and possibly reproduce symptoms.

Sciatic Nerve

Course: It originates from the nerve roots L4, L5, S1, S2, S3. It courses towards the pelvis through the iliolumbar ligament, anterior to the sacroiliac joint. It passes under the piriformis and exits through the sciatic notch. It rarely passes through the piriformis. It descends down the posterior lateral aspect of the thigh and above the knee divides into the tibial and common peroneal nerves (Fig. 19.5).

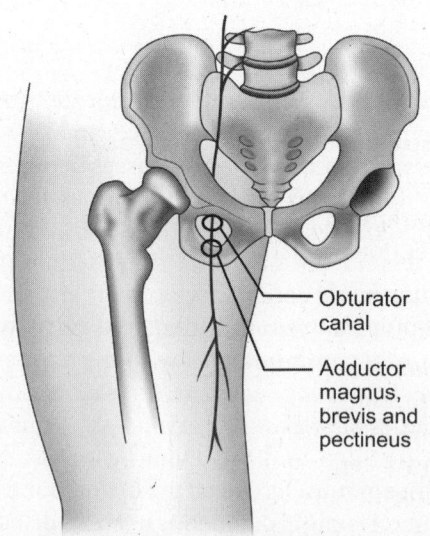

Fig. 19.4: Obturator nerve.

Relevant Anatomy

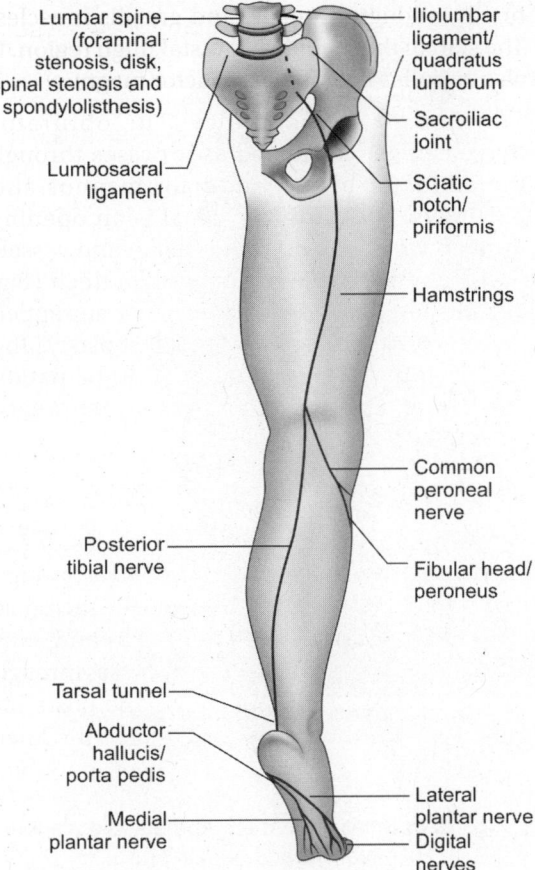

Fig. 19.5: Sciatic nerve and posterior branches.

Structures supplied: This nerve supplies the hamstrings and adductor magnus.

Entrapment etiopathology: The sciatic nerve can be entrapped the spine owing to the following conventional back dysfunctions.

Lumbar herniated disk: Herniation of the nucleus pulposis and secondary nerve irritation.

Lumbar stenosis: The spinal canal or the vertebral foramen may be narrowed secondary to degenerative changed and spur formation which causes a canal stenosis and entraps the nerve passing through.

Lumbar spondylosis/disk degeneration/facet syndrome: The facet joint being a synovial joint and the disk is subject to wear and tear with irritation of the facet capsule. Causes for nerve irritation maybe spur formation, narrowing of the intervertebral space and foramen, and effusion from the capsule.

Spondylolisthesis: Slippage of the body of the vertebra anteriorly secondary to a pars defect which narrows the spinal and foraminal canal irritating the nerve.

Quadratus lumborum syndrome: This condition occurs similar clinically to the Iliolumbar syndrome. The sciatic nerve is subject to entrapment here between iliac crest and the transverse processes of the L2-L5.

Iliolumbar syndrome: The sciatic nerve can get entrapped between the L5 transverse process and iliac crest. Occurs after strain injuries and present with pain and tenderness in the low back. Pain is worse bending away from the involved side. Examination reveals local tenderness at the insertion of the Iliolumbar ligament over the posterior iliac crest (Fig. 19.6).

Lumbosacral ligament: The lumbosacral ligament has been described to irritate the L5 nerve root although evidence is in adequate. It can also be seen with spondylolisthesis. This is also known as the transforaminal ligament.

Sacroiliac joint dysfunction: Sacral flexion and innominate dysfunctions can irritate the sciatic nerve which lies anterior to it it. Irritation of the

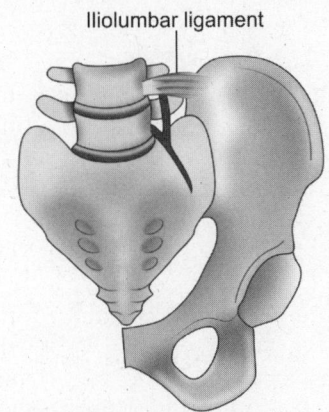

Fig. 19.6: Iliolumbar ligament.

sacroiliac joint capsule on the anterior aspect can also irritate the sciatic nerve (Fig. 19.7).

Piriformis syndrome: The piriformis originates from the S2-S4 vertebrae, sacrotuberous ligament, and the upper margin of the greater sciatic foramen passes laterally through the greater sciatic notch and inserts on the superior surface of the greater trochanter of the femur. Its function is to flex the sacrum acting bilaterally and cause a rotation, side bending torsional movement acting unilaterally. The muscle can be dysfunctional due to torsional dysfunctions or secondary to weakness of the gluteus medius wherein this muscle functions as an abductor, especially with the hip flexed. Dysfunctional states of this muscle may sometimes irritate the sciatic nerve.

Hamstring syndrome: Dysfunctional states of the hamstrings can irritate the sciatic nerve as it passes through them causing sciatic pain (Fig. 19.8). Prolonged direct compression is also a causative factor.

Posterior Tibial Nerve/Plantar Nerves

Course: The posterior tibial nerve is a branch of the sciatic nerve derived from the nerve roots (L4-S3). It enters the lower leg between the two heads of the gastrocnemius. It then passes between the tibialis posterior, flexor digitorum longus, and flexor hallucis longus and travels behind the medial malleolus. This is the location

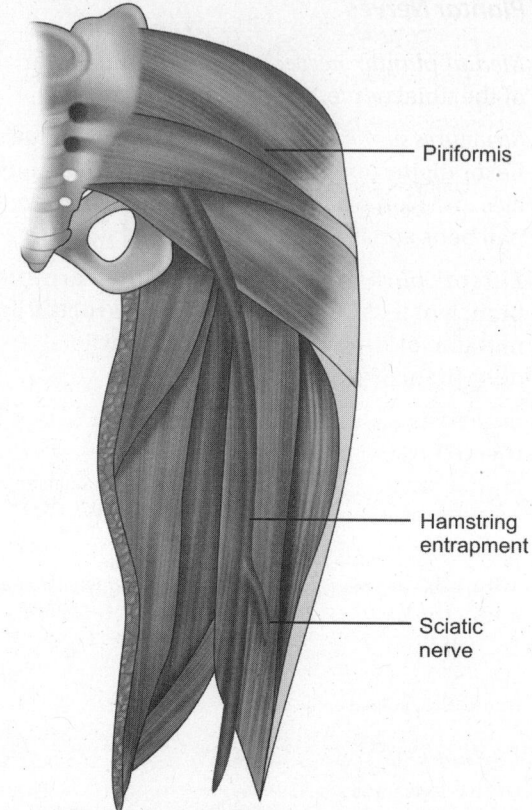

Fig. 19.8: Sciatic nerve entrapment sites at the piriformis and hamstrings.

of the proximal tarsal tunnel formed by the lancinate ligament. It subsequently divides into the medial and lateral plantar nerves.

Structures supplied: The posterior tibial nerve supplies the popliteus, gastrocnemius, soleus, plantaris, flexor hallucis longus (FHL), flexor digitorum longus (FDL) and tibialis posterior.

Entrapment etiopathology: The most common site of entrapment is the tarsal tunnel on the medial aspect of the rear foot. Prolonged pronation of the rearfoot can cause the lancinate ligament to compress the posterior tibial nerve causing symptoms. The other cause for entrapment is the soleus muscle at the popliteal fossa. Patients present with pain in the medial heel and foot with tingling and numbness. Aggravating factors are weight bearing for extended periods of time and local compression.

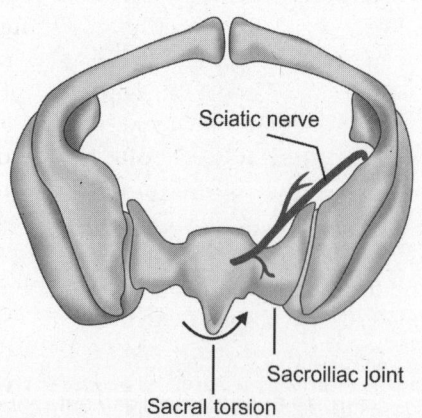

Fig. 19.7: Superior view of the pelvic inlet.

Plantar Nerves

Medial plantar nerve: It is the terminal branch of the tibial nerve.

Structures supplied: It supplies abductor hallucis, flexor digitorum brevis, and 1st lumbrical muscles and skin over the medial 3 and a half toes, nail beds and tips of the toes.

Lateral plantar nerve: It is also a terminal branch of the tibial nerve. At the base of the 5th metatarsal it divides into the superficial and deep branches.

Structures supplied: The main branch supplies the quadratus plantae, abductor digiti minimi and cutaneous branches to the lateral part of sole. The superficial terminal branch supplies the flexor digiti minimi and interosseous muscles of 4th space. The deep terminal branch supplies the adductor hallucis, 2nd, 3rd and 4th lumbricals, and all the interossei except the 4th. They offer sensory supply to the lateral part of the sole, lateral one and a half toes.

Entrapment etiopathology: Prolonged pronation of the foot can diminish the ability of the long toe flexors during push off. Instead, the head of the first metatarsal becomes the lever and push off occurs with the help of the abductor hallucis. Excessive contraction of the abductor hallucis and dysfunctional states of this muscle can entrap the medial plantar nerve.

Digital Nerve

Course and structures supplied: The common digital nerves originate from the medial and lateral plantar nerves. The medial plantar nerve divides into 3 common digital nerves which in turn bifurcate, supplying cutaneous branches to the medial 3.5 digits. The lateral plantar nerve gives rise to two common digital nerves, supplying cutaneous branches to the lateral one and a half digit.

Entrapment etiopathology: The shearing that occurs between the metatarsal heads is the cause. The mechanical cause is however the result of abnormal pronation during the propulsive phase of gait. During abnormal pronation, the 1st, 2nd and 3rd meatarsal heads move laterally and upwards, while the 5th metatarsal head moves downward and medially. This opposite movement of the metatarsal heads create a shear and irritate the tissue surrounding the neurovascular bundles resulting in fibrotic proliferations which are neuromas. The digital nerve gets irritable under the transverse intermetatarsal ligament and intermetatarsal head space especially 2-3 or 3-4. A cramping sensation on the plantar aspect with numbness, burning or shooting pain of either the second, third, or fourth interspace are the common symptoms. Compression of the metatarsals as in a positive 'Mulder click test' may be present.

Common Peroneal (Superficial and Deep) Nerve Entrapments

Course: The sciatic nerve divides into the posterior tibial nerve and the common peroneal nerve above the popliteal fossa with the common peroneal nerve on the lateral side. Prior to its division into the superficial and deep peroneal nerves it divides into the sural communicating branch and lateral cutaneous nerve of calf which provides cutaneous sensation to the proximal and lateral aspect of the leg. It also supplies the knees joint via its articular branches. The common peroneal nerve then courses around the fibular neck and passes through the fibroosseous opening in the superficial head of the peroneus longus muscle. This is a potential source of entrapment as this opening has an angulation combined with significant fibrous connective tissue that secures the nerve to this proximal portion of the fibula. Distal to this fibular tunnel, the common peroneal nerve divides into the superficial and deep peroneal nerves.

The superficial peroneal nerve travels down the leg to pierce an opening in the deep fascia at about the distal third of the anterior leg and runs down the lateral aspect of the ankle anterior to the lateral malleolus (Fig. 19.9).

The deep peroneal nerve descends along the leg, passes under the extensor retinaculum on the anterior aspect of the ankle mortise. Approximately 1 cm distal to the ankle mortise, the nerve divides into lateral and medial branches. It then divides into the dorsolateral cutaneous nerve of the great toe and the dorsomedial cutaneous nerve of the second toe.

Superficial Peroneal Nerve

Structures supplied: Peroneus longus and brevis and sensation over most of the dorsum of the foot, except for the region that lies between the first and second toes.

Deep Peroneal Nerve (Fig. 19.10)

Structures supplied: Tibialis anterior, extensor hallucis longus (EHL), extensor digitorum longus (EDL), peroneus tertius, extensor hallucis previs (EHB), extensor digitorum brevis (EDB), second and third dorsal interosseous, and sensation to the web space between the first and second toes, the adjacent metatarsophalangeal (MTP) and interphalangeal joints.

Entrapment etiopathology: Superficial: The most common site of irritation of the superficial peroneal nerve is the fibular head secondary to habitual leg positions and prolonged postures secondary to immobilization. The location of the nerve on the lateral aspect of the ankle makes it especially vulnerable to dysfunction secondary to repetitive lateral ankle sprains. Excessive overuse that results in compartment syndromes can also entrap neurovascular structures.

Deep: This nerve is vulnerable as it passes beneath the extensor retinaculum at the anterior ankle region due to chronic over activity, or compression as in tight shoe straps or shoelaces.

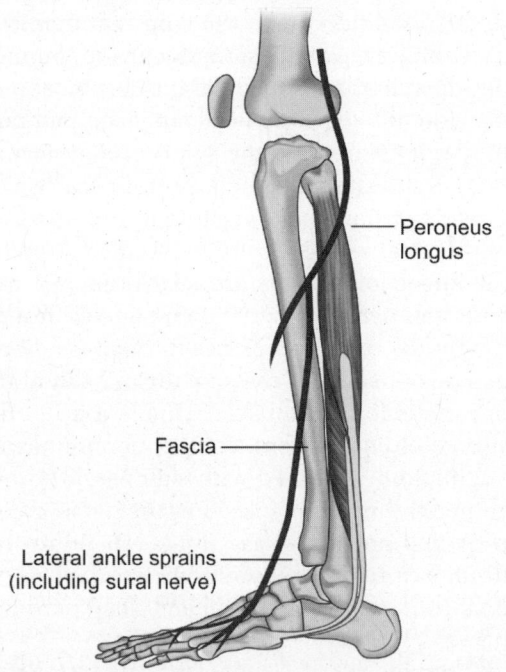

Fig. 19.9: Common peroneal nerve and superficial peroneal nerve.

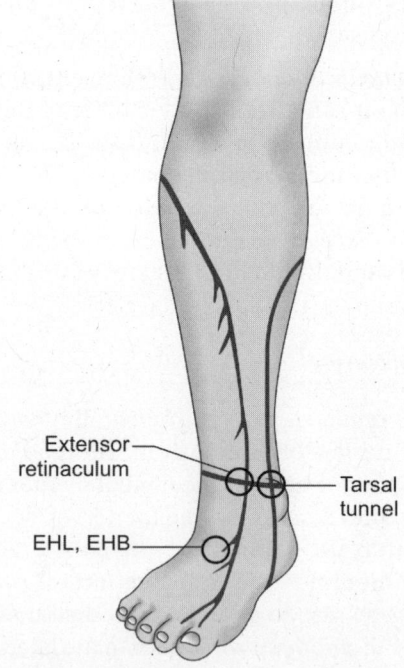

Fig. 19.10: Deep peroneal nerve. (EHL: extensor hallucis longus; EHB: extensor hallucis brevis)

Other causes are hypertrophied EHL and EHB tendons, prominent bony processes of the talus, navicular and cuneiform and exertional compartment syndromes. Symptoms include pain over the superolateral aspect of the lower leg with symptom reproduction on compression. Occasional weakness of ankle and toe dorsiflexion and ankle eversion may be evident.

Upper Limb[4]

Extraspinal nerve interfaces and radicular pain in the upper limb.

Median Nerve

Course: Formed by C5 to C7 roots from lateral cord of brachial plexus C8 and T1 roots from medial cord. After receiving inputs from both the lateral and medial cords of the brachial plexus, the median nerve courses with brachial artery on medial side of arm between biceps brachii and brachialis. It then crosses anteriorly to run medial to the artery in the distal arm and into the cubital fossa. There are no branches in the upper arm (Fig. 19.11).

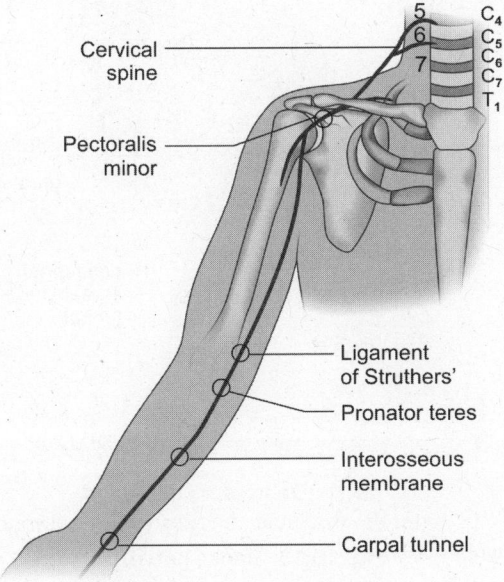

Fig. 19.11: Median nerve.

The median nerves arises from the cubital fossa and gives off two branches as it courses through the forearm which are as follows:
1. Anterior interosseous.
2. Palmar cutaneous (sensation of lateral palmar skin).

Structures supplied: Pronator teres, flexor carpi radialis, flexor digitorum sublimis, palmaris longus.

Anterior interosseous branch: Flexor pollicis longus, flexor digitorum profundus to 2nd and 3rd fingers, pronator quadratus.

Thenar eminence: Abductor pollicis brevis, opponens pollicis, flexor pollicis brevis, and 1st and 2nd lumbricals.

Sensation: Skin over thenar eminence and palmar surface of thumb, 2nd, 3rd and lateral 1/2 of 4th finger.

Entrapment etiopathology: The most common site of involvement is the cervical spine secondary to degenerative changes or discogenic pathology. The axilla is a potential site secondary to crutch compression, and anterior shoulder instability. The pectoralis has a notorious predisposition to compress the median nerve. At the elbow the most common cause is a hypertrophied and irritable pronator teres. An anomalous ligament of Struthers is a potential cause at the elbow level. The interosseous membrane in the forearm and the carpal tunnel at the wrist are the potential distal sites of entrapment.

Ulnar Nerve

Course: The ulnar nerve originates from the lower trunk of the brachial plexus C8, T1. As it exits from the brachial plexus it passes through the scalenes, the costoclavicular space, anterior to the shoulder and axilla on the posteriomedial aspect of the humerus inferiorly and behind the medial epicondyle at the elbow. It passes through the cubital tunnel formed by the flexor carpi ulnaris and enters the anterior side of the forearm, and runs parallel to the ulna. It then enters the palm of the hand superficial to the flexor retinaculum through the Guyon's canal and hypothenar eminence (Fig. 19.12).

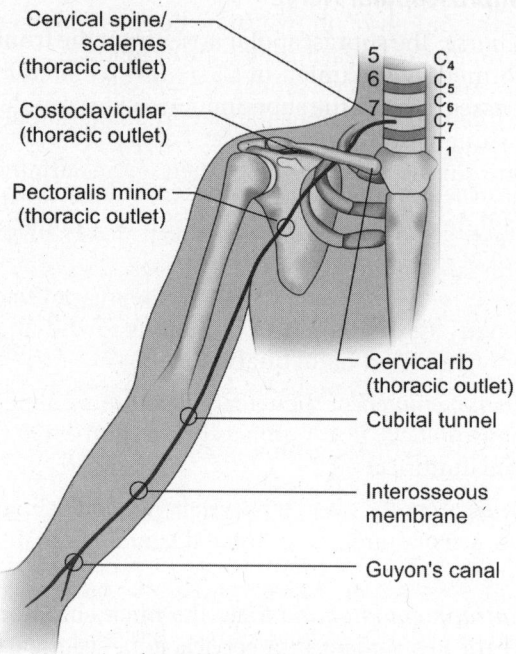

Fig. 19.12: Ulnar nerve.

to a hypertrophied flexor carpi ulnaris is a common presentation. Distally, the interroseous membrane and the Guyon's canal at the hook of the hammate secondary to a hypertrophied pisohammate ligament are potential sites of the entrapment.

Radial Nerve

Course: The radial nerve originates from the posterior cord of the brachial plexus C5,6,7,8,T1. From the brachial plexus, the radial nerve travels posteriorly through the triangular interval. It then enters the arm in the axilla and it then travels posteriorly on the medial side of the arm and winds around the radial groove. On emerging from the groove on the lateral aspect of the humerus, it passes through the radial tunnel on the lateral aspect of the elbow, and Arcade of Frohse. It subsequently descends down as the posterior interosseous nerve to the radial aspect of the wrist (Fig. 19.13).

Structures supplied: Above the elbow it supplies the triceps, anconeus. At or below elbow it

Structures Supplied: In the forearm it supplies the flexor carpi ulnaris, flexor digitorum profundus (4th and 5th fingers). In the hand (hypothenar eminence) the superficial branch of ulnar nerve supplies the palmaris brevis and the deep branch supplies the opponens digiti minimi, abductor digiti minimi, flexor digiti minimi brevis, adductor pollicis, third and fourth lumbrical muscles, dorsal and palmar interossei. It offers sensation to proximal ulnar palm, 5th and ulnar side of the 4th finger

Entrapment etiopathology: The most common site of entrapment of the ulnar nerve is the thoracic outlet, although the cervicothoracic junction is also a vulnerable site. The thoracic outlet is typically vulnerable secondary to a hypertrophied scalenes, elevated first rib and hypertrophied pectoralis minor. Occasionally, an anomalous cervical rib may be a source of pathology. A cubital tunnel syndrome at the medial aspect of the elbow secondary

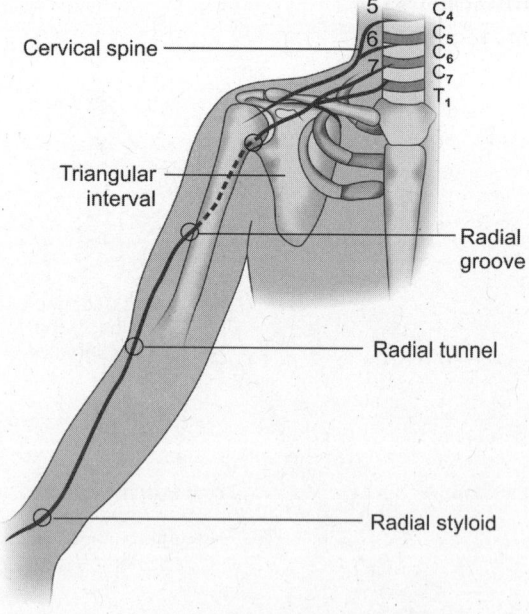

Fig. 19.13: Radial nerve.

supplies the brachioradialis, extensor carpi radialis longus and brevis, and supinator. After crossing the Arcade of Frohse (posterior interosseus nerve) supplies the extensor digitorum, extensor digiti minimi, extensor carpi ulnaris, abductor pollicis longus, extensor pollicis brevis, extensor pollicis longus, extensor indicis. The radial nerve provides sensory inervation to much of the back of the hand, including the web of skin between the thumb and index finger.

Entrapment etiopathology: It is commonly involved in the axilla secondary to pressure as a crutch palsy. A bigger source of pain and dysfunction occurs at the triangular interval on the superior lateral border of the scapula secondary to a hypertrophied triceps and teres major. The condition is called triangular interval syndrome (Fig. 19.14).[7] Severe triceps contractions make this nerve vulnerable at the midlevel of the medial aspect of the humerus. At the level of the elbow the extensor carpi radialis brevis and supinator can entrap the radial nerve. The radial styloid is the most distal, possible site of entrapment secondary to prolonged twisting movement of the forearm.

Suprascapular Nerve

Course: The suprascapular arises from the trunk formed by the union of C5, 6. It runs laterally passes through the superior transverse scapular ligament and suprascapular notch, and enters the supraspinous fossa. It then curves around the lateral border of the spine of the scapula passes through the spinoglenoid ligament to the infraspinous fossa (Fig. 19.15).

Structures supplied: Supraspinatus, Infraspinatus.

Entrapment etiopathology: The suprascapular nerve is most commonly entrapped by the spinoglenoid ligament and suprascapular notch of scapula secondary to repeated overhead activity or faulty posture as in excessive protraction. Direct trauma is yet another cause. Pain in the shoulder is a predominant symptom and is often mistaken for a rotator cuff syndrome. Tenderness is usually evident over the spinoglenoid ligament or suprascapular notch. The spinoglenoid ligament is more often involved. There is classical weakness of arm abduction and external rotation.

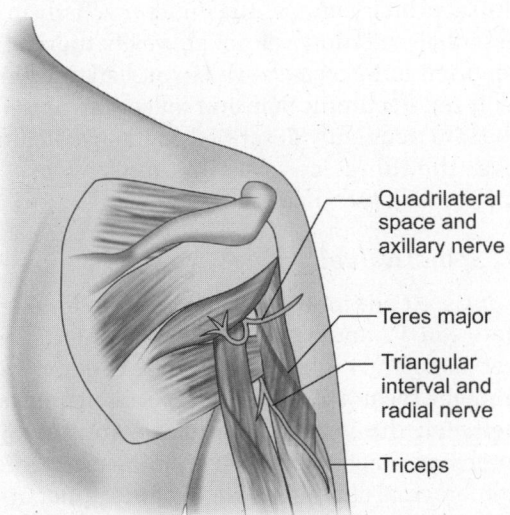

Fig. 19.14: Axillary and radial nerve.

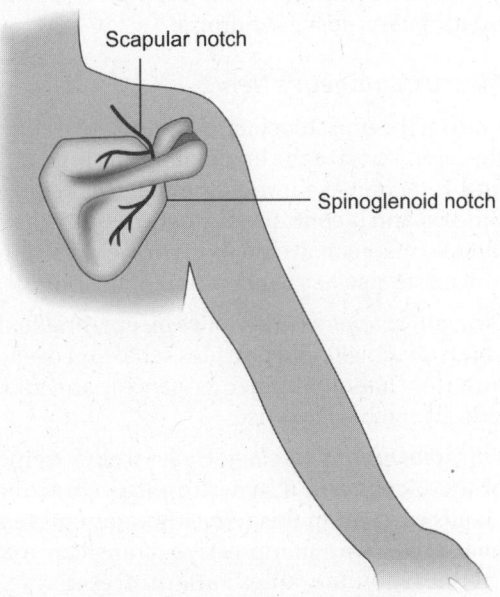

Fig. 19.15: Suprascapular nerve.

Wasting of the supraspinatus and infraspinatus may be a feature.

Axillary Nerve

Course: The axillary nerve arises from the posterior cord of the brachial plexus at the level of the axilla from C5 and C6. The axillary nerve travels through the quadrilateral space. It then divides into an anterior and posterior branch. The anterior branch supplies the deltoid and the posterior branch supplies the teres minor and posterior deltoid.

Structures supplied: It supplies the deltoid and teres minor. It offers sensory supply on the skin over lateral shoulder, and lateral forearm.

Entrapment etiopathology: The biggest source of pain and dysfunction from the axillary nerve is secondary to compression in the quadrilateral space (formed by teres minor, major and triceps) secondary to faulty posture. Prolonged direct compression secondary to prolonged overhead positions, rotator cuff tear and trauma are other causes. Pain is a predominant symptom and is often a poor indicator. Palpation of the quadrilateral space can appear tender and can reproduce symptoms. This condition is called quadrilateral space syndrome.

Musculocutaneous Nerve

Course: The musculocutaneous nerve arises from the lateral cord of the brachial plexus from C 5,6, and 7. It courses through the anterior aspect of the arm and is continued into the forearm as the lateral antebrachial cutaneous nerve (Fig. 19.16). The nerve also has a inervation to the bone.

Structures supplied: It supplies biceps, brachialis, coracobrachialis and provides sensation over the forearm (lateral cutaneous nerve), and radial side from elbow to wrist.

Entrapment etiopathology: Heavy weight training of the biceps and a hypertrophied coracobrachialis can entrap this nerve. Rotator cuff tears, heavy bags with compressive straps can make this nerve vulnerable. Patient presents with pain in the anterior upper arm with weakness of supination and elbow flexion. Symptoms

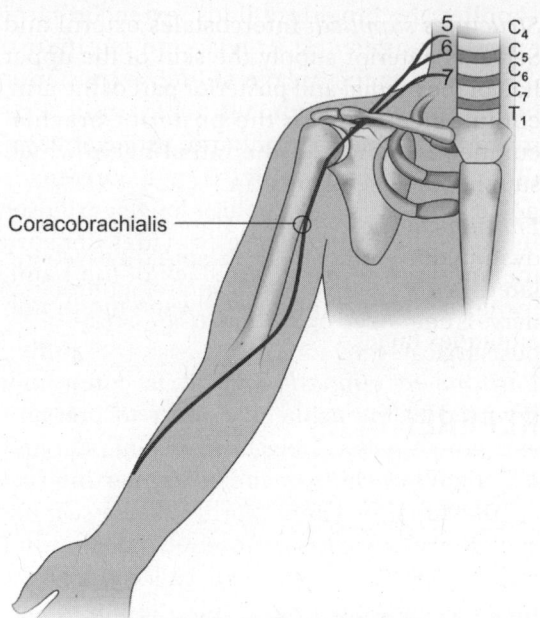

Fig. 19.16: Musculocutaneous nerve.

increase with repetitive elbow flexion and supination.

Thoracic Dorsal Ramus

Notalgia paresthetica: Notalgia paresthetica is thought to be caused by a lesion of a thoracic dorsal primary ramus. The injury mechanism is essentially unknown although weight training is reported to be a causative factor. Patients typically report chronic pain and sensory symptoms that are frequently described as intense itching over the thoracic paraspinal muscles at the inferomedial scapula.

T2 Spinal Nerve[5,6]

Course: Arises from the intervertebral foramen between T2 and T3 as the second intercostal nerve. Lateral cutaneous branches are derived from the second intercostal nerve about midway between the vertebrae and sternum as the intercostobracial nerve which joins the medial antebrachial cutaneous nerve of the upper arm and the posterior brachial cutaneous branch of the radial nerve of forearm.

Structures supplied: Intercostales externi and Serratus anterior supply the skin of the upper half of the medial and posterior part of the arm, communicating with the posterior brachial cutaneous branch of the radial nerve which supplies the lateral forearm.

Entrapment etiopathology: Upper thoracic facet dysfunction entraps the T2 spinal nerve. The lateral cutaneous branch, intercostobrachial nerve is entrapped by the direct trauma especially postsurgical scars, commonly, postmastectomy.

REFERENCES

1. Paris SV. Anatomy as related to function and pain. Orthop Clin North Am. 1983;14:475-89.
2. Gray H. Gray's Anatomy, 1999, Running press, Philadelphia.
3. McCluskey LF, Webb LB. Compression and entrapment neuropathies of the lower extremity. Clin Podiatr Med Surg. 1999;16:97-125.
4. Pratt N. Anatomy of nerve entrapment sites in the upper quarter. J Hand Ther. 2005;18:216-29.
5. Sebastian D. T2 radiculopathy: A differential screen for upper extremity radicular pain. Journal of manual and manipulative therapy. 2011; Abstracts of the American Academy of Orthopaedic Manual Physical Therapists (AAOMPT) annual conference, Anaheim, California.
6. Sebastian D. T2 radiculopathy: a differential screen for upper extremityradicular pain. Physiother Theory Pract. 2013;29:75-85.
7. Sebastian D.Triangular interval syndrome: A differential diagnosis for upper extremity radicular pain. Physiother Theory Pract. 2010; 26:113-9

CHAPTER 20

Understanding Mechanical Nerve Dysfunction

Peripheral nerves are not static tissues. As our limbs move, the nerves are expected to adapt to the changes in length. This is accomplished by a sliding or gliding motion of the nerve through the surface they pass through. When nerves glide through their respective surfaces they change in length up to several millimeters which prevents the nerve from being kinked and stretched. These surfaces through which the nerve glides are what are known as 'interfaces'. Typically the following are the types of interfaces that a nerve may encounter:
1. Muscle
2. Ligament
3. Fibrous bands
4. Fascia
5. Fibro-osseous tunnels (including the intervertebral foramen)
6. Disk

Since gliding motion has been described and the surfaces being varied as mentioned above, the possibility of friction of the nerve over the surface exists. To avoid excessive friction of these gliding nerves over the interfaces, an adaptive mechanism in the form of a smooth gliding surface exists. Surrounding the nerve trunk is a conjunctiva like adventia that permits excursion of the nerve trunk. This extraneural gliding surface is also called paraneurium. Within the nerve trunk the individual nerve fibers are grouped together in fascicles that are arranged either in a cable or plexiform manner. These fascicles during normal movement slide against each other. The paraneurium together with the normally occurring sliding of fascicles against each other in the deeper layers (intraneural gliding surfaces), makes the normal gliding of the nerve during joint motion possible. The second important structure that provides motion is the loose connective tissue between the fascicles, which also provides space filled with loose tissue for volume adaptation. This enables motion between the fascicles which is necessary to allow normal gliding.[1]

This normal gliding mechanism of the nerve has been compared with movement occurring in the joints. Recall from descriptions of normal joint movement that the gross range of motion that is viewed externally are what are known as 'osteokinematic' movements and the simultaneous movement that occurs within the joint is termed as 'arthrokinematic' motion. Similar descriptions have occurred for the peripheral nerves as well and the field being termed as 'neurobiomechanics'. All major nerves have been described to have a certain direction of movement where they are maximally stretched. These directions have been specifically described for every major nerves by the pioneers in the field of nerve mobilization. They call them 'tension tests'.[2] For example, movement or excursion of the nerves in the upper limb are called upper limb tension tests (ULTT). The descriptions are as follows:
- ULTT 1 and 2 (median)
- ULTT 3 (radial)
- ULTT 4 (ulnar)

Similarly for the lower limb:
- Passive neck flexion (PNF)
- Straight leg raise (SLR)

- Slump
- Prone knee bend (PKB).

The concept being, when these nerves are tested to tension, if no abnormal responses are elicited, be it pain or other obvious neural signs, then there is normal movement or gliding of the nerve. This gross gliding is termed as neurodynamic motion. This may be analogous to the osteokinematic motion of the joint where a gross motions is visualized. Taking it one step further, it has been described that if there was a restriction observed in this gross osteokinematic motion then a well informed clinician would suspect a restriction in the joint play 'inside of' or 'within' the joint. This is the normal roll and gliding that occurs in a joint. Mobilization and treatment procedures are focused on these arthrokinematic restriction before a gross osteokinematic test, or mobilization is performed.

Analogs to this scenario, the normal neurodynamic motion of a nerve is dependent on the interface mobility as in the muscle, ligament, fascia, fibrous bands, and fibro-osseous tunnels that the nerve passes through. Various dysfunctional situations can cause a restriction on the nerve in one of these interface sites. (These dysfunctions and sites of entrapment are described in subsequent chapters and are specific for each nerve). Ideally then, just as a clinician would determine the appropriate arthrokinematic motion for a restricted osteokinematic motion, an appropriate determination of nerve restriction in the specific interfaces should be done and managed before testing or treating with gross neurodynamic motion. This specific motion or restriction within the specific interface of the nerve is hypothetically termed as 'neurokinematic' motion or mobility.[3] Thus:

Joint mobility	Nerve mobility
Osteokinematic (gross flexion, extension, etc.)	Neurodynamic (ULTT, SLR, slump, PKB, etc.)
Arthrokinematic (inferior glide, posterior glide, etc.)	Neurokinematic (specific fibrous, muscular, osseous entrapment, etc.)
Mobilizing arthrokinematic restriction restores osteokinematic motion	Mobilizing neurokinematic restriction restores neurodynamic motion/gliding

(ULTT: upper limb tension tests; SLR: straight leg raise, PKB: prone knee band)

It should be noted that gross neural mobilization can also assist in mobilizing the paraneurium and fascicles within the nerve trunk.

Factors Influencing Nerve Mechanics and Effects of Restricted Gliding

As described earlier, the epineurium is the outermost layer of the peripheral nerve. It is also called epifascicular epineurium in contrast with the interfascicular epineurium between the fascicles. Above this epifascicular epineurium, a loose connective tissue fills the space between the nerve and surrounding tissue. This structure is called the paraneurium and it corresponds to the paratendinium as a gliding layer around tendons over sections without tendon sheaths.

The paraneurium fills the gap between the nerve and surrounding tissue. It is designed to allow motion and provide some space for caliber changes. It also causes some friction. The paraneurium may become fibrotic and form adhesions; it then becomes indistinguishable from the epifascicular epineurium. Shrinkage of the fibrotic paraneurium and/or the combined paraneurium and epineurium may cause compression of the entire nerve trunk like a stocking that is too tight. This causes an internal entrapment and may show as conduction changes along with pain. Fibrosis is a more difficult situation to deal with as far as nerve mobilization is concerned, whereas adhesions of the paraneurium respond well to nerve mobilization.

The second important structure that provides motion is the fascicles within the nerve trunks. Motion between the fascicles is necessary to allow mobility in the epifasicular epineurium and paraneurium. The fascicles can change position and consequently change the cross-sectional area of a nerve trunk without becoming compressed. This is achieved by the undulations seen in the fascicles which can adapt to changes in length, however, it becomes physiologically necessary for the fascicles to return to their original length. This ability of the fascicles to return to their original length is impeded in the presence of entrapment.

Motion between the fascicles is also necessary in a thick nerve trunk to compensate for the difference in distances to the plane of motion. When a nerve is shortened during flexion, the volume absorbing effect is necessary because flexion of the joint makes the nerve shorter and causes an increased volume of the shorter segment. If the joint is extended again and the shortened nerve is elongated, the volume decreases. With further elongation, if the length of a given fascicle is extended, the fascicle becomes more narrow along its course, particularly in its middle segment because of the transverse contraction.[1] With the above description it is obvious that there could be two possible types of entrapment, one being a nerve entrapment in relation to the surrounding tissue and two being the entrapment of the connective tissue within the nerve.

What Causes Pain?

Mechanosensitivity

It has been suggested that pain can occur following relatively minor nerve damage at a preneuropraxic level can occur secondary to inflammation of the nerve trunk. Studies in the rat have shown that a local neuritis can cause pain-related behavioral changes and that intact nerve fibers can become sensitive to pressure at the lesion site.[4] However, despite pain production no axonal damage was identified at the lesion site. In other words, there is often no obvious physical nerve injury. Inflammation of nerve trunks could play a major role in many widespread painful conditions such as radicular pain seen in the neck and back pain from nerve root irritation. In these conditions, inflammation could cause widespread changes to nerve fibers resulting in increased mechanosensitivity as well as dysfunction at the peripheral terminals. Both intact and damaged fibers can become mechanosensitive, and it is likely to be these fibers that contribute to mechanosensitive symptoms including nerve trunk tenderness and painful responses to nerve stretch during joint movements. This is what we may hypothesize as pathological neurodynamics. Although the percentage of fibers that develop mechanosensitive properties appears small, 4.0% of all C-fibers is in fact a large number of units especially when most of these are likely to be nociceptive.

The following are some mechanisms hypothesized as causes of nerve trunk mechanosensitivity:

- The accumulation of sodium channels at nerve fiber endings in neuromas is considered to play a major role in the development of spontaneous activity.
- The accumulation of channels at the endings of degenerated fibers is probably a major cause of the local mechanosensitivity.
- Disruption of axonal transport in intact fibers might also result in the accumulation of channels at the lesion site leading in the development of mechanosensitive properties.
- Studies in the rat have shown that a local neuritis can cause pain-related behavioral changes and that intact nerve fibers can become sensitive to pressure and movement at the lesion site.[4] However, despite pain production no axonal damage was identified at the lesion site. They concluded that inflammation of nerve trunks could play a major role in many widespread painful conditions such as radicular pain seen in the neck and back pain from nerve root irritation. This mechanosensitivity was due to the release of neuropeptides by the nervi nervorum[5] or due to the presence of mechanosensitive abnormal impulse-generating sites.[6]

Cross-sectional Stenosis and Decreased Vascularity (Ischemia)

If the nerve cannot move in the longitudinal direction because of adhesions of the surrounding tissues caused by fibrosis of the paraneurium, then the lack of movement at the level of a nerve trunk can be compensated by the increased longitudinal movement of the fascicles inside the trunk. This is a very important point to the physical therapist as this is the physiological implication to radicular pain. In addition, extraneural entrapment can occur if the surrounding interface is fibrotic or dysfunctional. This can also interfere with the gliding of the nerve and possible increase in longitudinal movement past the entrapment site. Note as mentioned earlier, conduction in a nerve strongly depends on vascularity and axonal transport. If a elastic structure like a nerve is stretched then the cross-sectional area of that elastic structure can decrease if the physiological limit is crossed. The peripheral nerve stretches to a certain length in all functional activities as a normal physiological function. As an example, consider the normal length of the sciatic nerve in standing. Now assume the leg is lifted up to kick a ball. In which case, the sciatic nerve, which is posterior to the thigh requires a certain degree of flexibility like the hamstrings to adapt to the function. This function is performed without any compromise to the cross-sectional area and subsequently to the vascularity and axonal transport. However, assume that the sciatic nerve is entrapped in one of its interfaces, say the hamstrings. While kicking the ball the nerve glides normally until the site of entrapment, however, since the action needs to be completed, it overstretches past the entrapment site to complete the function. When a circular elastic structure is overstretched, the cross-sectional area of the structure decreases leading to a disturbance in the circulation.[7,8] The nerve is made to adapt for changes without a disturbance in the intraneural circulation, however, pathological situations occur if the stretching is past physiological limits and prolonged. If the fascicles move in one direction but cannot easily return at an entrapment site, symptoms such as pain and paraesthesia develop and subside only if the fascicles are straightened again. If such an entrapment occurs in sequence, fibrosis develops in the fascicles within the nerve segment. Fibrosis of the interfascicular epineurium may also cause compression of the fascicles. All of the aforementioned factors can result in a decrease in intraneural circulation and ischemic pain. If such a restriction is appropriately mobilized at the interface level then the normal gliding of the nerve can be re-established with a decrease in the symptomatology. Controversy seems to exist as to whether pain arises from entrapment of tissue within the nerve (intraneural) or epineural tissue in relation to the surrounding tissues.

Intraneural vessels are arranged so that stretching has no immediate effect on the circulation. However, Lundborg and Rydevik[9] defined the lower stretching limit, as far as the circulation is concerned, as 8% elongation. Apparently, a 50% decrease of blood flow can occur with elongation of 8%, with associated fibrosis of interfascicular tissue. This explains clearly that normal physiology is maintained following stretching of nerves, as long as it occurs at a lesser degree of elongation. There is debate however, that when normal physiology is altered secondary to excessive elongation, and the symptoms are predominantly pain as opposed neurological deficits, it is the epineurial tissue that requires mobilization to restore the normal physiology.

REFERENCES

1. Topp KS, Boyd BS. Structure and biomechanics of peripheral nerves: nerve responses to physical stresses and implications to physical therapist practice. Phys Ther. 2006;86:92-109.
2. Butler D. Mobilisation of the Nervous System, 1st edition, 1991. Churchill Livingstone, Melbourne.
3. Sebastian D. Effects of neural interface mobilization on peripheral nerve mobility and pain: a single case design. Journal of Manual and Manipulative Therapy. 2005:3:185.
4. Dilley A, Lynn B, Pang SJ. Pressure and stretch mechanosensitivity of peripheral nerve fibres following local inflammation of the nerve trunk. Pain. 2005;117:462-72.
5. Chen Y, Devor M. Ectopic mechanosensitivity in injured sensory axons arises from the site of spontaneous electrogenesis. Eur J Pain. 1998; 2:165-78.
6. Sauer SK, Bove GM, Averbeck B, et al. Rat peripheral nerve components release calcitonin

gene-related peptide and prostaglandin E2 in response to noxious stimuli: evidence that nervi nervorum are nociceptors. Neuroscience. 1999; 92:319-25.
7. Kobayashi S, Shizu N, Suzuki Y, et al. Changes in nerve root motion and intraradicular blood flow during an intraoperative straight-leg-raising test. Spine. 2003;28:1427-34.
8. Millesi H, Zoch G, Reihsner R. Mechanical properties of peripheral nerves. Clin Orthop Relat Res. 1995;(314):76-83.
9. Lundborg G, Rydevik B. Effects of stretching the tibial nerve of the rabbit. A preliminary study of the intraneural circulation and the barrier function of the perineurium. J Bone Joint Surg Br. 1973;55:390-401.

CHAPTER
21

Examination

Examination in mechanical peripheral nerve pathology begins with routine evaluation of peripheral nerve integrity. All clinical tests for nerve conduction is performed in the order of motor, sensory and reflex testing. The clinician should always remember that the focus of this approach is for a condition where the nerve pathology is preneuropraxic and hypomobile. An outline for each level is as follows:

NEURAL REPRESENTATION

Lower Limb

Dermatomes and Myotomes

- L1 Inguinal
- L2 Middle and anterior thigh, hip flexion
- L3 Medial knee, knee extension
- L4 Medial lower ankle, ankle dorsiflexion
- L5 Web space of 1st and 2nd toes, great toe extension
- S1 Lateral border of foot, ankle plantarflexion, eversion
- S2 Popliteal space, knee flexion
- S3-4 Saddle area.

Reflexes

- L2,L3: Patellar
- S1: Achilles

Upper Limb

Dermatomes and Myotomes

- C1 Vertex, head flexion
- C2 Auricular, head extension
- C3 Lateral neck, head side bending
- C4 Shawl area, shoulder shrug
- C5 Lateral arm, shoulder abduction
- C6 Posterior thumb, elbow flexion, wrist extension
- C7 Posterior middle finger, elbow extension, wrist flexion
- C8 Posterior little finger, thumb extension
- T1 Medial forearm, finger abduction/adduction.
- T2 Medial arm and posterior forearm.

Reflexes

- C5: Biceps
- C6: Brachioradialis
- C7: Triceps

The standard neurological examination[1] helps to locate the level of lesion in the spine, however, may present as being normal even in the presence of mechanical nerve dysfunction. Hence, once routine peripheral neurological examination is complete, methods of identification converge to two components:

1. Identifying the presence of adverse neural tension.
2. Identifying the presence of extraspinal interface entrapment.

For the above two principles need to be adopted. They are as follows:

1. To identify adverse neural tension—the clinician performs routine adverse neural tension examination procedures, to identify and/or localize the presence of nerve entrapment.[2]

2. To identify the presence of extraspinal interface entrapment—the clinician localizes the possible area of entrapment and looks for 3 components that may further strengthen the evaluation.[3] This is done by observing for the presence of:
   - **A:** Alignment deviation of landmarks or unilateral weakness and tightness of soft tissue.
   - **R:** Restricted joint or tissue mobility.
   - **T:** Tenderness locally with pressure mechanosensitivity.

Lower Limb

Sciatic Nerve and its Branches

1. Identifying the presence of adverse neural tension

   The concept of adverse neural tension has been described earlier including the fact that inadequate gliding can be a source of pathology. However, identification of its source is important, as the possible cause for adverse neural tension may be any source in the course of the nerve. The methods described as nerve tension testing gives us an overall picture of the presence of tension and such a diagnosis should first be established. Localization would be the next step. The test described that holds quantitative value for establishing the presence of adverse neural tension in the sciatic continuum is called the slump test.

Slump

The following steps describe the method of execution of this test which are as follows:

Cervical and Thoracic Flexion
(Observe for Presence of Symptoms)

Reproduction of symptoms would indicate that the possible site of irritation is the thoracolumbar spine, if no symptoms are produced, proceed to.

Knee Extension
(Observe for Presence of Symptoms)

Reproduction of symptoms would indicate that the possible site of irritation is the lumbar spine or pelvic area, if no symptoms are produced, proceed to.

Foot Dorsiflexion
(Observe for Presence of Symptoms)

Reproduction of symptoms would indicate that the possible site of irritation is the posterior thigh or superior tibiofibular joint, if no symptoms are produced, proceed to.

Foot Dorsiflexion with Inversion/Eversion

Reproduction of symptoms would indicate that the possible site of irritation is the tarsal tunnel for eversion (tibial nerve at tarsal tunnel and plantar nerves at abductor hallucis) and lateral ankle for inversion (superficial peroneal nerve), if no symptoms are produced, then the test is negative. However, do not consider the test to be positive if the symptoms are reproduced. The possibly of muscle and fascia stretch versus nerve tension should be ruled out. Hence one should observe effects of.

Release of Cervical Flexion

If symptoms ease on release of neck flexion the possibility of nerve tension exists, however, if symptoms persist it maybe of a muscle/fascial origin. If at a specific stage of the slump test, symptoms are reproduced, release of neck flexion is done at that level to rule out myofascial versus nerve mediation (Figs. 21.1 and 21.2).

Identifying the Presence of Extraspinal Interface Entrapment

Recollect the possible interfaces of the sciatic nerve and its branches:

Intervertebral foramen

Erector spinae muscle: Flexible rotated side (FRS), extended rotated side (ERS), disk herniation,

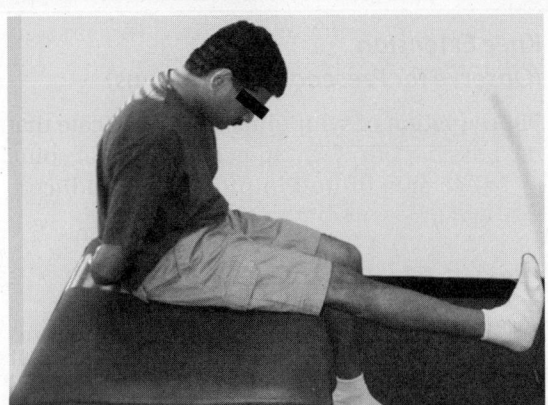

Fig. 21.1: Slump test.

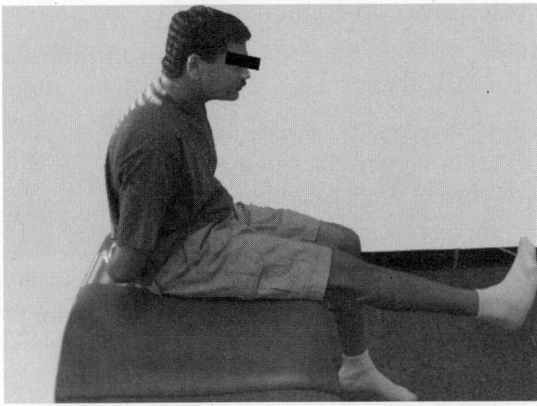

Fig. 21.2: Slump with release of neck exion.

tenderness over the facet articulation at the level of the transverse process, tenderness over the erector spinae.

Quadrartus lumborum
Iliolumbar ligament: No dysfunctional triad described, more secondary to soft tissue fibrosis.

Anterior sacroiliac joint
Piriformis: Presence of torsional sacral dysfunctions, irritability of the piriformis and tenderness/weakness of the gluteus medius, iliopsoas tightness as the piriformis works as an abductor in hip flexion.

Lower hamstrings: Hamstring tightness, prolonged knee flexion and tibial internal roation secondary to a pronated foot.

Popliteus/soleus: Prolonged tibial internal rotation secondary to a pronated foot. Achilles tendo tightness secondary to a pronated foot (plantarflexed calcaneus).

Superior tibiofibular joint: Hamstring tightness, prolonged knee flexion and tibial internal rotation secondary to a pronated foot. All components of a supinated foot with evertor weakness.

Lateral ankle: All components of a supinated foot with evertor weakness.

Tarsal tunnel: All components of a pronated foot.

Anterior ankle/extensor retinaculum
Abductor hallucis muscle: All components of a pronated foot with tenderness over the abductor hallucis.
Extensor hallucis brevis and digitorum longus.

Femoral Nerve and its Branches

1. Identifying the presence of adverse neural tension.

Side Lying Knee Bend

Patient in side lying with lumbar spine in neutral and adequate room for cervical and thoracic flexion.

Cervical and Thoracic Flexion
(Observe for Presence of Symptoms)

Reproduction of symptoms would indicate that the possible site of irritation is the thoracic spine, if no symptoms are produced, proceed to.

Hip Extension
(Observe for Presence of Symptoms)

Reproduction of symptoms would indicate that the possible site of irritation is the pelvis (inguinal ligament, psoas and iliacus muscles), if no symptoms are produced, proceed to.

Knee Flexion
(Observe for Presence of Symptoms)

Reproduction of symptoms would indicate that the possible site of irritation is the quadriceps muscle, sartorius and the vastus medialis oblique (VMO) if no symptoms are produced then the test may be considered negative. However, do not consider the test to be positive if the symptoms are reproduced. The possibly of muscle and fascia stretch versus nerve tension should be ruled out. Hence one should observe effects of.

Release of Cervical Flexion

If symptoms ease on release of neck flexion the possibility of nerve tension exists, however, if symptoms persist it maybe of a muscle/fascial origin. If at a specific stage of the side lying knee bend test, symptoms are reproduced, release of neck flexion is done at that level to rule out myofascial versus nerve mediation (Fig. 21.3).

Identifying the Presence of Extraspinal Interface Entrapment

Recollect the possible interfaces of the femoral nerve and its branches:

Intervertebral Foramen: FRS, ERS dysfunctions, disk herniation.

Psoas Major and Iliacus: Innominate dysfunctions/hip flexor tightness.

Inguinal Ligament: Innominate dysfunction.

Sartorius (saphenous nerve): Innominate and myofascial dysfunction.

VMO (saphenous nerve): Patellofemoral dysfunction.

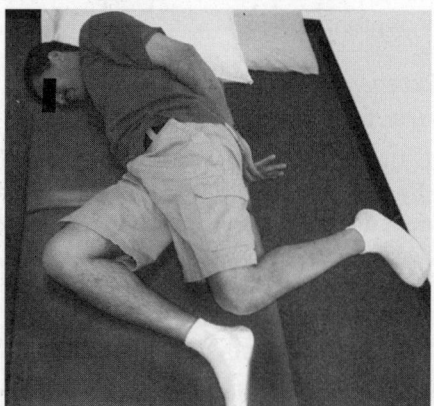

Fig. 21.3: Side lying knee bend test.

Other nerve entrapments that do not present with positive adverse neural tension.

Obturator

Pubic dysfunction, innominate dysfunction, tightness and irritability of the adductors.

Lateral Cutaneous

Innominate dysfunction, tenderness over the inguinal ligament and sartorius.

Iliohypogastric

Look for postsurgical scars and tenderness over the transverse abdominus.

Ilioinguinal

Look for postsurgical scars and tenderness over the external oblique muscle. Also look for the presence of thoracolumbar junction syndrome.

Genitofemoral

This is rare presentation and is most commonly seen as a postsurgical sequelae.

Upper Limb
Median Nerve Tension Test

Shoulder girdle Depression

Reproduction of symptoms would indicate that the possible site of irritation is the cervical spine, scalenes, if no symptoms are produced, proceed to shoulder abduction to 110°, external rotation of the shoulder.

Reproduction of symptoms would indicate that the possible site of irritation is the cervical spine, pectoralis minor, and medial musculature, if no symptoms are produced, proceed to elbow extension forearm supination and wrist and finger extension.

Reproduction of symptoms would indicate that the possible site of irritation is the pronator teres, and carpal tunnel, if no symptoms are produced, proceed to

Cervical side flexion away: This test can be considered positive if it reproduces the patient's symptoms.

However, do not consider the test to be positive if the symptoms are reproduced. The possibly of muscle and fascia stretch versus nerve tension should be ruled out. Hence one should observe effects of.

Release of cervical lateral flexion and depression: If symptoms ease on release of neck lateral flexion and shoulder depression the possibility of nerve tension exists in the cervical spine, however, if symptoms persist it maybe of a muscle/fascial origin.

Release of elbow extension with shoulder girdle depression and cervical side flexion maintained.

If symptoms ease on release of elbow extension with shoulder girdle depression and cervical side flexion maintained the possibility of nerve tension exists in the pronator teres, however, if symptoms persist it maybe of a muscle/fascial origin.

Release of wrist extension with elbow extension, shoulder girdle depression and cervical side flexion maintained.

If symptoms ease on release of wrist extension with elbow extension, shoulder girdle depression and cervical side flexion maintained the possibility of nerve tension exists in the carpal tunnel, however, if symptoms persist it maybe of a muscle/fascial origin (Figs. 21.4 and 21.5).

Identifying the Presence of Extraspinal Interface Entrapment

Recollect the possible interfaces of the median nerve and its branches:

Intervertebral foramen: ERS, FRS dysfunctions, disk herniation.

Scalenes, pectoralis major: Tightness and myofascial dysfunction.

Pronator teres: Tightness and myofascial dysfunction.

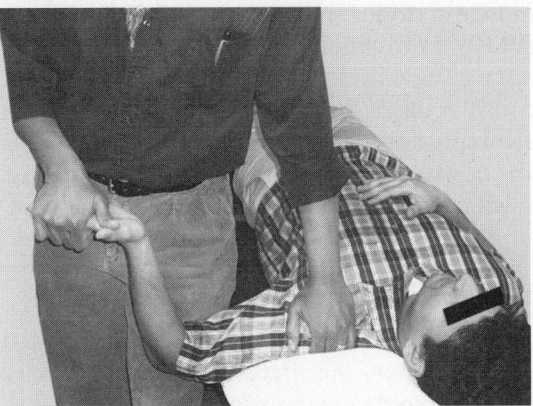

Fig. 21.4: Medial nerve tension test starting position.

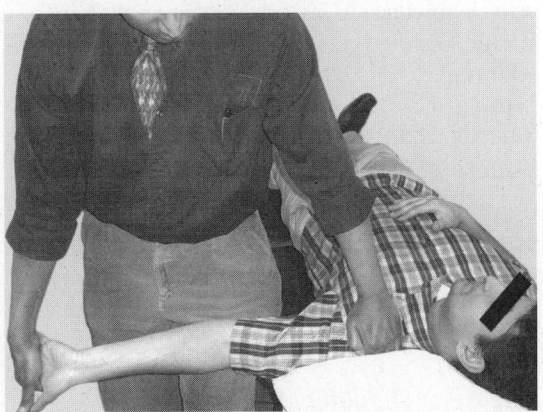

Fig. 21.5: Median nerve tension test and elbow extension.

Carpal tunnel: Carpal bone hypomobility, transverse carpal ligament inflammation.

Radial Nerve Tension Test

Shoulder girdle Depression

Reproduction of symptoms would indicate that the possible site of irritation is the cervical spine, if no symptoms are produced, proceed to.

Shoulder Medial Rotation/Horizontal Adduction

Reproduction of symptoms would indicate that the possible site of irritation is the triangular interval (triceps and teres major), if no symptoms are produced, proceed to.

Elbow Extension/Forearm Pronation

Reproduction of symptoms would indicate that the possible site of irritation is the radial tunnel (supinator), if no symptoms are produced, proceed to.

Wrist/Finger Flexion with Ulnar Deviation

Reproduction of symptoms would indicate that the possible site of irritation is the radial styloid, if no symptoms are produced the test is negative.

However, do not consider the test to be positive if the symptoms are reproduced. The possibly of muscle and fascia stretch versus nerve tension should be ruled out. Hence one should observe effects of.

Release of Shoulder Depression/or Ipsilateral Side Bending

If symptoms ease on release of shoulder depression or with ipsilateral side bending the possibility of nerve tension exists in the cervical spine, however, if symptoms persist it maybe of a muscle/fascial origin.

Release of Shoulder Medial Rotation, Horizontal Adduction, Elbow Extension/ Forearm Pronation

If symptoms ease on release of shoulder medial rotation, horizontal adduction, elbow extension/ forearm pronation with shoulder girdle depression maintained the possibility of nerve tension exists in the triangular interval, radial tunnel (supinator), however, if symptoms persist it maybe of a muscle/fascial origin.

Release of Wrist/Finger Flexion with Ulnar Deviation

If symptoms ease on release of wrist/finger flexion with ulnar deviation, shoulder girdle depression maintained the possibility of nerve tension exists in the radial styloid, however, if symptoms persist it maybe of a muscle/fascial origin.

Identifying the Presence of Extraspinal Interface Entrapment

Recollect the possible interfaces of the median nerve and its branches:

Intervertebral foramen: ERS, FRS dysfunctions, disk herniation

Radial groove: Medial intermuscular septum, myofasical dysfunction

Triangular interval: Hypertrophy and myofascial dysfunction of triceps, and teres major.

Supinator: Radial dysfunctions, supinator hypertrophy.

Radial styloid: Repetitive activity

Ulnar Nerve Tension Test

Wrist Extension Radial Deviation with Forearm Supination

Reproduction of symptoms would indicate that the possible site of irritation is the Guyon's canal, if no symptoms are produced, proceed to.

Elbow Flexion

Reproduction of symptoms would indicate that the possible site of irritation is the cubital tunnel, if no symptoms are produced, proceed to.

Shoulder Depression/Lateral Rotation

Reproduction of symptoms would indicate that the possible site of irritation is the scalenes, if no symptoms are produced, proceed to.

Shoulder Abduction

Reproduction of symptoms would indicate that the possible site of irritation is the pectoralis minor, if no symptoms are produced, proceed to.

Neck Side Flexion Away

Reproduction of symptoms would indicate that the possible site of irritation is the scalenes/ intervertebral foramen, if no symptoms are produced, the test is negative.

However, do not consider the test to be positive if the symptoms are reproduced.

The possibly of muscle and fascia stretch versus nerve tension should be ruled out. Hence one should observe effects of.

Release of Wrist Extension, Radial Deviation with Forearm Supination

If symptoms ease on release of wrist extension, radial deviation with forearm supination the possibility of nerve tension exists in the Guyon's canal, however, if symptoms persist it maybe of a muscle/fascial origin (Figs. 21.6A and B and 21.7).

Release of Elbow Flexion

If symptoms ease on release of elbow flexion the possibility of nerve tension exists in the cubital tunnel, however, if symptoms persist it maybe of a muscle/fascial origin.

Release of Shoulder Depression/Lateral Rotation

If symptoms ease on release of shoulder depression/lateral rotation the possibility of nerve tension exists in the scalenes/costoclavicular space however, if symptoms persist it maybe of a muscle/fascial origin.

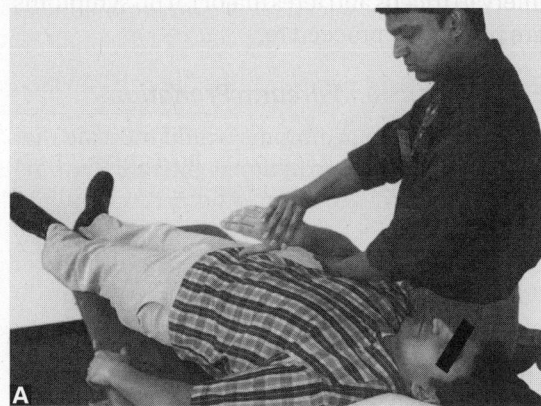
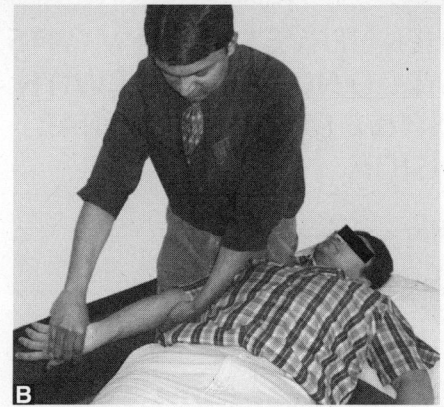

Fig. 21.6A and B: Radial nerve tension test.

Release of Shoulder Abduction

If symptoms ease on release of shoulder abduction the possibility of nerve tension exists in the pectoralis minor however, if symptoms persist it maybe of a muscle/fascial origin.

Release of Neck Side Flexion Away

If symptoms ease on release of neck side flexion away the possibility of nerve tension exists in the cervical spine/scalenes, however, if symptoms persist it maybe of a muscle/fascial origin.

Identifying the Presence of Extraspinal Interface Entrapment

Recollect the possible interfaces of the median nerve and its branches:

Intervertebral foramen: ERS, FRS dysfunctions, disk herniation.

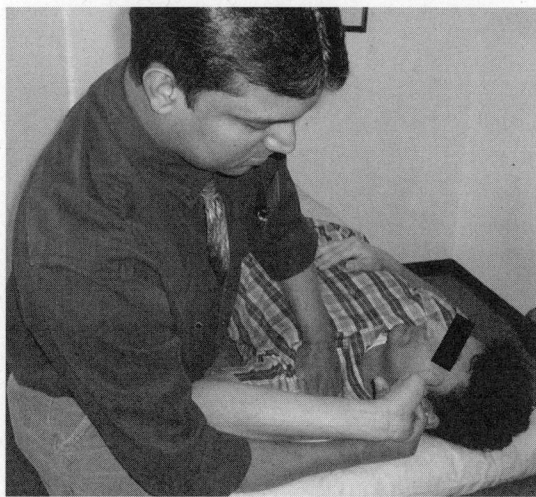

Fig. 21.7: Ulnar nerve tension test with radial deviation and forearm supination.

Thoracic outlet (scalenes): Hypertrophied scalenes

Thoracic outlet (costoclavicular space): Elevated 1st rib, tight subclavius.

Thoracic outlet (pectoralis minor): Hyperabduction, hypertrophy/tightness, rounded shoulders.

Cubital tunnel: Tensile valgus stresses, flexor carpi ulnaris (FCU) irritability secondary to overuse.

Guyon's canal: Compression, repetitive wrist motion.

OTHER NERVE ENTRAPMENTS THAT DO NOT PRESENT WITH POSITIVE ADVERSE NEURAL TENSION

Axillary

- Quadrilateral space syndrome
- Scapula dysfunctions
- Hypertrophic teres.

Musculocutaneous

Hypertrophic coracobrachialis and pectoralis minor.

Thoracic Dorsal Ramus

Hypertrophy/tissue texture abnormality paraspinals in inferomedial scapular area.

T2 Spinal Nerve

Pressure mechanosensitivity just lateral to T2, T3 with upper thoracic facet dysfunction.

REFERENCES

1. Hoppenfield S. Physical Examination of the Spine and Extremities, 1976, Connecticut: Appleton and Lange, Norwalk.
2. Butler D. Mobilisation of the Nervous System, 1st edn, 1991. Churchill Livingstone, Melbourne.
3. Greenman PE. Principles of manual medicine, 2nd edn, 1996, Williams and Wilkins, Baltimore.

CHAPTER 22

Treatment

INTRODUCTION AND PRINCIPLES OF MANAGEMENT

Management of mechanical radicular pain will not differ much in the initial management from the principles of application in joint dysfunction. The joint retains its priority as it is the main component of a motion segment, and that the nerve is irritated secondary to an aberrance of joint mechanics with its associated muscular component. Conventional principles of management of nerve dysfunction focus attention on the dynamic gliding ability of the nerve. This, without doubt is the mainstay of management of nerve dysfunction. However, the newer speculation is to normalize the milieu of the nerve from a mechanical perspective (neurokinematics)[1] prior to attention to gliding (neurodynamics).[2]

While addressing the milieu of the nerve 3 factors need to be addressed from a mechanical perspective which is very much the anthem of the application principles.[3]

- **A:** Alignment deviation of landmarks or unilateral weakness and tightness of soft tissue.
- **R:** Restricted joint or tissue mobility.
- **T:** Tenderness locally with pressure mechanosensitivity.

It is speculated that these three factors can collectively entrap a nerve anywhere along its course in the form of interfaces. Dysfunction then can occur at the location and distal to that site of entrapment as the entrapment not only affects the ability of the nerve to glide but can overstretch the nerve distal to the site of entrapment as it is a compensation to maintain the length of the nerve, proportional to the activity in question. Hence, gross gliding can only further encourage this overstretching and may be an erroneous approach if initiated without addressing the interfaces first. The principles of management enumerated below will follow the same principle and one should understand that the techniques described in the regional application chapters are not only addressing the joint dysfunction in question but also addressing the interfaces of the nerve entrapment at hand.

LOWER EXTREMITY MECHANICAL RADICULAR PAIN FROM THE LUMBOPELVIC HIP REGION

Sciatic Nerve

Neurokinematic Restriction

- Intervertebral foramen
- *Erector spinae muscle:* Causes for restriction are flexed rotated side (FRS), extended rotated side (ERS) closing and opening restrictions. There may be palpable tenderness over the facet articulation at the level of the transverse process with tenderness over the erector spinae. Treatment addresses appropriate management for the above restrictions with soft tissue mobilization. The discogenic

component and core stability cannot be overlooked.
- *Iliolumbar ligament:* No dysfunctional triad described, more secondary to soft tissue fibrosis and hence soft tissue mobilization is indicated.
- *Anterior sacroiliac joint*
- *Piriformis:* Presence of anterior torsional sacral dysfunctions may be sources of irritation. Patients present with landmark deviation of the sacral base and inferior lateral angles with irritability of the piriformis and tenderness/weakness of the gluteus medius. Treatment includes appropriate maneuvers to address anterior torsional sacral dysfunctions, soft tissue mobilization of the piriformis and gluteus medius with gluteus medius strengthening and piriformis stretching. The piriformis is rendered dysfunctional in the presence hip flexor and hip capsule tightness. With the femur in relative flexion, the piriformis functions as an abductor during stance and hence chronically irritated and potentially irritating the sciatic nerve if it passes through it. Hence, additionally, stretching the iliopsoas and hip capsule, and strengthening the gluteus maximus is recommended.

Gross Neural Mobilization

Once interface restriction is addressed, gross neural mobilization is done in a sidelying modified slump position. This repeated sliding motion done based on tolerance of the level of irritability may assist gross mobility of the nerve without overstretching.

Femoral Nerve

Neurokinematic Restriction

- *Intervertebral foramen:* Causes for restriction are FRS/ERS, closing and opening restriction. There may be palpable tenderness over the facet articulation at the level of the transverse process, with tenderness over the erector spinae. Treatment addresses appropriate management for the above restrictions with soft tissue mobilization. The discogenic component and core stability cannot be overlooked.
- *Psoas major and iliacus*
- *Inguinal ligament:* The presence of anterior innominate dysfunction has a tendency to shorten the iliopsoas muscle group and move the inguinal ligament posteriorly, and the iliopectineal eminence anteriorly. This may entrap the femoral nerve causing symptoms. Treatment typically addresses stretching of the iliopsoas and correction of anterior innominate dysfunction.
- *Sartorius (saphenous nerve):* Soft tissue dysfunction of the subsartorial canal (Hunter's canal) can irritate the saphenous nerve. The canal is formed by the adductors medially, the vastus medialis laterally and the sartorius as the roof. Treatment is most effectively addressed with the soft tissue mobilization.

Gross Neural Mobilization

Once interface restriction is addressed, gross neural mobilization is done in a sidelying knee bend position. This repeated sliding motion done based on tolerance of the level of irritability may assist gross mobility of the nerve without overstretching.

MECHANICAL RADICULAR PAIN FROM THE KNEE

Sciatic Nerve

Neurokinematic Restriction

- *Lower hamstrings:* Hamstring tightness and dysfunction can entrap the sciatic nerve resulting in a hamstring syndrome. Prolonged tibial internal rotation secondary to a pronated foot creates a knee flexion moment causing aberrant activity in the hamstrings. Previous trauma or tightness may be predisposing factors as well. Treatment addresses components of a pronated foot

including soft tissue mobilization for the hamstrings with stretching.
- *Popliteus/soleus:* Prolonged tibial internal rotation secondary to a pronated foot and gastrosoleus tightness can entrap the tibial nerve. All components of a pronated foot with soft tissue mobilization of the popliteus and stretching of the soleus is recommended.

Gross Neural Mobilization

Once interface restriction is addressed, gross neural mobilization is done in a side lying modified slump position. However, the proximal component is maintained, while the knee extension component is reinforced.

Superior Tibiofibular Joint

Neurokinematic Restriction

Dysfunction of the superior tibiofibular joint is commonly associated with dysfunctions of the foot. Prolonged pronation causes a compromise of the posterior tibial nerve at the tarsal tunnel, however, it also shortens the peroneus and can cause dysfunction at the level of the superior tibiofibular joint. Treatment best addresses all components of a pronated foot with joint mobilization at the superior tibiofibular joint.

Gross Neural Mobilization

Once interface restriction is addressed, gross neural mobilization is done in a side lying modified slump position. However, the proximal component is maintained while the knee extension component is reinforced with the foot in inversion for the superficial peroneal nerve and the eversion for the tibial nerve. This procedure is repeated for entrapments occurring at the ankle and foot.

Femoral Nerve

Neurokinematic Restriction

- *Vastus medialis obliquus (VMO) (saphenous nerve):* Irritability and hypertrophy of the vastus medialis obliquus can irritate the saphenous nerve giving rise to medial knee pain. Patellofemoral dysfunction is common precursor. Tracking dysfunctions of the patella or weakness of the VMO are causes. Treatment may effectively address patellar tracking dysfunction and soft tissue mobilization of the VMO followed by strengthening.

MECHANICAL RADICULAR PAIN FROM THE ANKLE AND FOOT

Lateral Ankle (Superficial Peroneal Nerve)

Neurokinematic restriction: Repeated lateral ankle sprains are a common sequelae in the chronically supinated foot, however, the superficial peroneal nerve has a tendency to develop irritability secondary to its close proximity to the ligament. Treatment addresses all components of a supinated foot including strengthening of the peronei and gastrosoleus.

Tarsal Tunnel (Posterior Tibial Nerve)

Abductor Hallucis Muscle (Plantar Nerve)

Neurokinematic restriction: Entrapment of the posterior tibial nerve and the plantar nerves are commonly associated with dysfunctions of the foot. Prolonged pronation causes a compromise of the posterior tibial nerve at the tarsal tunnel, however, it also shortens the peroneus and can cause dysfunction at the level of the superior tibiofibular joint. While the abductor hallucis overworks during push off it can, in dysfunctional states cause medial heel pain and entrap the plantar nerve. Treatment best addresses all components of a pronated foot including strengthening of the tibialis posterior with soft tissue mobilization of the abductor hallucis.

Gross neural mobilization: Once interface restriction is addressed, gross neural mobilization is done in a side lying modified slump position. However, the proximal component is maintained while the knee extension component is reinforced with the foot in inversion for the superficial peroneal nerve and the eversion for the tibial nerve.

OTHER NERVE ENTRAPMENTS THAT DO NOT PRESENT WITH POSITIVE ADVERSE NEURAL TENSION

Obturator

Obturator nerve entrapments are seen secondary to pubic dysfunction, innominate dysfunction, and tightness and irritability of the adductors.

Lateral Cutaneous Nerve

Lateral cutaneous nerve entrapments are seen secondary to innominate dysfunction, and irritability of the sartorius.

Medial Cutaneous Nerve

This nerve can cause medial thigh pain secondary to an entrapment at the Hunter's canal.

Posterior Cutaneous Nerve

This nerve can be entrapped at the sciatic notch as it exists with the sciatic nerve.

Iliohypogastric

Look for postsurgical scars and tenderness over the transverse abdominus.

Ilioinguinal

Look for postsurgical scars and tenderness over the external oblique muscle. Also look for the presence of thoracolumbar junction syndrome.

Genitofemoral

This is rare presentation and is most commonly seen as a postsurgical sequelae.

UPPER EXTREMITY MECHANICAL RADICULAR PAIN FROM THE CERVICOTHORACIC REGION

Median Nerve

Neurokinematic Restriction

- *Intervertebral foramen:* Causes for restriction are FRS/ERS, closing and opening restriction. There may be palpable tenderness over the facet articulation at the level of the transverse process, with tenderness locally. Treatment addresses appropriate management for the above restrictions with soft tissue mobilization. The discogenic component and core stability should be addressed. The subcranial component should also be addressed.
- *Scalenes, pectoralis major:* Tightness of the scalenes and pectoralis major are common and hence soft tissue mobilization and stretching is advocated. Core stability cannot be overlooked.

Ulnar Nerve

Neurokinematic Restriction

- *Intervertebral foramen*: Causes for restriction are FRS/ERS, closing and opening restriction. There may be palpable tenderness over the facet articulation at the level of the transverse process, with tenderness locally. Treatment addresses appropriate management for the above restrictions with soft tissue mobilization. The discogenic component and core stability should be addressed. The subcranial component should be addressed.

The scalenes are accessory muscles of respiration and can be tightened posturally as well. This can entrap the lower trunk of the brachial plexus causing ulnar nerve symptoms. Treatment addresses appropriate management for the scalenes with soft tissue mobilization and stretching. Core stability cannot be overlooked.

Radial Nerve

Neurokinematic Restriction

- *Inervertebral foramen:* Causes for restriction are FRS/ERS, closing and opening restriction. There may be palpable tenderness over the facet articulation at the level of the transverse process, with tenderness locally. Treatment addresses appropriate management for the above restrictions with soft tissue mobilization. The discogenic component and core stability should be addressed. The subcranial component should be addressed.

Gross Neural Mobilization

Gross neural mobilization of the medial, ulnar, radial nerve for entrapments at the cervicothoracic region incorporates gentle passive shoulder girdle depression with the neck in contralateral side bending. Other methods may be cervical side glides or soft tissue mobilization with shoulder girdle depression maintained.

T2 Thoracic Spinal Nerve

Upper thoracic closing manipulation. Soft tissue mobilization of the upper thoracic paraspinals. The subcranial component and core weakness should also be addressed.

MECHANICAL RADICULAR PAIN FROM THE SHOULDER

Ulnar Nerve

Neurokinematic Restriction

The thoracic outlet is a common site of entrapment of the ulnar nerve in the shoulder region. Causes are tight subclavius muscle with an elevated first rib, and tightness of the pectoralis minor. These are first treated appropriately with mobilization and stretching.

Gross Neural Mobilization

Gross neural mobilization of the ulnar nerve for entrapments at the shoulder (thoracic outlet) region continues to incorporate gentle passive shoulder girdle depression with the neck in contralateral side bending. However, horizontal abduction is added.

Radial Nerve

Neurokinematic Restriction

The radial nerve can be entrapped at the triangular interval secondary to a protracted and downward rotated scapula and hypertrophy of the triceps. Treatment addresses scapular upward rotation, retraction and soft tisse mobilization of the triceps and teres major.

Gross Neural Mobilization

Gross neural mobilization of the radial nerve at the shoulder region continues to incorporate gentle passive shoulder girdle depression with the neck in contralateral side bending. However, horizontal adduction with internal rotation is added.

OTHER NERVE ENTRAPMENTS THAT DO NOT PRESENT WITH POSITIVE ADVERSE NEURAL TENSION

Musculocutaneous

A hypertrophic coracobrachialis secondary to vigorous contraction is the most common cause. Soft tissue mobilization with minimizing stress of contraction may be appropriate management with cessation of strengthening activity.

Thoracic Dorsal Ramus

Hypertrophy/tissue texture abnormality of the paraspinals in inferomedial scapular area can irritate the thoracic dorsal ramus resulting in notalgia paresthetica. Soft tissue mobilization of the paraspinals in the inferomedial scapular area may be the treatment of choice.

Axillary

Hypertrophy of the teres muscles secondary to a protracted and downward rotated scapula can compromise the quadrilateral space. Treatment addresses scapular upward rotation and retraction, soft tissue mobilization of the teres major and minor.

MECHANICAL RADICULAR PAIN FROM THE ELBOW, WRIST AND HAND

Median Nerve

Neurokinematic Restriction

The median nerve is commonly entrapped at the elbow by a hypertrophied pronator teres. Since many functional activities involve wrist flexion with pronation of the forearm, there is a tendency for dysfunction. Appropriate treatment is soft tissue mobilization.

The carpal tunnel is the next common site of entrapment. Carpal bone hypomobility with inflammation of the transverse carpal ligament are common causes. Inflammation reduction modalities, carpal mobilization and tendon gliding are appropriate measures.

Gross Neural Mobilization

Gross neural mobilization of the median nerve for entrapments at the elbow incorporates the upper limb tension tests (ULTT) are position for median nerve. However, repeated cyclic elbow flexion and extension with wrist flexion and extension is done to tolerance.

Ulnar

Neurokinematic Restriction

The cubital tunnel on the medial aspect of the elbow boundaried by the flexor carpi ulnaris (FCU) is a common cause. Tensile valgus stresses secondary to throwing, FCU irritability secondary to overuse of wrist flexion and ulnar deviation are causes. The Guyon's canal formed by the pisiform, hamate and pisohamate ligament are entrapment sites. Compression, repetitive wrist motion, ligamentous irritability are causes. Treatment consists of addressing mechanics of throwing and wrist flexion with soft tissue mobilization of the FCU and pisohammate ligament.

Gross Neural Mobilization

Gross neural mobilization of the ulnar nerve for entrapments at the elbow incorporates the ULTT position for ulnar nerve. However, repeated cyclic elbow flexion and extension with wrist radial and ulnar deviation are done to tolerance.

Radial

Neurokinematic Restriction

The supinator muscles form the radial tunnel and since supination is a repetitive activity done by the forearm, hypertrophy and secondary entrapment is observed. Mobility of the radial head is also an influence. The effects are also felt at the radial styloid. Treatment addresses soft tissue mobility of the supinator, and mobility of the radial head.

Gross Neural Mobilization

Gross neural mobilization of the radial nerve for entrapments at the elbow incorporates the ULTT position for radial nerve. However, repeated cyclic elbow flexion and extension with pronation and supination of the forearm with wrist flexion are done to tolerance.

REFERENCES

1. Sebastian D. Effects of neural interface mobilization on peripheral nerve mobility and pain:a single case design. Journal of Manual and Manipulative Therapy. 2005;3:185.
2. Butler D. Mobilisation of the Nervous System, 1st edition, 1991, Churchill Livingstone, Melbourne
3. Greenman PE. Principles of manual medicine, 2nd edn, 1996, Williams and Wilkins, Baltimore.

PART 3

Regional Conditions and Relevant Manual Therapy Intervention

Chapter 23: Cervical Region
Chapter 24: Thoracic Region
Chapter 25: Lumbopelvic Region
Chapter 26: Hip Region
Chapter 27: Knee Region
Chapter 28: Ankle and Foot Region
Chapter 29: Shoulder Region
Chapter 30: Elbow, Wrist and Hand Region

INTRODUCTORY NOTE

This is an overview to give the clinician an idea and direction and by no means suggested as a cook book interpretation. All conditions are not mentioned, rather, ones that may indicate manual intervention are described. The clinician is advised that in the indicated conditions, manual therapy is only a part, but an integral and important part of intervention. It is recommended that all other adjunct and pertinent interventions as in (most importantly) exercise prescription, orthotic management, taping, electrotherapy, activity modification, etc. be considered. It is wise to remind ourselves that conditions can occur together. Additionally, all standard precautions and contraindications should be considered. The signs and symptoms described are somatic and not complete examination findings and other literature is suggested for a broader overview. It might be interesting to note the similarity in intervention for many conditions in a certain region. This simply means that regional mechanical dysfunction is a result of faulty baseline mechanics and any structure in that functional chain, that is in harm's way, is the vulnerable structure and the resultant lesion.

Note: The clinician is reminded that manual therapy intervention for mechanical somatic dysfunction may prove futile first without an accurate diagnosis, second without adequate exercise prescription and activity modification. An effective outcome is strongly dependent on the appropriate interplay of the above combined with clinical experience and an intuitive sense that results from repeated practice.

CHAPTER 23

Cervical Region

Note: Many of the conditions described under the spine section require adequate manual intervention, however, the most effective maintenance of objectives achieved by manual intervention is good exercise prescription. Hence, the value of core strengthening cannot be undermined.

CERVICAL SPONDYLOSIS

Cervical spondylosis is a disorder caused by abnormal wear on the cartilage and bones of the cervical vertebrae with degeneration and mineral deposits in the intervertebral disks. It is about time that we understood that cervical spondylosis is a movement disorder secondary to faulty movement patterns in the cervical complex.[1-4] Aging and deficiency are an added factor. The cervical complex is appropriately designed to distribute movement which is hindered during restrictive situations. This occurs predominantly in the upper cervical spine. The result is a compensatory hypermobility in the midcervical spine resulting in wear and tear. It is common to see wear in the midcervical spine compared to the upper cervical spine. These accumulated changes caused by the degeneration can wear the facet joint and the capsule with subsequent narrowing of the intervertebral formen. These accumulated changes caused by degeneration and the narrowing of the foramen can gradually compress one or more of the exiting nerve roots.

This can lead to increasing pain in the neck and arm, with motor weakness, and changes in sensation. In advanced cases, the spinal cord becomes involved and is called cervical myelopathy. This can affect not just the arms, but the legs as well with positive long tract signs as in hyperreflexia, Hoffman and Babinski.

It comprises all aspects of the above description and commonly occurs secondary to faulty mechanics with hypermobility of the midcervical spine as a compensation to upper cervical hypomobility. When the degenerative changes extend to the facet joint and capsule, the resultant dysfunction is broadly known as *facet joint degeneration, facet capsule impingement*. This classically leads to opening and closing restrictions. When a restriction persists in the joint and overactivity occurs on the opposite side the result is excessive shearing of the interposed annular fibers and may lead to a *Disk Herniation* (Fig. 23.1). The narrowing of the foramen secondary to wear and tear and the protruding disk from a herniation can impinge on the exiting cervical nerve roots resulting in *Nerve root irritation and radicular pain*. This nerve root pain can occur without the presence of a disk herniation, secondary to wear and tear and subsequent narrowing of the intervertebral foramen. A situation as this can compress or irritate the nerve root exiting out of the foramen resulting in *Cervical Radiculopathy* (Fig. 23.2).[4]

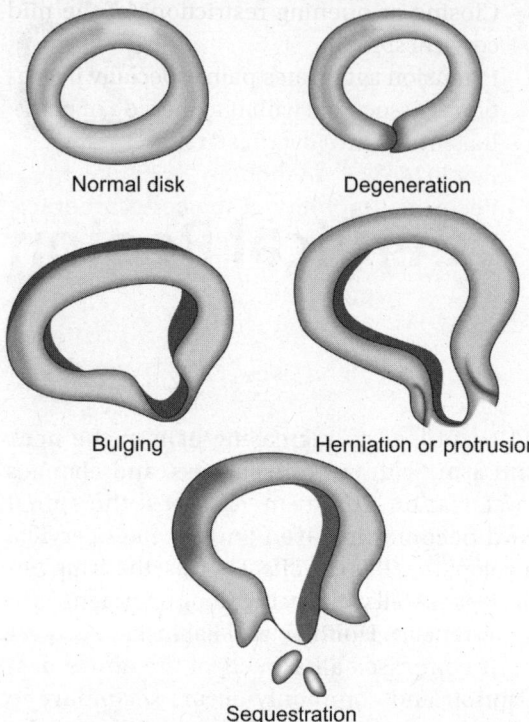

Fig. 23.1: Types of disc pathology.

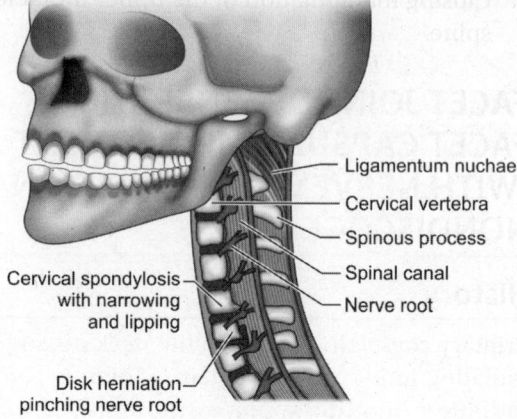

Fig. 23.2: Lesions.

FACET JOINT DEGENERATION, FACET CAPSULE IMPINGEMENT (WITHOUT NERVE ROOT IRRITATION)

History

Primary complaint is pain in the neck possibly radiating into the scapular area. There is no pain radiating into the upper extremities. There is difficulty in moving the neck freely with restricted range of motion.[1,2] There may be a sensation of popping and cracking of the joints on movement. A sensation of tightness of the cervical musculature may be evident. There may be a painful catching sensation in certain parts of the range of motion. Occupation may include prolonged periods of desk work, cradling the phone, overhead activity or lifting overhead.

Possible Somatic Findings

Forward Head Posture

- Tight suboccipitals, occipito-atlantal (OA) stuck in backward bending
- Restricted range of motion with painful muscle trigger points (commonly levator scapula, upper and middle trapezius)
- Muscle tightness may be evident especially by the superficial groups (upper trapezius, levator scapula, sternocleidomastoid, scalenes)
- Closing or opening restrictions of the mid-cervical spine
- Restricted OA/atlantoaxial (AA) mobility
- Restricted mobility of the cervicothoracic junction.

Manual Therapy Intervention

Suboccipital Release

- Stretch upper trapezius, levator scapula, sternocleidomastoid, scalenes
- Trigger point compression of levator scapula, upper and middle trapezius
- OA forward nodding
- AA rotation if restriction is present
- Midcervical opening or closing if present

- Closing manipulation of the upper thoracic spine.

FACET JOINT DEGENERATION, FACET CAPSULE IMPINGEMENT (WITH NERVE ROOT IRRITATION/ NONDISCOGENIC)

History

Primary complaint is pain in the neck possibly radiating into the scapular area. There is pain radiating into the upper extremities.[3] If the radiation is appendicular skeleton (arms) then the possible lesion is the nerve. If the pain radiation is axial skeleton (trunk) especially the upper, middle and lower parts of the scapula, then the possible tissue lesion is the facet joint capsule. The facet capsule of the upper levels C5, C6 radiate pain into the scapula above the scapular spine and the lower levels as in C7, radiate pain into the body and inferior angle of the scapula. There is difficulty in moving the neck freely with restricted range of motion. There may be a sensation of popping and cracking of the joints on movement. A sensation of tightness of the cervical musculature may be evident. There may be a painful catching sensation in certain parts of the range of motion. There is no pain on coughing or sneezing. There is relief of symptoms when the arm is held overhead. Occupation may include prolonged periods of desk work, cradling the phone, overhead activity or lifting overhead. There may be loss of sensation with a history of dropping objects secondary to a weak grip.

Possible Somatic Findings

Forward Head Posture

- Restricted range of motion with painful muscle trigger points (commonly levator scapula, upper and middle trapezius)
- Muscle tightness may be evident especially the superficial groups (upper trapezius, levator scapula, sternocleidomastoid, scalenes)
- Closing or opening restrictions of the mid cervical spine
- Extension aggravates pain especially if rotation is associated with it to the side of pain
- Raising the arm overhead relieves pain
- Restricted OA/AA mobility
- Restricted mobility of the cervicothoracic junction
- Positive finding on upper limb tension test (ULTT)
- Positive finding for the clinical prediction rule (CPR) for cervical radiculopathy.

Manual Therapy Intervention (Following traction)

Suboccipital Release

- Stretch upper trapezius, levator scapula, sternocleidomastoid, scalenes
- Trigger point compression of levator scapula, upper and middle trapezius
- OA forward nodding
- AA rotation if restriction is present
- Midcervical opening or closing if present
- Closing manipulation of the upper thoracic spine
- Neural interface mobilization for the appropriate nerve followed by the gross neural mobilization.

DISK HERNIATION

History

Primary complaint is pain in the neck possibly radiating into the scapular area. There is pain radiating into the upper extremities. Onset may be secondary to lifting a heavy weight, especially overhead, or a violent cough or sneeze. There is difficulty in moving the neck freely with restricted range of motion. There may be a sensation of popping and cracking of the joints on movement. A sensation of tightness of the cervical musculature may be evident. There may be a painful catching sensation in certain parts of the range of motion. There is pain on coughing or sneezing. There may be loss of sensation with a history dropping objects secondary to a weak grip. Occupation may include prolonged periods of desk work, cradling the phone, overhead activity or lifting overhead. Although, the history describes a single lift or sneeze causing the problem, one should understand that individual annular tears have been occurring in a cumulative fashion over a period of time.

Possible Somatic Findings

Forward Head Posture

- Restricted range of motion with painful muscle trigger points (commonly levator scapula, upper and middle trapezius)
- Muscle tightness may be evident especially the superficial groups (upper trapezius, levator scapula, sternocleidomastoid, scalenes)
- Closing or opening restrictions of the midcervical spine
- Restricted OA/AA mobility
- Restricted mobility of the cervicothoracic junction
- Positive finding on upper limb tension test
- Positive finding for the CPR for cervical radiculopathy
- Flexion aggravates symptoms and extension alleviates.

Manual Therapy Intervention

Distraction always precedes manual intervention, provided all contraindications are considered

Suboccipital Release

- Stretch upper trapezius, levator scapula, sternocleidomastoid, scalenes
- Trigger point compression of levator scapula, upper and middle trapezius
- OA forward nodding
- AA rotation if restriction is present
- Midcervical opening or closing if present (preferably side gliding)
- Closing manipulation of the upper thoracic spine
- Neural interface mobilization for the appropriate nerve followed by the gross neural mobilization.

The direction and types of herniation are varied. Commonly, they are either in the posterolateral direction or central. When the herniation is posterolateral, the direction is towards the intervertebral foramen (lateral canal or lateral recess). This will involve the spinal nerve root. However, when the herniation is central, its direction is towards the spinal canal. Hence, the cord is involved with the exception of the lower lumbar region where the cauda equina is involved. So additionally the clinician may observe bladder bowel dysfunction or positive Babinski. When present, it represents the signs of myelopathy or cauda equina compression and hence, manual therapy is contraindicated.

Bladder Bowel Dysfunction

Positive Babinski

When present, it represents the signs of myelopathy and hence, manual therapy is contraindicated.

CERVICAL MYELOPATHY

History

Primary complaint is pain in the neck possibly radiating into the scapular area. There is pain radiating into the upper extremities, bilaterally. Onset may be secondary to lifting a heavy weight, especially overhead, or a violent cough or sneeze. There is difficulty moving the neck freely with restricted range of motion. There may be a sensation of popping and cracking of the joints on movement. A sensation of tightness of the cervical musculature may be evident. There may be pain on coughing or sneezing. There may be loss of sensation with a history dropping objects secondary to a weak grip. There may be a history of loss of balance and involuntary movements of the extremities which may be a characteristic finding of this condition.[6,7]

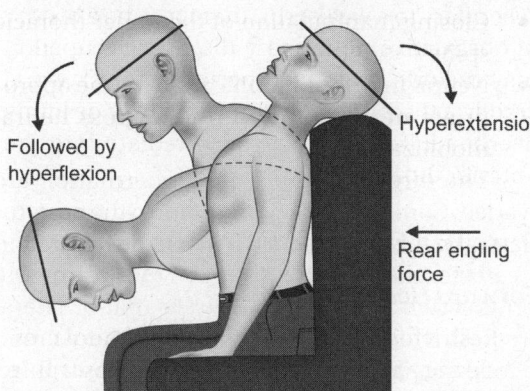

Fig. 23.3: Whiplash injury mechanism.

Possible Somatic Findings

Although somatic findings are present in this presentation, if signs of myelopathy are present, especially a positive Babinski with hyperreflexia, manual therapy is contraindicated.

WHIPLASH INJURIES

Whiplash is an injury to the neck resulting from a sudden extension and then a flexion contraction of the neck (Fig. 23.3). Whiplash injury is most commonly the result of the motion caused by an automobile accident. In a sudden stop, the head is usually thrown forward and then backwards violently, putting a brief but major strain on the neck. The reverse happens if rear ended. This stretches muscles and ligaments in the anterior aspect of the neck. The principal structures are sternomastoid, deep cervical flexors and upper cervical ligaments. This is immediately followed by a reflex contraction of the muscles, joint restriction and pain. Other causes are sports injuries and physical abuse. The musculature and upper cervical joints are commonly involved.[8] In addition there are autonomic signs secondary to a stretch of the cervical sympathetic ganglion. Rarely a concussion may be evident.

History

There is a history of motor vehicle accident, hit on the head or being punched on the face, being tackled in sport. There may be previous history of neck pathology. There may be a report of no immediate pain but exacerbation of symptoms the next day with progressive pain and increased stiffness.

Possible Somatic Findings

The subcranial spine is usually the most involved.

Forward Head Posture

- Restricted range of motion with painful spasms
- Muscle tightness may be evident especially by the superficial groups (upper trapezius, levator scapula, sternocleidomastoid, scalenes)
- Restricted OA/AA mobility with local tenderness
- Closing or opening restrictions of the mid-cervical spine
- Restricted mobility of the cervicothoracic junction
- May or may not have a positive finding on upper limb tension Test
- May or may not have a positive finding for the CPR for cervical radiculopathy.

Manual Therapy Intervention

If protective spasm and guarding in all directions is detected, and this patient has not had an emergency room evaluation or an X-ray, it raises a red flag concern and manual therapy is contraindicated unless proven otherwise. The same concern applies if Babinski or Hoffman test is positive. When contraindications in a fracture or ligamentous instability has been ruled out, manual therapy may be appropriate.

Suboccipital Release

- Stretch upper trapezius, levator scapula, sternocleidomastoid, scalenes
- Trigger point compression of levator scapula, upper and middle trapezius
- OA forward nodding
- AA rotation if restriction is present
- Midcervical opening or closing if present

- Closing manipulation of the upper thoracic spine
- Neural interface mobilization for the appropriate nerve.

THORACIC OUTLET SYNDROME

Thoracic outlet syndrome is a condition whereby symptoms are produced from compression of nerves or blood vessels, or both, because of an inadequate passageway through the thoracic outlet between the base of the neck and axilla. The thoracic outlet is surrounded by the muscle, bone, and other tissues (Fig. 23.4). Any condition that results in enlargement or movement of the tissues of, or near the thoracic outlet can cause the thoracic outlet syndrome. The structures most commonly involved is the lower trunk of the brachial plexus. Often the vascular structures as in the subclavian may also be involved. The common causes are:

History

Primary complaint may be pain in the lateral aspect of the neck and radiating into the upper extremities. The pain specifically radiates to the ring and little fingers. A sensation of tightness of the cervical musculature may be evident. There is no pain on coughing or sneezing. There is an increase in symptoms when the arm is held overhead for a period of time which is characteristic of this condition.[9] There may be loss of sensation with a history dropping objects secondary to a weak grip. There may be a history of obstructive pulmonary disease. Occupation may include prolonged periods of desk work, cradling the phone, overhead activity or lifting overhead. The pain may also radiate into the anterior thoracic area.

Possible Somatic Findings

Forward Head Posture

- Restricted range of motion with painful muscle trigger points (commonly levator scapula, upper and middle trapezius and scalenes)
- Muscle tightness may be evident especially by the superficial groups (mainly the scalenes, pectoralis minor)
- Closing or opening restrictions of the midcervical spine
- Restricted OA/AA mobility
- Restricted mobility of the cervicothoracic junction
- Positive finding on upper limb tension Test of the ulnar nerve
- Tight scalenes
- Elevated 1st rib or tight subcalvius
- Tight pectoralis minor
- Overhead activity aggravates pain.

Manual Therapy Intervention

Suboccipital Release

- OA forward nodding
- Stretch scalenes and pectoralis minor
- First rib depression
- Trigger point compression of levator scapula, upper and middle trapezius
- AA rotation if restriction if present
- Midcervical opening or closing if present
- Closing manipulation of the upper thoracic spine
- Neural interface mobilization for ulnar nerve.

MUSCLE PATHOLOGIES

The one finding in a muscle in conjunction with a mechanical neck dysfunction is tenderness with soft tissue thickening of the musculature. Tenderness in a muscle can lead to an assumption

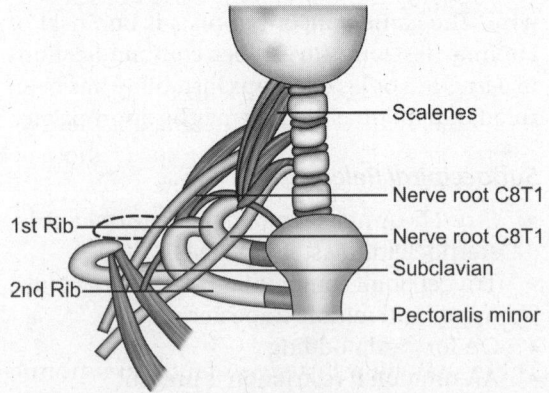

Fig. 23.4: Sites of entrapment in the thoracic outlet.

that the muscle is the source of the dysfunction. This may be the case but not always. Every joint or motion segment has a corresponding muscle that helps to effect movement. Dysfunctional states of the joint can cause additional stress on the supporting soft tissue and result in muscle guarding. This can lead to an accumulation of metabolites in the involved muscle and result in local tenderness with hypertrophy due to guarding. Common causes for soft tissue pathology are prolonged faulty postures or overuse.[5] Several theories exist as to why a soft tissue lesion can occur secondary to prolonged faulty postures or overuse. The three most common theories are as follows:

1. Prolonged and excessive contraction as would occur with overuse or faulty postures may induce fatigue in a muscle. The muscle contracts in response to fatigue by excessive and prolonged actin and myosin cross-bridging and persists to create a local soft tissue dysfunction with localized tender point called 'trigger points'.
2. Excessive and faulty muscle contraction, or direct trauma can cause injury to the myofibrils of the muscle bulk which may heal with scarring. This scarring can inhibit normal physiological contraction and deprive the area of nutrition and encourage chemical accumulation causing pain. In addition possible nerve endings in the healed scar may also be pain sensitive.
3. Faulty activity can influence the muscle at an intrafusal level creating constant aberrant gamma motor activity which renders the soft tissue dysfunctional.

Muscle attachments to the vertebra in dysfunctional states as mentioned above can stress the bony vertebral attachments and result in alignment dysfunctions of the vertebra.

History

Primary complaint is pain in the neck possibly radiating into the scapular area. There may or may not be a history of pain radiating into the upper extremities. There is difficulty in moving the neck freely with restricted range of motion. There may be a sensation of popping and cracking of the joints on movement. A sensation of tightness of the cervical musculature may be evident. There is no pain on coughing or sneezing. There is relief of symptoms when laying down or resting. Occupation may include prolonged periods of desk work, cradling the phone, overhead activity or lifting overhead.

Possible Somatic Findings

- May or may not present with a forward head posture
- Restricted range of motion with painful muscle trigger points (commonly levator scapula, upper and middle trapezius)
- Muscle tightness may be evident especially by the superficial groups (upper trapezius, levator scapula, sternocleidomastoid, scalenes, pectoralis minor)
- Closing or opening restrictions of the mid-cervical spine may or may not be present
- May or may not present with restricted mobility of the cervicothoracic junction
- May or may not present with restricted OA/AA mobility.

Manual Therapy Intervention

Soft tissue mobilization:

Suboccipital Release

- Stretch upper trapezius, levator scapula, sternocleidomastoid, scalenes
- Trigger point compression of levator scapula, upper and middle trapezius
- OA forward nodding
- AA rotation if restriction is present
- Midcervical opening or closing if present
- Closing manipulation of the upper thoracic spine if present.

MYOGENIC HEADACHES

History

There may be a history of faulty ergonomic postures of the neck or a history of whiplash

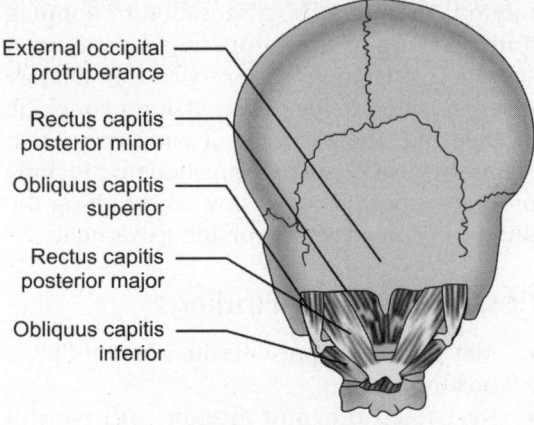

Fig. 23.5: Suboccipital muscles.

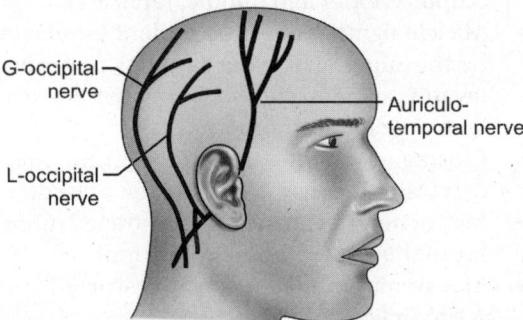

Fig. 23.6: Occipital nerves.

injury. The forward head posture is seen either as a habit, natural tendency, slouching or wearing bifocals. It is also seen in individuals who function looking down as in a desk job. As a result, subcranial backward bending occurs. This can cause a shortening of the soft tissue structures including the suboccipital muscles (Fig. 23.5).

Restriction can occur in the OA and AA joints. The greater occipital nerve (Fig. 23.6) can be irritated causing occipital and temporal headaches.[10] A similar situation can occur secondary to a whiplash injury and subsequent dysfunction of the OA and AA joints. A restricted upper thoracic segment can cause a dysfunction of the semispinalis muscle which can irritate the greater occipital nerve. Dysfunctional states of the guy ropes of the cervical spine namely sternocleidomastoid (SCM) and trapezius can also trigger muscular headaches.

Possible Somatic Findings

Forward Head Posture

- Restricted range of motion with painful muscle trigger points (commonly levator scapula, upper and middle trapezius, SCM)
- Muscle tightness may be evident especially the superficial groups (upper trapezius, levator scapula, sternocleidomastoid, scalenes, pectoralis minor)
- Restricted OA/AA mobility
- Closing or opening restrictions of the mid-cervical spine and upper thoracic spine
- Restricted mobility of the cervicothoracic junction.

Manual Therapy Intervention

Suboccipital Release

- Stretch upper trapezius, levator scapula, sternocleidomastoid, scalenes
- Trigger point compression of levator scapula, upper and middle trapezius
- Soft tissue mobilization of the sternocleidomastoid
- OA forward nodding
- AA rotation
- Midcervical opening or closing if present
- Closing manipulation of the upper thoracic spine.

REFERENCES

1. Lippitt AB. The facet joint and its role in spine pain. Management with facet joint injections. Spine. 1984;9:746-50.
2. Mooney V, Robertson J. The facet syndrome. Clin Orthop Relat Res. 1976;115:149-56.
3. Waldrop MA. Diagnosis and treatment of cervical radiculopathy using a clinical prediction rule and a multimodal intervention approach: a case series. J Orthop Sports Phys Ther. 2006;36:152-9.
4. Porterfield JA, DeRosa C. Mechanical neck pain. Perspectives in functional anatomy. 1994, WB Saunders, Philadelphia,pp.47-81.
5. Travell JG, Simons DG, Simons LS. Travell and Simson's Myofascial pain and dysfunction: The trigger point Manual. Volume 1st and 2nd,1999, Williams and Wilkins Baltimore.

6. Kawabori M, Hida K, Akino M, et al. Cervical myelopathy by C1 posterior tubercle impingement in a patient with DISH. Spine. 2009;34;E709-11.
7. Tang JG, Hou SX, Shang WL, et al. Cervical myelopathy caused by anomalies at the level of atlas. Spine. 2010;35(3):E77-9.
8. Woodhouse A, Liljebäck P, Vasseljen O. Reduced head steadiness in whiplash compared with non-traumatic neck pain. J Rehabil Med. 2010; 42:35-41
9. Gilbert A. [Thoracic outlet syndromes] Neurochirurgie. 2009;55:432-6.
10. Biondi DM. Cervicogenic Headache: a review of diagnostic and treatment strategies. J Am Osteopath Assoc. 2005;10:16-22S.

CHAPTER 24

Thoracic Region

MYOGENIC HEADACHES

See cervicogenic headaches in the cervical section.

Possible Somatic Findings

- Same as in cervicogenic headaches
- Closing restriction of the upper thoracic spine.

Manual Therapy Intervention

- Same as in cervicogenic headaches
- Closing manipulation of the upper thoracic spine.

INTERCOSTAL NEURALGIA

It is a neuralgia of one or more of the intercostal nerves.[1] The intercostal nerves are 12 in number and consist of an anterior and posterior rami. These nerves run in a groove in the lower edge of the ribs called the intercostal groove. Common causes are anemia, cold exposure, pressure from tumors, postherpetic neuralgia from shingles or an aortic aneurysm. Clinical relevance to the physical therapist is that it can arise from dysfunctions of the thoracic vertebrae. In mechanical dysfunctions of the thoracic vertebrae, associated rib dysfunctions can occur. Additionally, faulty postures and muscle imbalances secondary to weakness of the serratus anterior can cause rib dysfunctions[2] and associated intercostal neuralgic pain. Often the sympathetic nervous system is also addressed via the thoracic region in conditions like sympathetic dystrophy.[3]

Possible Somatic Findings

The pain is sharp shooting and can wind around the rib cage:
- Usually in the area of the fifth nerve
- Presence of thoracic or rib dysfunction.

Manual Therapy Intervention

Intercostal Space Stretching

- Closing or opening manipulation of the thoracic segments
- Muscle energy for rib dysfunction, anterior and posterior.

T2 RADICULOPATHY

T2 radiculopathy is a condition where the second thoracic nerve is entrapped in the intervertebral foramen between T2, T3 resulting in upper extremity radicular pain.

The anterior divisions of the thoracic spinal nerves, intercostal nerves exit from the thoracic spinal column beneath their corresponding vertebra. They differ from the anterior divisions of the other spinal nerves in that each pursues an independent course without plexus formation. Lateral cutaneous branches are derived from the intercostal nerves about midway between the vertebrae and sternum; they pierce the intercostales externi and serratus anterior, and divide into anterior and posterior branches. The lateral cutaneous branch of the second intercostal nerve which exits between T2, T3, does not divide like the other thoracic nerves into an anterior and posterior branch; but midway anterior to the axilla, gives off a branch the intercostobrachial nerve (ICBN). It pierces the intercostalis externus, serratus anterior, crosses the axilla to the medial side of the arm, and joins with a filament from the medial brachial cutaneous nerve. It then pierces fascia, and supplies the skin of the upper half of the medial and posterior part of the arm, communicating with the posterior brachial cutaneous branch of the radial nerve which supplies the lateral forearm. The ICBN is the communicating link between the T2 spinal nerve and upper extremity (Fig. 24.1). Thus, the sequence of events resulting in a T2 radiculopathy involve the T2 spinal nerve, adjoining intercostobrachial nerve, medial antebrachial cutaneous nerve and the posterior brachial cutaneous branch of the radial nerve.

The vulnerability of the upper thoracic spine to mechanical dysfunction is described to be secondary to facet restriction, degeneration, faulty posture and muscle imbalances. The key contributor to dysfunction is the forward head posture which comprises upper cervical extension, lower cervical flexion, upper and lower thoracic kyphosis. This could lead to considerable hypomobility of the thoracic spine. The above factors collectively favor the presence of degenerative and mechanical dysfunction of the upper thoracic region. While the upper thoracic spine is vulnerable for degenerative and mechanical dysfunction, the potential for irritation of the second thoracic spinal nerve exists, if the T1, T2, T2, T3 segments are involved, resulting in upper extremity radicular pain. The author is credited for having been the first to describe this condition.[4,5]

Possible Somatic Findings

The presence of upper thoracic somatic dysfunction, restricted cervical mobility (especially extension) and pressure mechanosensitivity over the lateral aspect of the thoracic vertebrae may be diagnostic indicators.

Manual Therapy Intervention

Soft tissue mobilization of the upper and midthoracic region:
- Closing manipulation of upper thoracic segments
- Cervical components to be addressed if present.

COSTOCHONDRITIS

It is a painful condition characterized by the inflammation of the costochondral articulations. It is often difficult to identify a single cause of costochondritis. This condition is thought to be commonly secondary to repetitive microtrauma, or overuse. The most frequently affected age group is young adults between 20 and 40 years old. Costochondritis can also occur as an overuse injury in athletes. In particular this condition has been identified in competitive rowers or activities that involve frequent repetitive horizontal adduction. It can also be found after a traumatic injury. Commonly secondary to a car accident where the driver's chest strikes the steering wheel and injuring the ribs and cartilage in the costochondral area. Viral infections, usually upper respiratory infections have also been identified as a cause of costochondritis.

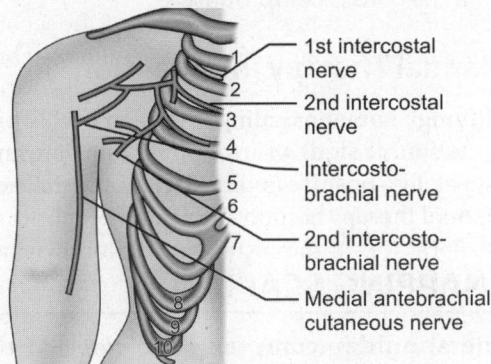

Fig. 24.1: T2 Radiculopathy.

Individuals with rheumatological pathology are also susceptible.

Possible Somatic Findings

- Local tenderness in the costochondral area
- Muscle imbalance as in strong powerful anterior groups (pectorals) and weak posterior and lateral groups (lower trapezius, rhomboids, serratus anterior)
- Rib dysfunction, anterior and posterior.

Manual Therapy Intervention

Ideally besides a less aggressive method of correcting anterior and posterior rib dysfunctions, as in muscle energy, a more symptomatic approach with muscle strengthening is recommended for these patients.

T4 SYNDROME

Although, the existence of this entity is often refuted by authorities it is still worth knowing its existence. T4 syndrome is a condition characterized by the midthoracic pain and symptoms associated with, usually, a hypomobility lesion at T4 and a level above or below.[6] The condition is characterized by the complaints of arm pain or vague discomfort in the arm accompanied by the parasthesia that does not follow any dermatomal patterns. There may also be associated hand symptoms which are considered to be an integral part of this condition. The mechanism of pain production is unknown, but it is postulated that autonomic nerve control may be compromised. The cause is usually mechanical secondary to overuse of arm movements, static postures of the trunk and arm movement (driving, computer work) or trauma.

Possible Somatic Findings

- Nonneutral dysfunction (opening and closing restriction) of the T4,5,6 segments with associated local tenderness
- Radicular symptoms into the arm but dermatomal and myotomal representations may be normal

- Poor posture with muscle imbalance and weakness of core cervicothoracic musculature.

Manual Therapy Intervention

Closing or opening manipulation of the thoracic segments.

THORACIC DISK HERNIATION

The mechanism of disk herniation in the thoracic region is the same as mentioned in the cervical region but there seems an important and serious clinical implication. The spinal canal in the thoracic region is much narrower than the other regions and hence the risk of the herniated disk compromising the cord. Many herniated thoracic disks are shown to be calcified and they typically occur from the third to fifth decade. The perception of pain maybe due to the presence of unmyelinated, free nerve root endings seen in structures surrounding the intervertebral disk which include ligaments, synovial capsule, and vertebral periosteum. For obvious reasons the nerve exiting out of the foramen may also be compromised resulting in pain.

Somatic Findings

- Local pain in the thoracic region
- Pain may radiate into the intercostal region
- May have a positive Babinski or hyperreflexia if the cord is compromised.

Manual Therapy Intervention

Although somatic findings are seen in this presentation, if signs of myelopathy are present, especially a positive Babinski with hyperreflexia, manual therapy is contraindicated.

SNAPPING SCAPULA

The shoulder complex comprises of the scapulothoracic and glenohumeral articulations, principally and in addition to the acromioclavicular and sternoclavicular. The normal scapulohumeral rhythm is a harmonious interplay of the scapulothoracic and glenohumeral articulations. In situations where the glenohumeral articulation is hypomobile, the scapula tends to be rendered hypermobile causing excessive friction of the scapula over the rib cage. Alternately, excessive and repetitive motion of the scapula can also cause excessive friction of the scapula over the rib cage.[7] Changes in the alignment or contour of the bones of the scapula or ribs can also cause snapping scapula. As an example, a fractured rib or scapula that heals in a malaligned position can alter the normal mechanics of the scapulothoracic articulation resulting in friction and pain.[11] The structure on the anterior surface of the scapula is the subscapularis and bursa exists between the subscapularis and rib cage called the subscapularis bursa. The source of pain is usually from these structures.

Somatic Findings

- Grating, grinding, or snapping may be heard or felt along the edge or undersurface of the scapula as it moves along the chest wall.
- Pressure on the scapula and gliding along the rib cage will reproduce symptoms
- Presence of hypomobile, capsular pattern of the shoulder (adhesive capsulitis, etc.)
- Weakness of scapula stabilizers namely serratus anterior and trapezius.

Manual Therapy Intervention

The indication is most at the glenohumeral joints followed by the stabilization exercises of the scapula.

SHOULDER PATHOLOGY/HYPOMOBILITY

This is an entity that all clinicians treating musculoskeletal disorders should recognize as the scapula is the integral component of shoulder alignment and stability. Scapulohumeral rhythm describes normal rhythm as being a ratio of 2:1 of humeral and scapular movement. However, in situations of shoulder pathlogy leading to hypomobile situations of the glenohumeral joint, the scapula moves excessively stressing the muscle attachments of the thoracic spine and scapula. When prolonged, this can lead to pain and dysfunction of the thoracic region.

Examination Findings

- Shoulder pathology with capsular pattern of restriction
- Scapula and humeral dysfunction (see shoulder section)
- Faulty posture of the cervicothoracic region as in forward head with core weakness.

Manual Therapy Intervention

The indication is most at the glenohumeral joints.

MUSCLE PATHOLOGY (INCLUDING NERVE MEDIATED PAIN)

The following are nerves causing pain in the thoracic region, their anatomical location and possible pain mediation:

- Dorsal scapular nerve 5th cervical—supplies rhomboids 3rd, 4th cervical—supplies levator scapula. The above can occur secondary to cervical dysfunctions
- Thoraco dorsal—supplies lattismus dorsi. Lattismus dorsi pain secondary to thoraco dorsal nerve compression is relatively rare.
- Long thoracic nerve—supplies serratus anterior. The long thoracic nerve arises from the C 5,6,7. It runs beneath the subscapularis muscle and terminates in the serratus anterior muscle. Causes of injury to this nerve usually occurs from a direct blow or from compression, heavy packs or surgery. Burning scapular pain and winging are noted although the latter is more common.[8,11]

Somatic Findings

As in cervical spondylosis with nerve root irritation. Tenderness and myofascial dysfunction of the corresponding serratus anterior.

Manual Therapy Intervention

As in cervical spondylosis with nerve root irritation. In addition, if the long thoracic nerve is involved, treatment is as outlined in the serratus anterior section. Although this is a nerve root irritation presentation, the symptoms are not appendicular (extremities) but axial (trunk). Hence neural tension tests are negative.

LEVATOR SCAPULA SYNDROME

The levator scapula muscle is often predisposed to pain and dysfunction, or be a potential mediator of pathology in other areas.[9,10] The following are some of the possible reasons:

Subcranial Dysfunction

Owing to its attachment to the upper cervical spine and superomedial border of the scapula, dysfunctional situations of this muscle can predispose to subcanial dysfunction and resultant myogenic headaches.

Variation of Insertion

A unique insertion variant of this muscle can potentially cause a change in the mechanics and result in myofascial pain syndromes. The levator scapulae muscle may give rise to an accessory head that can insert by way of a flat aponeurotic band to the ligamentum nuchae, tendon of the rhomboideus major and the superior aspect of the serratus posterior superior muscle. The innervation being provided by a branch of the dorsal scapular nerve. They exert a unilateral traction on the vertebrae and surrounding musculature resulting in clinical consequences including scoliosis and movement abnormalities of the head and neck as well as myofascial pain syndrome.

Nerve Mediation

The 3,4th cervical branches of the dorsal scapular nerve supplies the levator scapula. Dysfunctional situations of these cervical segments can cause pain in the levator scapula.

Impingement Tendonitis

The levator scapula is prone for tightness, being a postural muscle. Tightness can encourage a downward rotation of the scapula wich brings the acromion relatively lower narrowing the subacromial space. This can predispose to impingement tendonitis of the supraspinatus.

Somatic Findings

- Forward head posture with core weakness
- Local tenderness over the levator scapula
- Tightness of the levator scapula
- Scapula dysfunction (see shoulder section)
- OA-and AA dysfunction
- C3, C4 nerve root involvement.

Manual Therapy Intervention

Suboccipital Release

- Stretch upper trapezius, levator scapula
- Trigger point compression of levator scapula, upper and middle trapezius
- OA forward nodding
- AA rotation if restriction is present
- Midcervical opening or closing if present
- Scapula retraction and upward rotation (see shoulder section)
- Neural interface mobilization for the appropriate nerve if radicular symptoms are present.

RHOMBOID STRAIN

A rhomboid muscle strain or spasm is usually caused by the overuse of the shoulder and arm, especially during overhead activities like serving a tennis ball or reaching to put objects on a high shelf. Besides repetitive activity, the other common cause of rhomboid strains are static and prolonged faulty postures as in sitting in front of a computer or driving, and faulty alignment.[11] Carrying a heavy backpack especially over one shoulder could also be a causative factor.

Somatic Findings

- Pain and tenderness in the interscapular area
- A spasm feels like tightness in the interscapular area
- Pain on movement of the shoulders (lifting and pulling), or on breathing
- Forward head posture with core weakness, including rhomboids
- Opening and closing restrictions of the thoracic spine.

Manual Therapy Intervention

Distraction precedes if the origin is from the dorsal scapular nerve at C5.

Suboccipital Release

- Stretch upper trapezius, levator scapula
- Soft tissue mobilization at the midthoracic level
- Trigger point compression of levator scapula, upper and middle trapezius, rhomboids
- OA forward nodding
- AA rotation if restriction is present
- Midthoracic opening or closing if present, with instability being considered
- Scapula retraction (see shoulder section).

SERRATUS ANTERIOR/ INTERCOSTALS

The serratus anterior is a common source of lateral thoracic pain in excessively active individuals. The serratus anterior is often called the "boxer's muscle" because it assists in protraction of the scapula which is essential during punching. The serratus anterior also helps to stabilize the scapula against the rib cage and is an important contributor of maintaining the subacromial space when an individual is vulnerable to impingement tendinitis. In addition, it assists in rotating the scapula upward. There is controversy as to whether this muscle plays a role in respiration, however, rib dysfunctions/stress fractures can cause pain in this muscle.

Somatic Findings

- Pain and tenderness in the lateral rib area
- Pain on movement of the shoulders (lifting and pulling), or on breathing
- Forward head posture with core weakness
- Opening and closing restrictions of the thoracic spine
- Rib dysfunctions, anterior or posterior.

Manual Therapy Intervention

Suboccipital Release

- Stretch upper trapezius, levator scapula
- Trigger point compression of levator scapula, upper and middle trapezius, rhomboids
- OA forward nodding
- Scapula retraction (see shoulder section)
- Opening and closing manipulation of the thoracic spine with caution to first rule out stress fractures of the rib.
- Muscle energy for rib dysfunctions, anterior or posterior.

SERRATUS POSTERIOR SUPERIOR

The serratus posterior superior muscles are located in the same region as the rhomboids. The difference is that the rhomboids have a thoracic and scapular attachment and the serratus posterior superior has a thoracic and rib attachment. Often this muscle can be involved in direct trauma as in a fall on the back of the trunk. Individuals may report a sensation of gasping for breath as this involves the ribs with a spasm of the serratus posterior superior. Other causes are similar to a rhomboid strain. There is controversy that this muscle has a repiratory function. Literature describes the serratus posterior superior have been implicated in the myofascial pain syndromes.[12]

Somatic Findings

- Pain and tenderness in the interscapular area
- A spasm feels like tightness in the interscapular area
- Pain on movement of the shoulders (lifting and pulling), or on breathing
- Forward head posture with core weakness including the rhomboids
- Opening and closing restrictions of the thoracic spine.

Manual Therapy Intervention

Suboccipital Release

- Stretch upper trapezius, levator scapula
- Soft tissue mobilization in the interscapular area
- Trigger point compression of levator scapula, upper and middle trapezius, rhomboids
- OA forward nodding
- Scapula retraction (see shoulder section)
- Opening and closing manipulation of the thoracic spine
- Muscle energy for rib dysfunction, anterior or posterior.

REFERENCES

1. Gonzalez-Darder JM. Thoracic dorsal ramus entrapment. Case report. J Neurosurg. 1989; 70:124-5.
2. Leong JC, Lu WW, Luk KD, et al. Kinematics of the chest cage and spine during breathing in healthy individuals and in patients with adolescent idiopathic scoliosis. Spine. 1999;24:1310-5.
3. Menck JY, Requejo SM, Kulig K. Thoracic spine dysfunction in upper extremity complex regional pain syndrome type I. J Orthop Sports Phys Ther. 2000;30:401-9.
4. Sebastian D. T2 radiculopathy: A differential screen for upper extremity radicular pain. Journal of manual and manipulative therapy. 2011; Abstracts of the American Academy of Orthopaedic Manual Physical Therapists (AAOMPT) annual conference, Anaheim, California.
5. Sebastian D. T2 radiculopathy: a differential screen for upper extremity radicular pain. Physiother Theory Pract.2013;29:75-85.
6. McGuckin N. The T4 syndrome. In: Grieve GP, editor. Modern Manual Therapy of the Vertebral Column.1986, Churchill Livingstone, New York.
7. Lazar MA, Kwon YW, Rokito AS. Snapping scapula syndrome. J Bone Joint Surg Am. 2009; 91:2251-62.
8. Flynn TW. (Ed). The Thoracic Spine and Chest Wall. Boston, MA: Butterworth-Heinemann; 1996;171-210.
9. Norlander S, Gustavsson BA, Lindell J, et al. Reduced mobility in the cervico-thoracic motion segment--a risk factor for musculoskeletal neck-shoulderpain: a two-year prospective follow-up study. Scand J Rehabil Med. 1997;29:167-74.
10. Norlander S, Nordgren B. Clinical symptoms related to musculoskeletal neck-shoulder pain and mobility in the cervicothoracic spine. Scand J Rehabil Med. 1998;30:243-51.
11. Home Study Course 16.2: Current concepts in orthopedic physical therapy. La Crosse, WI: Orthopaedic Section, APTA, Inc; 2006.
12. Joel A. Vilensky, Marsha Baltes, Laura Weikel, et al. Serratus posterior muscles: anatomy, clinical relevance, and function. Clin. Anat. 2001; 14:237-41.

CHAPTER 25

Lumbopelvic Region

LUMBAR SPONDYLOSIS

Lumbar spondylosis like cervical spondylosis is a disorder caused by abnormal wear on the cartilage and bones of the lumbar vertebrae with degeneration and mineral deposits in the intervertebral disks.

Lumbar spondylosis similar to cervical spondylosis, is a movement disorder predominanly secondary to faulty movement patterns in the lumbar complex. The lumbar complex is appropriately designed to distribute movement which is hindered during restrictive situations. This occurs predominantly in the junctions where the thoracic spine meets the lumbar (thoracolumbar junction) and the lumbar spine meets the sacrum (lumbosacral junction). Emprical evidence suggests that thoracolumbar junction is often restricted due to its transitional nature. The result is a compensatory hypermobility in the lumbosacral junction resulting in wear and tear. It is common to see wear in the lumbosacral junction and L4, L5 junctions compared to the thoracolumbar junction. Additionally, when capsular restriction prevails in the hip joints, the result is compensatory hypermobility at the lumbosacral junction resulting in wear and tear.

These accumulated changes caused by degeneration can wear the facet joint and intervertebral disk and the capsule with subsequent narrowing of the intervertebral for men. These accumulated changes caused by the degeneration and narrowing of the foramen can gradually compress one or more of the exiting nerve roots (Fig. 25.1). This can lead to increasing pain in the back and legs, with motor weakness, and changes in sensation. *Lumbar spondylosis* comprises all aspects of the above description and commonly occurs secondary to faulty mechanics with hypermobility of the lower lumbar levels (L4, L5) as a compensation to thoracolumbar hypomobility. When the degenerative changes extend to the facet joint and capsule, the resultant dysfunction is broadly known as *facet joint degeneration, facet capsule impingement*. This classically leads to opening and closing restrictions. When a restriction persists in the joint and overactivity occurs on the opposite side the result is excessive shearing of the annular fibers and may lead to a *Disk Herniation* (Fig. 25.2). This is further aggravated by the faulty body mechanics as in excessive bending and twisting. The narrowing of the foramen secondary to wear and tear and the protruding disk from a herniation can impinge on the exiting lumbar nerve roots resulting in *nerve root irritation and radicular pain*. This nerve root pain can occur without the presence of a disk herniation, secondary to wear and tear and subsequent narrowing of the intervertebral foramen. A situation as this can compress or irritate the nerve root exiting out of the foramen, resulting in *lumbar radiculopathy*.[1-4]

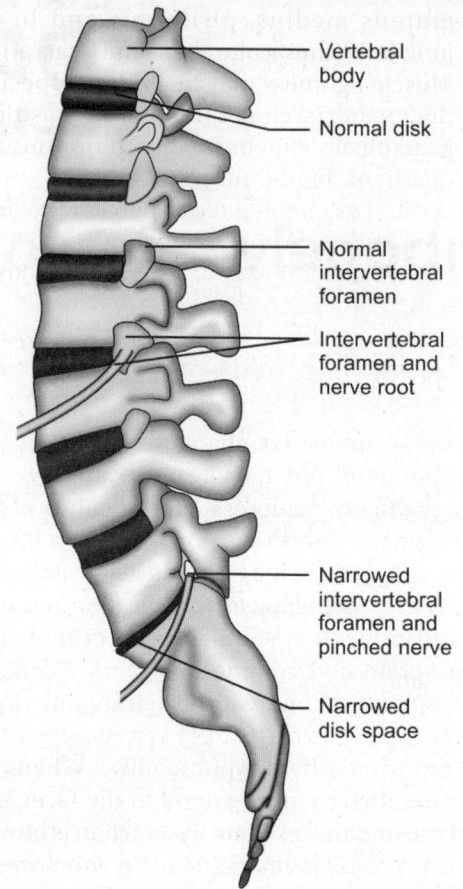

Fig. 25.1: Lumbar spondylosis and radiculopathy.

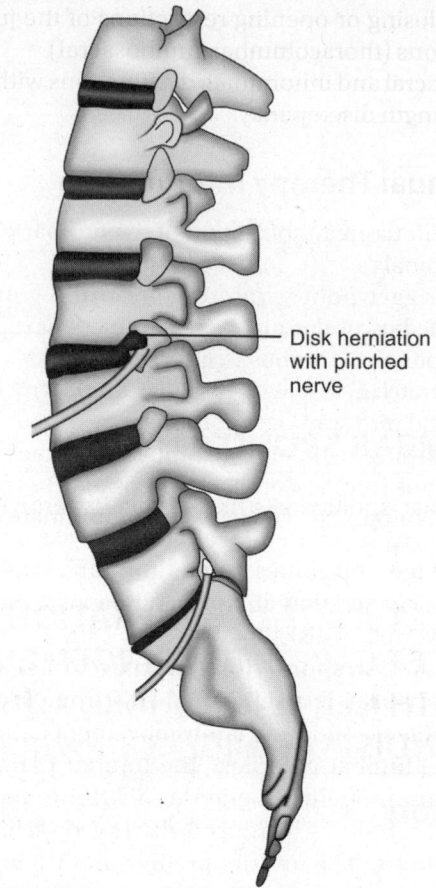

Fig. 25.2: Disk herniation and radiculopathy.

FACET JOINT DEGENERATION, FACET CAPSULE IMPINGEMENT (WITHOUT NERVE ROOT IRRITATION)

History

Primary complaint is pain in the back possibly radiating into the buttock area. There is no pain radiating into the lower extremities. There is difficulty in moving the back freely with restricted range of motion. There may be a sensation of popping and cracking of the joints on movement. A sensation of tightness of the lumbopelvic musculature may be evident. There may be a painful catching sensation in certain parts of the range of motion if instability is prevalent. Occupation may include prolonged periods of physical activity, driving, riding, bending, twisting and lifting.

Somatic Findings

Changes in Lumbar Lordosis

- Restricted range of motion with painful muscle trigger points (commonly in the gluteus medius, piriformis and in the junctions (thoracolumbar, lumbosacral)
- Muscle tightness may be evident especially by the superficial groups (Iliopsoas, hamstrings, paraspinals, gluteus medius, piriformis and quadratus lumborum)

- Closing or opening restrictions of the junctions (thoracolumbar, lumbosacral)
- Sacral and innominate dysfunctions with leg length discrepancy.

Manual Therapy Intervention

- Soft tissue mobilization of the lumbar paraspinals
- Trigger point compression to the gluteus medius, piriformis and in the junctions (thoracolumbar, lumbosacral)
- Stretch iliopsoas, hamstrings, gluteus medius and piriformis as appropiate
- Closing or opening manipulation of the junctions (thoracolumbar, lumbosacral)
- Manipulation of sacral and innominate dysfunctions.

FACET JOINT DEGENERATION, FACET CAPSULE IMPINGEMENT (WITH NERVE ROOT IRRITATION, NONDISCOGENIC)

History

Primary complaint is pain in the back possibly radiating into the buttock area. There is pain radiating into the lower extremities. There is difficulty in moving the back freely with restricted range of motion.[5] There may be a sensation of popping and cracking of the joints on movement. A sensation of tightness of the lumbo-pelvic musculature may be evident. There may be a painful catching sensation in certain parts of the range of motion. Occupation may include prolonged periods of physical activity, driving, riding, bending, twisting and lifting. Extension, standing and walking with aggravates the pain, while flexion, sitting, alleviates the pain.

Somatic Findings

Changes in Lumbar Lordosis

- Restricted range of motion with painful muscle trigger points (commonly in the gluteus medius, piriformis and in the junctions (thoracolumbar, lumbosacral)
- Muscle tightness may be evident especially the superficial groups (Iliopsoas, hamstrings, paraspinals, gluteus medius, piriformis and quadratus lumborum)
- Closing or opening restrictions of the junctions (thoracolumbar, lumbosacral)
- Sacral and innominate dysfunctions with leg length discrepancy
- Weakness of core musculature (transversus abdominis, gluteus medius, pelvic floor and multifidus)
- A pinching sensation in a specific point of the range of motion
- Positive finding on lower limb tension test [straight leg raise (SLR), SLUMP].

Manual Therapy Intervention

Distraction precedes provided there are no signs of instability:

- Soft tissue mobilization of the lumbar paraspinals
- Trigger point compression to the gluteus medius, piriformis and in the junctions (thoracolumbar, lumbosacral)
- Stretch iliopsoas, hamstrings, gluteus medius and piriformis as appropiate
- Closing or opening manipulation of the junctions (thoracolumbar, lumbosacral)
- Manipulation of sacral and innominate dysfunctions
- Neural interface mobilization followed by the sliders and tensioners.

DISK HERNIATION

History

Primary complaint is pain in the back possibly radiating into the buttock area. There is pain radiating into the lower extremities. Onset may be secondary to lifting a heavy weight especially overhead, or a violent cough or sneeze. There is difficulty in moving the back freely with restricted range of motion. A sensation of tightness of the lumbopelvic musculature may be evident more in this clinical situation than any other. There may be a painful catching sensation in certain parts of the range of motion and often intense spasms. Patient may wake up in the morning with a tight spasm like feeling in the lumbar area. There is pain on coughing or sneezing (valsalva). There may be motor loss knee (L2,3) ankle (L4,S1) and foot [extensor hallucis longus (EHL), L5] and loss of sensation. Occupation may include prolonged periods of physical activity, driving, riding, bending, twisting and lifting. Extension, standing and walking alleviates pain while flexion, sitting, aggravates the pain.

Somatic Findings

Changes in Lumbar Lordosis

- Restricted range of motion with painful muscle trigger points (commonly in the gluteus medius, piriformis and in the junctions (thoracolumbar, lumbosacral)
- Muscle tightness may be evident especially hyper the superficial groups (iliopsoas, hamstrings, paraspinals, gluteus medius, piriformis and quadratus lumborum)
- Closing or opening restrictions of the junctions (thoracolumbar, lumbosacral)
- Sacral and innominate dysfunctions with leg length discrepancy
- Weakness of core musculature (tranversus abdominis, gluteus medius, pelvic floor and multifidius)
- A pinching sensation in a specific point of the range of motion
- Positive finding on lower limb tension test (SLR, SLUMP).

Manual Therapy Intervention

Distraction precedes provided there are no signs of instability.
- Soft tissue mobilization of the lumbar paraspinals
- Trigger point compression to the gluteus medius, piriformis and in the junctions (thoracolumbar, lumbosacral)
- Stretch iliopsoas, hamstrings, gluteus medius and piriformis as appropiate
- Mobilization or manipulation in closing to facilitate extension is preferred as this may assist the centralization process. It is done with caution in acute discogenic situations. Thrust manipulation is not preferred in the lumbosacral area
- Manipulation of sacral and innominate dysfunctions
- Neural interface mobilization followed by sliders and tensioners.

The direction and types of herniation are varied. Commonly, they are either in the posterolateral direction or central. When the herniation is posterolateral, the direction is towards the intervertebral foramen (lateral canal or lateral recess). This will involve the spinal nerve root. However, when the herniation is central, its direction is towards the spinal canal. Hence, the cord is involved. So additionally the clinician may observe.

Bladder Bowel Dysfunction

Positive Babinski:
However, note that the cord ends at L1 and if cord signs are evident then the central herniation is probably not at the lumbar level, but the thoracic and cervical regions require attention. It may be wise to always consider the possibility of disk herniations at the thoracolumbar junction, sometimes with cord compromise.

Hence in any routine examination, if the clinician observes motor loss, bladder bowel dysfunction and a positive babinski it is a red flag which contraindicates manual therapy and warrants an immediate surgical consult.

MUSCLE PATHOLOGIES

The one finding in a muscle in conjunction with a mechanical back dysfunction is tenderness with soft tissue thickening of the musculature. Tenderness in a muscle can lead to an assumption that the muscle is the source of the dysfunction.

This may be the case but not always. Every joint or motion segment has a corresponding muscle that helps to effect movement. Dysfunctional states of the joint can cause additional stress on the supporting soft tissue and result in muscle guarding. This can lead to an accumulation of metabolites in the involved muscle and result in local tenderness with hypertrophy due to guarding. Common causes for soft tissue pathology are prolonged faulty postures or overuse. Several theories exist as to why a soft tissue lesion can occur secondary to prolonged faulty postures or overuse. The three most common theories are as follows:

1. Prolonged and excessive contraction as would occur with overuse or faulty postures may induce fatigue in a muscle. The muscle contracts in response to fatigue and persists to create a local soft tissue dysfunction with localized tender point called 'trigger points'.
2. Excessive and faulty muscle contraction can cause injury to the myofibrils of the muscle bulk which may heal with scarring. This scarring can inhibit normal physiological contraction and deprive the area of nutrition and encourage chemical accumulation causing pain. In addition possible nerve endings in the healed scar may also be pain sensitive.
3. Faulty activity can influence the muscle at an intrafusal level creating constant aberrant gamma motor activity which renders the soft tissue dysfunctional.

History

Primary complaint is pain in the back possibly radiating into the buttock area. There may or may not be a history of pain radiating into the lower extremities. There is difficulty moving the back freely with restricted range of motion. There may be a sensation of popping and cracking of the joints on movement. A sensation of tightness of the lumbo-pelvic musculature may be evident. There is no pain on coughing or sneezing. There is relief of symptoms when laying down or resting. Occupation may include prolonged periods of physical activity, driving, riding, bending, twisting, long-standing and lifting.

Somatic Findings

Changes in Lumbar Lordosis

- Restricted range of motion with painful muscle trigger points (commonly in the gluteus medius, piriformis and in the junctions (thoracolumbar, lumbosacral)
- Muscle tightness may be evident especially the superficial groups (Iliopsoas, hamstrings, paraspinals, gluteus medius, piriformis and quadratus lumborum)
- May or may not present with closing or opening restrictions of the junctions (thoracolumbar, lumbosacral)
- May or may not present with sacral and innominate dysfunctions with leg length discrepancy
- Weakness of core musculature (transversus abdominus, gluteus medius, pelvic floor and multifidi)
- A pinching sensation in a specific point of the range of motion.

Manual Therapy Intervention

- Soft tissue mobilization of the lumbar paraspinals
- Trigger point compression to the gluteus medius, piriformis and in the junctions (thoracolumbar, lumbosacral)
- Stretch iliopsoas, hamstrings, gluteus medius and piriformis as appropiate
- Closing or opening manipulation of the junctions (thoracolumbar, lumbosacral) if present
- Manipulation of sacral and innominate dysfunctions if present.

Commonly muscle pathologies may have associated joint dysfunction going with it, however, there is controversy as to where the dysfunction begins. The reason being activity involves in the joint and muscle equally.

STENOSIS

A stenotic situation is one where a certain defined space is narrowed. On reviewing the anatomy of the spinal canal there are two distinct

openings, one for the cord and one for the exiting nerve roots. The central opening that houses the cord is called the spinal canal and the lateral opening where the nerve roots from the cord exit is the intervertebral foramen or lateral recess. Hence, two types of stenotic situations can occur:
1. Foraminal stenosis
2. Central canal stenosis

Foraminal Stenosis

The foramen can become narrow for several reasons. They are as follows:
- Opening and closing restrictions of the joint can cause changes in the patency of the foramen
- Disk and facet joint degeneration approximates the vertebral bodies together. This can narrow the foramen. This situation is seen in cervical spondylosis with nerve root irritation
- When a ruptured disk herniates posterolaterally towards the foramen it can pour its contents into the foramen causing stenosis.

All of the above three situations can cause radicular pain. Hence adverse neural tension is positive, but since the cord is not involved Babinski may be negative. However, although the cord is not involved, the situation is considered serious if the nerve root compression is severe enough to cause motor loss (e.g. foot drop) or involves the sacral roots causing bladder, bowel dysfunction. If such a situation arises it is considered a red flag and requires an immediate surgical consult.

History

Primary complaint is pain in the back possibly radiating into the buttock area. There is pain radiating into the lower extremities. Onset may be gradual over time (degenerative) or secondary to lifting a heavy weight, especially overhead, or a violent cough or sneeze (discogenic). There is difficulty moving the back freely with restricted range of motion. A sensation of tightness of the lumbopelvic musculature may be evident. There may be a painful catching sensation in certain parts of the range of motion and often intense spasms. There is pain on coughing or sneezing (valsalva). There may be motor loss knee (L2,3) ankle (L4,S1) and foot (EHL,L5) and loss of sensation. Occupation may include prolonged periods of physical activity, driving, riding, bending, twisting and lifting. These patients typically present with an increase in symptoms on prolonged standing and walking with relief of symptoms in sitting. This finding is very obvious in central canal stenosis, but can also occur with foraminal stenosis.

Somatic Findings

Changes in Lumbar Lordosis

- Restricted range of motion with painful muscle trigger points (commonly in the gluteus medius, piriformis and in the junctions (thoracolumbar, lumbosacral)
- Muscle tightness may be evident especially the superficial groups (Iliopsoas, hamstrings, paraspinals, gluteus medius, piriformis and quadratus lumborum)
- Closing or opening restrictions of the junctions (thoracolumbar, lumbosacral)
- Sacral and innominate dysfunctions with leg length discrepancy
- Weakness of core musculature (transversus abdominus, gluteus medius, pelvic floor and multifidi)
- A pinching sensation in a specific point of the range of motion
- Positive finding on lower limb tension testing (SLR, SLUMP).

Manual Therapy Intervention

Distraction precedes provided there are no signs of instability:
- Soft tissue mobilization of the lumbar paraspinals
- Trigger point compression to the gluteus medius, piriformis and in the junctions (thoracolumbar, lumbosacral)
- Stretch iliopsoas, hamstrings, gluteus medius and piriformis as appropiate

- Closing or opening manipulation of the junctions (thoracolumbar, lumbosacral) Thrust is not preferred in disk pathology
- Specific opening manipulation or mobilization if a particular nerve root is involved. For example, in L4 radiculopathy opening the facet between L4, 5 is preferred as the L4 nerve root exits between L4, 5.
- Neural interface mobilization followed by sliders and tensioners.

Central Canal Stenosis

Visualize the spine as concentric rings arranged on top of each other. Imagine if one individual ring translates forward. It is going to narrow the canal. This condition is called spondylolisthesis and is one of the causes for spinal stenosis. A herniated disk that protrudes centrally can head straight into the central spinal canal causing stenosis. A calcified and protruding ligament inside the canal as in the ligamentum flavum can cause stenosis. In central canal stenosis it is the cord that is being compromised. So if the patient presents with balance issues, bladder bowel dysfunction and a positive Babinski, it is a red flag and requires an immediate surgical consult.

History

Primary complaint is pain in the back possibly radiating into the buttock area. There is pain radiating into the lower extremities. Onset may be secondary to long standing or walking with obvious relief on sitting. There may be a history of fall or direct trauma, or periods of extension type of activity. There is difficulty moving the back freely with restricted range of motion. A sensation of tightness of the lumbo-pelvic musculature may be evident. There may be a painful catching sensation in certain parts of the range of motion and often intense spasms. There is pain on coughing or sneezing (valsalva). There may be motor loss knee (L2,3) ankle (L4,S1) and foot (EHL,L5) and loss of sensation. Occupation may include prolonged periods of physical activity, driving, riding, bending twisting and lifting. These patients typically present with an increase in symptoms on prolonged standing and walking with relief of symptoms in sitting. This finding is very obvious in central canal stenosis.

Somatic Findings

Findings may be similar to what is seen in a foraminal stenosis, but the risk of ivolving the cord (upper lumbar) and cauda equina (mid-and lower lumbar) prevails as the compromise is now in the spinal canal and not in the intervertebral foramen.

Changes in Lumbar Lordosis

- Faulty gait pattern secondary to intense pain or a previous pathology in the hip, knee and ankle
- Restricted range of motion with painful spasms (commonly in the gluteus medius, piriformis) and in the junctions (thoracolumbar, lumbosacral)
- Muscle tightness may be evident especially the superficial groups (iliopsoas, hamstrings, paraspinals, gluteus medius, piriformis and quadratus lumborum)
- Closing or opening restrictions of the junctions (thoracolumbar, lumbosacral)
- Sacral and innominate dysfunctions with leg length discrepancy
- Weakness of core musculature (transversus abdominus, gluteus medius, pelvic floor and multifidius)
- A pinching sensation in a specific point of the range of motion
- Positive finding on lower limb tension testing (SLR, SLUMP)
- A step deformity at the level if spondylolisthesis is the cause for stenosis.

Manual Therapy Intervention

This condition may indicate soft tissue mobilization and manual intervention of the pelvic complex, but manual intervention of the lumbar spine is contraindicated, especially if spondylolisthesis is the cause for the central stenosis.

INSTABILITY

Instability of the spinal column is a situation where the joint, muscle and ligamentous structures are unable to support a spinal motion segment in the appropriate anatomical position.[4] The concept of inner (core) and outer muscle groups needs to be enumerated. In a spinal motion segment from a mechanical sense, two aspects prevail. There is stability and mobility. Spinal musculature execute this function appropriately by first stabilizing the segment, and then moving it with the stability maintained. The stabilizing muscles are the core muscles and current research has greatly emphasized the transversus abdominis, multifidus, pelvic floor and gluteus medius as the key musculature that stabilize the spinal motion segment. The next common reason for instability is a loosening of the joint by excessive lengthening of the joint capsule secondary to repetitive motion past the normal physiological range or connective tissue laxity. The pathological cause for spinal instability is a defect in the pars interarticularis and subsequent slippage of the entire vertebral body, a condition is called spondylolisthesis.

The causes for instability are as follows:
- Due to excessive physical activity, sometimes beyond physiologic ranges.
- Repeated manipulations of the spine. Some individuals are habitual 'self crackers'.
- Systemic laxity, secondary to connective tissue or collagen disorders, or just the nature of the individual.
- Hormonal, as seen in women of childbearing age.
- Spondylolysis and spondylolisthesis.
- Inherent core weakness and repeated excessive physical activity over it.
- Following laminectomy (postlaminectomy syndrome).
- Wear and tear of the facet joints and the intervertebral articulations.

History

The patient typically reports of difficulty sustaining one position for too long (creep). Any static posture for extended periods of time, aggravates symptoms. There is a tendency for painful catching spasms as the musculature is doing much to protect the unstable segments. This is most apparent with sudden movements, turns, etc. There is a history of heavy physical activity sometimes beyond physiological limits as in gymnastics. The patient may be a habitual 'self cracker' of the spinal joints. They typically 'thigh climb' with their hands to come up to stand after a period of sitting.

Somatic and Examination Findings

Changes in Lumbar Lordosis

- Normal gait pattern, or faulty gait pattern secondary to a previous pathology in the hip, knee and ankle
- Increased range of motion with painful muscle trigger points (commonly in the gluteus medius, piriformis) and in the junctions (thoracolumbar, lumbosacral)
- Closing or opening restrictions of the junctions (thoracolumbar, lumbosacral)
- Sacral and innominate dysfunctions with leg length discrepancy
- Weakness of core musculature (transversus abdominus, gluteus medius, pelvic floor and multifidi)
- A pinching catching spasm in a specific point of the range of motion
- May or may not have a positive finding on lower limb tension test (SLR, SLUMP)
- Positive CPR for instability[6]
- Systemic laxity tests are positive.

The clinician is advised that instability is a feature that can be seen in association with lumbar spondylosis, disk herniation, spondylolysis and spondylolisthesis.

INSTABILITY (SPONDYLOLYSIS/SPONDYLOLISTHESIS)

The area between the superior and inferior articulations of the spinal motion segment is called pars interarticularis. A defect in the pars interarticularis is called spondylolysis. So spondylolysis means a defect in the thin isthmus of bone connecting superior and inferior facets, and could be unilateral or bilateral. Although the defect can be found at any level, the most common vertebra involved is the 5th lumbar vertebra (or L5). In cases of bilateral spondylolysis, the posterior articulations can no longer provide the posterior stability, and anterior slipping of the L5 vertebra over the sacrum could result. Visualize the spine as concentric rings arranged on top of each other. Imagine if one individual ring translates forward, it is going to narrow the canal. This condition is called spondylolisthesis and is one of the causes for spinal stenosis.

Causes of Spondylolisthesis

- Congenital
- Infection or tumor
- Trauma which typically begins as a stress fracture of the pars due to repetitive activity (especially extension).

History

Although some patients can be asymptomatic, back pain is probably the most common symptom, and presents during the adolescent growth spurt. There is often a history of trauma at sports (gymnastics, wrestling, weight training), slip and fall or a history of excessive physical activity. Standing, walking and arching the back may aggravate symptoms but sitting may relieve it. Radicular symptoms may prevail.

Somatic and Examination Findings

- All signs of central canal stenosis as described
- Changes in the lumbar lordosis
- Faulty gait pattern secondary to intense pain or a previous pathology in the hip, knee and ankle
- Restricted range of motion with painful spasms (commonly in the gluteus medius, piriformis and in the junctions (thoracolumbar, lumbosacral)
- Muscle tightness may be evident especially by the superficial groups (iliopsoas, hamstrings, paraspinals, gluteus medius, piriformis and quadratus lumborum)
- Closing or opening restrictions of the junctions (thoracolumbar, lumbosacral)
- Sacral and innominate dysfunctions with leg length discrepancy
- Diminished reflexes in the relevant nerve root involved
- Diminished sensation in the relevant dermatome
- Diminished strength in the relevant myotome
- Weakness of core musculature (transversus abdominis, gluteus medius, pelvic floor and multifidius)
- A pinching sensation in a specific point of the range of motion
- Positive finding on lower limb tension testing (SLR, SLUMP)
- A step deformity at the level
- Active extension aggravates symptoms
- Bicycle test may be positive.

Manual Therapy Intervention

As in stenosis, this condition may indicate soft tissue mobilization and manual intervention of the pelvic complex, but manual intervention of the lumbar spine is contraindicated especially if spondylolisthesis is the cause for the instability. Manual intervention may be indicated for other types of instability as in a postlaminectomy syndrome but should be used sparingly as the bigger indication for treatment is core strengthening.

WHIPLASH INJURIES

Whiplash is an injury to the neck, but can also occur in the back resulting from a sudden extension and then flexion contraction of the back. Whiplash injury is most commonly the result of the motion caused by an automobile accident. In a sudden stop, the trunk is usually thrown forward and then backward violently, putting a brief but major strain on the back. The reverse happens if rear ended. This stretches muscles and ligaments in the back. This is immediately followed by a reflex contraction of the muscles, joint restriction and pain. Other causes are sports injuries and physical abuse. The musculature and lumbar facet joints are commonly involved. One has to be constantly aware of a chance fracture or abdominal injuries secondary to a tight seat belt.

History

There is a history of motor vehicle accident, or being tackled in sport. There may be previous history of back pathology. There may be a report of no immediate pain but exacerbation of symptoms the next day with progressive pain and increased stiffness.

Somatic Findings

Changes in Lumbar Lordosis

- Faulty gait pattern secondary to intense pain or a previous pathology in the hip, knee and ankle
- Restricted range of motion with painful spasms (commonly in the gluteus medius, piriformis) and in the junctions (thoracolumbar, lumbosacral)
- Muscle tightness may be evident especially the superficial groups (Iliopsoas, hamstrings, paraspinals, gluteus medius, piriformis and quadratus lumborum)
- Closing or opening restrictions of the junctions (thoracolumbar, lumbosacral)
- Sacral and innominate dysfunctions with leg length discrepancy
- Weakness of core musculature (transversus abdominus, gluteus medius, pelvic floor and multifidi)
- A pinching sensation in a specific point of the range of motion
- May or may not have a positive finding on lower limb tension test (SLR, SLUMP)
- Tenderness in the thoracolumbar junction.

Manual Therapy Intervention

Provided a chance fracture has been ruled out:
- Distraction precedes if radicular symptoms prevail, provided there are no signs of instability
- Soft tissue mobilization of the lumbar paraspinals
- Trigger point compression to the gluteus medius, piriformis and in the junctions (thoracolumbar, lumbosacral)
- Stretch iliopsoas, hamstrings, gluteus medius and piriformis as appropiate
- Closing or opening manipulation of the junctions (thoracolumbar, lumbosacral)
- Manipulation of sacral and innominate dysfunctions
- Neural interface mobilization followed by sliders and tensioners if nerve root irritation is evident.

THORACOLUMBAR JUNCTION SYNDROME

The thoracolumbar junction is a transition zone between two regions, lumbar and thoracic T12/L1. In the T12 vertebra the superior facet is inclined as in the thoracic spine in a more frontal plane and in the inferior vertebra, as in the lumbar spine in a more sagittal plane. Since most of the thoracic rotation is restricted by the presence of the ribs, and mid lumbar area by the sagittal orientation of the facet joints, thoracolumbar junction is described as being one that possesses a significant amount of rotation. In the lumbosacral junction the orientation of the facet joints are in the frontal plane as opposed to the mid lumbar articulations which are more in the sagittal plane. Hence, a considerable amount of rotation also occurs in the lumbosacral junction. Pain from a thoracolumbar dysfunction is seldom felt in the thoracolumbar region. The primary site of referral is the iliac crest and gluteal region with the trochanteric and groin areas being other sites. The reason being the nerve representation. The posterior primary rami of the thoracolumbar spinal nerves innervate the skin of the back and intrinsic muscles of the apophyseal joints and supra- and interspinous ligaments. The cutaneous branches penetrate the lumbar fascia, descend in the subcutaneous tissue and end in the skin of the lower lumbar area. Cutaneous innervation also represents the gluteal region and is derived from the higher levels of the thoracolumbar region, T11, T12, L1.[7]

The thoracolumbar junction is described as being mostly hypomobile due to its transitory anatomy. Hence, the presence of an extended rotated side, (ERS) or flexor rotated side (FRS) dysfunction with local tenderness is possible and should be examined. The reason for mandatory assessment and treatment of the thoracolumbar junction is more than addressing symptoms locally. Hypomobility of the thoracolumbar articulation may cause a compensatory increase in mobility and stress in the lumbosacral junction and subsequent dysfunction. Assessment and treatment are similar to that done in the lower thoracic spine except that the focus is the T12, L1 segment. Again, the possibility of a disk herniation at the junction with a possible cord compromise warrants caution.

History

The individual may present with buttock, trochanteric or groin pain in an isolated presentation, however, the clinician should be aware of the fact that this may occur in conjunction with other low back syndromes, including whiplash sequelae. The pain is seldom felt in the thoracolumbar junction although there have been reports of local pain secondary to a disk herniation of the thoraco-lumbar junction. If pain is felt in the thoraco-lumbar junction a systemic source or a red flag should be suspected.

Somatic Findings

Changes in Lumbar Lordosis

- Faulty gait pattern secondary to intense pain or a previous pathology in the hip, knee and ankle
- Tenderness over the gluteus medius, piriformis and in the thoracolumbar junction
- Tenderness over the posterior-lateral iliac crest
- Closing or opening restrictions in the thoracolumbar junction
- Weakness of core musculature (transversus abdominis, gluteus medius, pelvic floor and multifidus)
- May or may not have a positive finding on lower limb tension testing (SLR, SLUMP)
- Tenderness in the thoracolumbar junction.

Manual Therapy Intervention

Soft tissue mobilization of the lumbar paraspinals
- Trigger point compression to the gluteus medius, piriformis and in the junctions (thoracolumbar, lumbosacral)
- Stretch Iliopsoas, hamstrings, gluteus medius and piriformis as appropiate
- Closing or opening manipulation of the junctions (thoracolumbar, lumbosacral), with a more obvious indication at the thoracolumbar junction
- Manipulation of sacral and innominate dysfunctions
- Neural interface mobilization followed by sliders and tensioners.

POSTLAMINECTOMY SYNDROME

A laminectomy is the removal of the lamina which is located in the back. This type of surgery is done for a herniated intervertebral disk pressing on a nerve root. The lamina is the very small plate that is located in the back of each vertebra. A full or even partial removal of the lamina can allow access to the patient's intervertebral disk. The surgical procedure can also alleviate any spinal pressure it may be causing. Postlaminectomy syndrome is also termed failed back syndrome however, the exact cause is not well described in most texts. Dr Paris describes it in an award winning paper.[8] The primary cause is described as an instability, as the ligamentum flavum is sacrificed when the lamina is removed and the posterior primary ramus is denervated with subsequent weakness of one of the key core stabilizers of the spine, multifidus. The ligamentum flavum and multifidus help to retract the facet capsule during facet movement. When this is lost secondary to the posterior denervation, the facet capsule is pinched and its inflammatory contents are poured into the foramen causing nerve pain. Additionally, due to faulty mechanics, the disk above or below the level of involvement may be stressed. The history and examination may be similar to that seen in instability.

History

The patient reports of having had a laminectomy in the past and has not kept up with core stabilization and has been indulging in heavy physical activity. The patient typically reports of difficulty sustaining one position for too long (creep). Any static posture for extended periods of time, aggravates symptoms. There is a tendency for painful catching spasms as the musculature is doing much to protect the unstable segments. This is most apparent with sudden movements, turns, etc. There is a history of heavy physical activity sometimes beyond physiological limits as in gymnastics. The patient may be a habitual 'self cracker' of the spinal joints. They typically 'thigh climb' with their hands to come up to stand, after a period of sitting.

Somatic and Examination Findings

Changes in Lumbar Lordosis

- Normal gait pattern, or faulty gait pattern secondary to pain and spasms or a previous pathology in the hip, knee and ankle
- Increased range of motion with painful muscle trigger points (commonly in the gluteus medius, piriformis) and in the junctions (thoracolumbar, lumbosacral)
- Decreased range of motion secondary to guarding and spasms
- Closing or opening restrictions of the junctions (thoracolumbar, lumbosacral)
- Sacral and innominate dysfunctions with leg length discrepancy
- Weakness of core musculature (transversus abdominus, gluteus medius, pelvic floor and multifidi)
- A pinching, catching spasm in a specific point of the range of motion
- May or may not have a positive finding on lower limb tension test (SLR, SLUMP)
- Positive CPR for instability.

Manual Therapy Intervention

The same consideration for instability, apply for a postlaminectomy syndrome.

S1 STRAIN/PIRIFORMIS SYNDROME

The pelvic complex consists of three bones and nine joints (2 articulating facets of L5, S1, 1 intervertebral disk, 2 sacroiliac, 2 coxafemoral (hip), 1 sacrococcygeal and 1 symphysis pubis) and hence highly mobile. The sacrum which is placed in the center is formed by the fused elements of S1 to S5. It articulates superiorly with the lumbar spine and inferiorly with the coccyx. They are termed as the lumbosacral and sacrococcygeal joints, respectively. Laterally, the sacrum articulates with the ilia or innominate bones to form the sacroiliac joints. The two innominates are joined anteriorly by the symphysis pubis joint.

The greater clinical significance of the pelvic complex originates at the lumbosacral junction. Most dysfunctions of the pelvic complex are viewed as dysfunctions at the sacroiliac joints and may be erroneous. As most times dysfunctions of the sacroiliac joint are caused by a dysfunction that occurs at the lumbosacral junction. The reason being that the lumbar spine is one that determines the mechanics of the sacrum at the lumbosacral joint which in turn determines the mechanics of the ilium or innominate at the sacroiliac joint. Hence, the clinician should always remember that when addressing dysfunctions of the pelvic complex, to first consider mechanics at the lumbosacral joint prior to addressing the sacroiliac joint which are mechanically two different areas but complimentary in causing a dysfunction. Dysfunctions in the pelvic complex occur in three regions. They occur either in the pubic symphysis, sacrum or ilium. Hence, they are classified as pubic, sacral and ilial dysfunctions.

The sacrum is probably the most important component of the pelvic complex and is often missed out in a sacroiliac dyfunction as the ilia receive more attention. The sacrum is the direct link of the lumbar spine to the pelvic complex and plays an important role in the walking cycle. The movements available in the sacrum are very limited for the fact that the center of gravity is located here and would make sense to have one that is stable. If this negligible movement of the sacrum is altered then a dysfunction would result. The sacrum has been described as a significant contributor to back pain and radicular pain. The reason being the close proximity of nerve structures to the sacroiliac joint, the ala of the sacrum and piriformis muscle as this muscle attaches to the lateral border of the sacrum. The mechanics of the sacrum has to be maintained for normalcy from a mechanical perspective. Dysfunctional mechanics can cause the piriformis to be hyperirritable. The common reason for piriformis irritability is hip flexion tightness and abductor weakness. When the femur is relatively flexed in weight bearing, the piriformis begins to work as an abductor. If one recalls the function of the abductors in stance phase to stabilize pelvis, then the piriformis tends to overwork during stance, in the presence of hip flexor tightness, and is hence rendered dysfunctional. In addition, as an anatomic variant, the sciatic nerve passes through the piriformis in a small population and hence becomes a causative factor for sciatic pain. The clinician should remember that sacroiliac pathology can occur alongside most lumbar dysfunctions.

History

Literature suggests that the sacroiliac joint is more vulnerable in the female[9] and hence should be looked for. The individual may have an associated lumbar dysfunction and hence all findings relevant a lumbar dysfunction should be looked for. In an isolated sacroiliac dysfunction, the pain is unilateral with/without radicular pain. Pain is localized to the buttock and increased with prolonged periods of sitting, driving with some relief, on standing and walking. However, in unstable situations, prolonged standing and walking may be uncomfortable. There may be a history of a fall on the buttock, surgeries around the abdomen and flank area, and multiple pregnancies.

Somatic and Examination Findings

Changes in Lumbar Lordosis

- Faulty gait pattern secondary to intense pain or a previous pathology in the hip, knee and ankle
- Restricted range of motion with pain and tenderness (commonly in the gluteus medius, piriformis) and in the lumbosacral junctions.
- Muscle tightness may be evident especially the superficial groups (Iliopsoas, hamstrings, paraspinals, gluteus medius, piriformis and quadratus lumborum), more so the iliopsoas.
- Thomas test is positive
- Closing or opening restrictions of the junctions (thoracolumbar, lumbosacral)
- Sacral and innominate dysfunctions with leg length discrepancy
- Weakness of core musculature (transversus abdominus, gluteus medius, pelvic floor and multifidi)
- May or may not have a positive finding on lower limb tension testing (SLR, SLUMP)
- Tenderness in the sacroiliac joint secondary to an irritable posterior sacroiliac ligament.
- CPR for sacroiliac dysfunction is positive.[10]

Manual Therapy Intervention

- Soft tissue mobilization of the lumbar paraspinals
- Trigger point compression to the gluteus medius, piriformis and in the junctions (thoracolumbar, lumbosacral)
- Deep frictions to the posterior sacroiliac ligament at the sacroiliac joint
- Stretch iliopsoas, hamstrings, gluteus medius and piriformis as appropiate
- Closing or opening manipulation of the junctions (thoracolumbar, lumbosacral)
- Manipulation of sacral and innominate dysfunctions
- Neural interface mobilization followed by sliders and tensioners
- Routine assessment of the hip for pathology, especially capsular restriction, if present, should be addressed first.

REFERENCES

1. Porterfield JA, DeRosa C. Mechanical neck pain. Perspectives in Functional anatomy, 1995, WB Saunders, Philadelphia, p.41.
2. Sedaghat N, Latimer J, Maher C, et al. The reproducibility of a clinical grading system of motor control in patients with low back pain. J Manipulative Physiol Ther. 2007;30:501-8.
3. Brennan GP et al. Identifying subgroups of patients with acute/subacute 'nonspecific' low back pain: results of a randomized clinical trial. Spine. 2006;31:623-31.
4. Fritz JM, George S. The use of a classification approach to identify subgroups of patients with acute low back pain. interrater reliability and short-term treatment outcomes. Spine. 2000; 25:106-14.
5. Mooney V, Robertson J. The facet syndrome. Clin Orthop Relat Res. 1976;115:149-56.
6. Hicks GE, Fritz JM, Delitto A, et al. Preliminary development of a clinical prediction rule for determining which patients with low back pain will respond to a stabilization exercise program. Arch Phys Med Rehabil. 2005;86:1753-62.
7. Sebastian D. Thoraco lumbar junction syndrome: a case report. Physiother Theory Pract. 2006; 22:53-60.
8. Paris SV. Anatomy as related to function and pain. Orthop Clin North Am. 1983;14:475-89.
9. Sebastian D. The Anatomical and physiological variations in the sacroiliac joints of the male and female: clinical implications. The Journal of Manual and Manipulative Therapy. 2000;8: 127-34.
10. Home Study Course 16.2: Current concepts in orthopedic physical therapy. La Crosse, WI: Orthopaedic Section, APTA, Inc; 2006.

CHAPTER 26

Hip Region

ANTERO-MEDIAL HIP PAIN/ GROIN PAIN

OSTEOARTHRITIS

Osteoarthritis describes a wear and tear of the interposing cartilage in a joint. The cause for wear and tear is multi-factoral,[1] however, the predominant cause is mechanical. Previous trauma, extreme changes in the angulation of the neck of femur, overuse, and obesity are dominant factors. More recently, genetics and the chemical composition of the human body including diet are also gaining importance. Certain foods as in refined sugars, processed meats, enriched flour and hydrogenated food are considered pro-inflammatories and predisposers of wear and tear. The subchondral bone is the underlying bone of the cartilage. Repeated stress is said to create microtrauma and microfractures of this subchondral bone, making the bed for the cartilage harder. This is considered a major predisposing factor. The head of the femur forms two-third of a sphere and is completely covered with articular cartilage except for a slight depression to which yet another ligament, the ligamentum teres is attached. The cartilage is the thickest on the medial central surface where it makes contact with the acetabulum and is thinnest on the periphery. The head of the femur, hence, faces the acetabulum in a medial position. This medial congruence is alternated by lateral and medial rotation of the hip during the swing and the stance phases of gait. This way the load of weight bearing is distributed. This mechanism is lost during capsular tightening of the hip. The femoral head may then hypothetically stay restricted in lateral rotation and cause excessive shearing in that position as it does not alternate positions. In other words, the load is not distributed and focused on the medial aspect which is where the articular cartilage is the thickest, predisposing to articular wear and tear and osteoarthritis (Fig. 26.1).

Somatic Findings

- Groin pain, increased with loading as in standing and walking
- Decreased internal rotation and extension of the hip

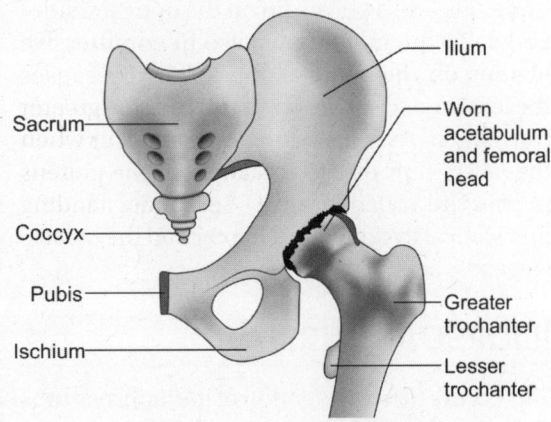

Fig. 26.1: Osteoarthritis hip.

- Pain and tenderness on palpation of the anterior rim of the acetabulum
- Supratrochanteric shortening.

Manual Therapy Intervention

- Hip distraction (long axis and lateral)
- Stretch internal rotators and hip flexors (exercise caution for myositis ossificans of iliopsoas in the elderly)
- Manipulation of sacral and innominate dysfunctions
- Trigger point compression of piriformis.

TROCHANTERIC BURSITIS

The mechanical causes for trochanteric bursitis may be faulty alignment or muscle weakness. Faulty alignment is more in the frontal plane. Any condition that causes leg length asymmetry can be a predisposition. This can range from a dysfunction of L5 or sacrum or the innominates, etc. Hence, a detail examination of the entire alignment of the lower extremity chain is essential.

Sacral torsion and anterior innominate dysfunctions can cause the leg to be longer on one side and it is usually the side of the long leg that is more prone for irritation. The reason being that the hip abductors on the long side are placed in a lengthened position (as weight bearing on a long leg creates a relative adduction on the same side and a pelvic dip on the opposite side) and subsequently an increase in compressive loading on the bursa as the pelvic dip causes the lengthened soft tissue to rub over the greater trochanter.[2] A similar situation can occur when the pelvis dips due to weakness of the gluteus medius (trendelenburg gait). See 'understanding mechanical dysfunction' chapter and the muscle weakness section.

ILIOPSOAS BURSITIS

This occurs when the tendon of the iliopsoas rubs over the iliopsoas bursa over the iliopectineal eminence. This occurs in situations of an anterior pubis or a posterior rotation of the innominate which brings the iliopectineal eminence closer to the tendon (Fig. 26.2). Repetitive activity can result in friction.[2]

Somatic Findings

- Clicking, grinding sensations are noted. This snapping sensation will classify this condition as an intra-articular anterior snapping hip syndrome. In the presence of posterior hip capsule tightness or dynamic valgus, the greater trochanter is prominent, favoring a similar friction syndrome. The IT band and gluteal tendons snap over the greater trochanter. This condition is called extra-articular snapping hip syndrome.
- Local tenderness around the greater trochanter
- Hip flexor tightness or positive Thomas test
- Sacral and innominate dysfunctions
- Weak gluteus medius
- Capsular pattern of restriction at the hip.

Manual Therapy Intervention

- Hip distraction if capsular tightness is present (long axis and lateral)
- Stretch internal rotators
- Stretch hip flexors
- Manipulation of sacral and innominate dysfunctions.

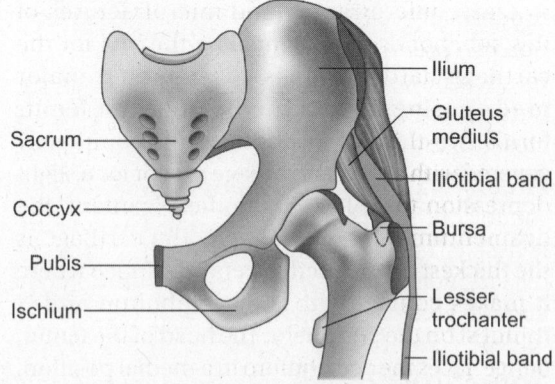

Fig. 26.2: Trochanteric bursitis.

TENDINITIS (ADDUCTORS/ILIOPSOAS)

The following muscles are prone for strain around the hip joint.[3]

Adductors: Muscles that cross a triplanar joint tend to change their function depending on the position of the joint. This phenomenon is called 'inversion of muscle action'. The adductors in the neutral position are also flexors, and in the flexed position can work as extensors. The adductors are commonly strained due to sudden stretching as in a slip and fall with the legs apart (on ice) or in sports due to a rapid change in direction where the adductors are used for propulsion as extensors. Strain is usually at the musculotendinous junction or at the teno-osseous junction near the symphysis pubis. Sports related adductor strains are referred as Gilmore's groin. The adductors originate from the ischium and pubis and insert into the medial aspect of the femur. Dysfunctions of the innominate or pubis and faulty alignment of the femoral shaft secondary to rotation as seen in capsular tightening can alter the length tension of these muscles. With this, sudden movement or overuse can predispose to a strain.

Iliopsoas: The iliopsoas is often prone to tightening as it is a postural muscle. While the length tension is altered due to tightness, a sudden extension of the knee with the hip flexed as in a start for a sprint run can strain this muscle. Innominate dysfunctions as in an anterior rotation can predispose to a shortening. A posterior rotation however can predispose to a iliopsoas bursitis, and a tendonitis as the tendon is brought closer to the iliopectineal eminence.

Piriformis: The piriformis is primarily an external rotator of the hip, however in a flexed position it assists in abduction. This poses a risk for dysfunction especially if the hip flexors are tight and the gluteus medius is weak.

Somatic Findings

Local tenderness over the adductors, iliopsoas and piriformis:

- Positive Thomas test (iliopsoas)
- Pain on resisted adduction (adductors)
- Presence of sacral and pubic dysfunctions (piriformis).

Manual Therapy Intervention

Manipulation of pubic, sacral and innominate dysfunctions:
- Stretch hip flexors
- Trigger point compression to piriformis
- Deep frictions to adductors.

NERVE ENTRAPMENT (OBTURATOR/ILIOINGUINAL)

Obturator: The obturator nerve runs downward from the lumbar spine to supply the adductors and are in close proximity to the iliopectineal eminence. Dysfunctions of the innominate, pubis and the iliopsoas can cause inflammation of the bursa. The nerve can be irritated in the process due the effusion from the inflammatory process and present as anterior hip and thigh pain. Additionally, the adductor magnus, brevis and pectineus are interfaces for the obturator nerve in hypertrophied states resulting in an entrapment dysfunction (Fig. 26.3).

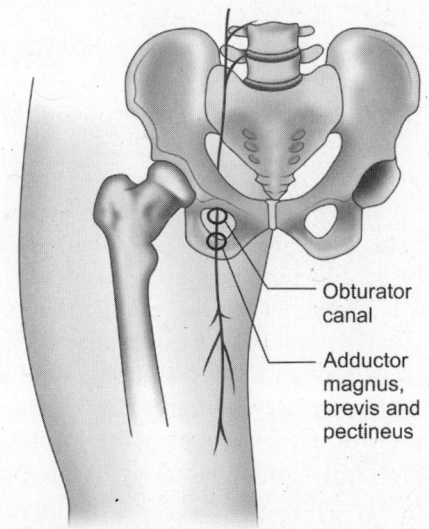

Fig. 26.3: Sites of obturator nerve entrapment.

Ilioinguinal: This nerve also passes under the inguinal ligament and can also be stressed by dysfunctional states of the innominate and pubis. Since it passes through the transverse abdominis it can also be compressed by vigorous contraction or a spasm of this muscle. A thoracolumbar dysfunction can entrap the corresponding segment and cause symptoms. The symptoms are sensory however can extend upto the genitalia on that side.

What to Look For

- Thoracolumbar junction dysfunction
- Scarring or tenderness of the transversus abdominis in the right lower quadrant
- Innominate and pubic dysfunctions
- Tightness, tenderness of the adductor magnus, brevis and pectineus.

Manual Therapy Intervention

- Manipulation of pubic, sacral and innominate dysfunctions
- Manipulation of the thoracolumbar junction
- Stretch hip flexors
- Trigger point compression to piriformis
- Deep frictions to adductors
- Deep friction to the transversus abdominis in the lower quadrants.

SYMPHYSITIS/OSTEITIS PUBIS

Osteitis pubis is a condition involving inflammatory and mechanical conditions of the symphysis pubis.[4] Causes are repeated trauma as in excessive impact loading, training errors and biomechanical aberrations, pelvic surgeries and childbirth. Infectious causes are also described. The symptoms include dull aching pain in the groin, loss of mobility in the groin region, and in more severe cases a sharp stabbing pain when attempting activity. Irregularity of the joint surface with tenderness over the joint, pubic tubercles, adductor and transversus muscles are common presentations. Capsular tightness of the hip joints can potentially lead to a compensatory overuse of the symphysis. Associated back and pelvic dysfunction may be evident. The contrasting presentation to this condition is a pubic separation or instability with warrants more of a stabilization approach.

Somatic Findings

- Groin pain, increased with loading as in standing and walking
- Decreased internal rotation and extension of the hip
- Pain and tenderness on palpation of the pubic tubercles and adductors
- Pubic, innominate or sacral dysfunctions.

Manual Therapy Intervention

- Hip distraction if capsular tightness is present (long axis and lateral)
- Stretch internal rotators
- Stretch hip flexors
- Shotgun for symphysis pubis
- Manipulation of sacral and innominate dysfunctions
- Soft tissue, trigger point approach to adductors and transversus.

LATERAL HIP PAIN

Trochanteric Bursitis/Extra-articular Lateral Snapping Hip Syndrome See Previous Section Under Iliopsoas Bursitis

TENDINITIS (TENSOR FASCIA LATA)

The tensor fascia lata (TFL) arises from the anterior part of the iliac crest and inserts between the two layers of the iliotibial band of the fascia lata about the junction of the middle and upper third of the thigh.[5] It works to tense the fascia lata and enables it to abduct the thigh and assists with internal rotation. Weakness of the gluteus medius has been noted for various reasons. Tracing evolution, the medius did not do much to stabilize the pelvis, as our ancestors walked on fours. Erect upright postures have considerably increased the demands on them. But since the demand is stabilizing more than dynamic abduction, it does not work in full range during gait. This may predispose to inherent weakness. Also a lesion of the L5 nerve root may weaken this muscle. In the elderly, asymptomatic gluteus medius tears have been described. For the above mentioned reasons, if the medius is weak the tensor fascia lata tries to take up the work of abduction. This is further complicated in the presence of hip flexor tightness as most of us tend to be tight secondary to prolonged sitting, driving, etc. This may also call in the piriformis to work as an abductor. As abduction is an important activity in closed chain as in gait, these muscles can be chronically irritated.

Somatic Findings

- Tenderness over the TFL
- Gluteus medius tenderness and weakness
- Signs of L5 nerve root compression
- Iliopsoas tightness.

Manual Therapy Intervention

- Manipulation of pubic, sacral and innominate dysfunctions
- Stretch hip flexors
- Trigger point compression of TFL
- Trigger point compression and soft tissue mobilization of gluteus medius
- Opening or closing restriction of L5.

TENDINITIS (GLUTEUS MEDIUS)

A tear in the gluteus medius muscle often occurs at its tendinous insertion on to the greater trochanter of the femur bone and can be a major cause of lateral hip pain.[6] Gluteus medius tears may be acute, traumatic or degenerative. Spontaneous degenerative tears are seen in the elderly. The majority of gluteus medius tears are degenerative caused by chronic inflammation of the gluteus medius tendon (tendinopathy) that results from many small tears overtime from overuse, repetitive movements, or friction from a tight iliotibial band. In many cases, degeneration of the gluteus medius tendon is associated with greater trochanteric bursitis, a condition called greater trochanteric pain syndrome. Risk factors for gluteus medius tears are overuse combined with an altered gait pattern from associated back pain, hip osteoarthritis, and gluteus medius weakness. They can collectively cause friction on the gluteus medius tendon and subsequent tears.

Somatic Findings

Tenderness over the gluteus medius:
- Gluteus medius tenderness and weakness
- Signs of L5 nerve root compression
- Decreased internal rotation and extension of the hip secondary to osteoarthritis
- Lumbar sacral and innominate dysfunctions
- Iliopsoas tightness.

Manual Therapy Intervention

Hip distraction if capsular tightness is present (long axis and lateral)
- Stretch internal rotators
- Stretch hip flexors
- Manipulation of lumbar, sacral and innominate dysfunctions
- Soft tissue, trigger point approach to gluteus medius
- Opening or closing restriction of L5.

MERALGIA PARESTHETICA

The lateral cutaneous nerve may be compressed under the inguinal ligament and sartorius muscle secondary to hypertrophy, and pressure from tight garments. Other causes for entrapment are diabetes, growths, obesity and surgical scarring. Patients present with pain in the anterolateral thigh with burning and tingling which increases with standing and walking. Symptoms may be reproduced by the pressure over the medial aspect of the anterior superior iliac spine (ASIS)

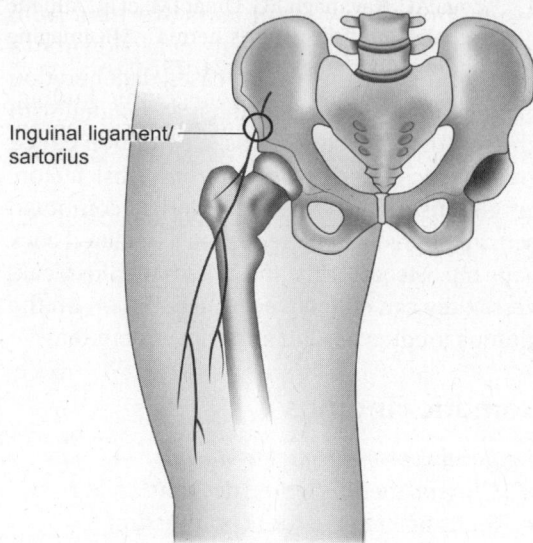

Fig. 26.4: Right thigh anterior view.

and over the origin of the sartorius (Fig. 26.4). This entrapment syndrome is described as 'meragia paresthetica'.[7]

Somatic Findings

- Possible pain and dysfunction over the origin of the sartorius under the ASIS with reproduction of symptoms on compression.
- Sacral and innominate dysfunctions.

Manual Therapy Intervention

- Manipulation of sacral and innominate dysfunctions
- Stretch hip flexors
- Deep frictions to sartorius under the ASIS and mid thigh.

POSTERIOR HIP PAIN

PIRIFORMIS SYNDROME

The piriformis originates from the S2-S4 vertebrae, sacrotuberous ligament, and the upper margin of the greater sciatic foramen, passes laterally through the greater sciatic notch and inserts on the superior surface of the greater trochanter of the femur. Its function is to flex the sacrum acting bilaterally and cause a rotation, side bending torsional movement, acting unilaterally. The muscle can be dysfunctional due to torsional dysfunctions or secondary to weakness of the gluteus medius wherein this muscle functions as an abductor, especially with the hip flexed. This can be seen in chronic hip flexor tightness. Lack of internal rotation of the hip as in a capsular restriction can cause a prolonged contraction on this muscle secondary to persistent lateral rotation. Dysfunctional states of this muscle may sometimes irritate the sciatic nerve.[8]

Somatic Findings

- Local tenderness over the piriformis
- Sacral, lumbar and innominate dysfunctions
- Positive Thomas test or tight hip flexors
- Weak gluteus medius
- Capsular hip restriction
- Pain reproduction on flexion, adduction, internal rotation.

Manual Therapy Intervention

- Manipulation of sacral and innominate and lumbar dysfunctions
- Stretch hip flexors
- Trigger point compression to piriformis.

NERVE ENTRAPMENT (SCIATIC/SUPERIOR GLUTEAL)

Sciatic/Superior gluteal: The mechanism of sciatic pain secondary to a piriformis dysfunction has been described earlier. Another nerve that is in close proximity is the superior gluteal nerve which passes between the piriformis and the inferior border of the gluteus minimus. A piriformis dysfunction can irritate this nerve as well giving rise to posterior hip or acute gluteal pain. The piriformis is in close proximity to the sciatic nerve only in a small population and hence increasing their vulnerability. Hyperactivity of the gluteus medius or an entrapment in the sciatic foramen may irritate the superior gluteal nerve. Refer lumbopelvic section for examination and intervention.

SACROILIAC DYSFUNCTION

See lumbopelvic section

REFERENCES

1. Valdes AM, Spector TD. The genetic epidemiology of osteoarthritis. Curr Opin Rheumatol. 2010;22: 139-43.
2. Rowand M, Chambliss ML, Mackler L. Clinical inquiries. How should you treat trochanteric bursitis? J Fam Pract. 2009;58:494-500.
3. Tibor LM, Sekiya JK. Differential diagnosis of pain around the hip joint. Arthroscopy. 2008;24: 1407-21.
4. Zoga AC, Kavanagh EC, Omar IM, et al. Athletic pubalgia and the "sports hernia": MR imaging findings. Radiology. 2008;247:797-807.
5. Bass CJ, Connell DA. Sonographic findings of tensor fascia lata tendinopathy: another cause of anterior groin pain. Skeletal Radiol. 2002;31:143-8.
6. Bunker TD, Esler CAN, Leac WJ. Rotator cuff tear of the hip. J Bone Joint Surg Br. 1997;79:618-20.
7. Erbay H. Meralgia paresthetica in differential diagnosis of low-back pain. Clin J Pain. 2002;18:132-5.
8. Tonley JC, Yun SM, Kochevar RJ, et al. Treatment of an individual with piriformis syndrome focusing on hip muscle strengthening and movement reeducation: a case report. J Orthop Sports Phys Ther. 2010;40:103-11.

CHAPTER 27

Knee Region

ANTERIOR KNEE PAIN
PATELLAR COMPRESSION
(Global/Lateral)/Patella Tracking Dysfunction

Patella compression[1] denotes the posterior aspect or retropatellar area compressing on the trochlea of the femur and causing pain. This typically occurs when there is a general or specific medial and lateral soft tissue tightness that results in the patella being excessively compressed within the trochlea. The soft tissue tightness of particular concern are the medial and lateral retinaculum. Moreover, direct trauma, immobilization, or knee surgery will encourage the development of arthrofibrosis and loss of patella mobility. This is also a precursor for global patella compression.

When the lateral structures as in the lateral retinaculum is tight it causes a lateral tilt of the patella causing lateral compression and pain. Tightness of the laterally placed iliotibial (IT) band also contributes to lateral compression. Internal rotation of the tibia causes the lateral portion of the patella to move against the femoral trochlear groove during weight bearing. Chronic irritation of the lateral patellar facet can also add to the lateral patellar compression syndrome.

Patellar Tracking: The analogy to describe this condition is to visualize the patella as a train and the trochlea groove as a track. Ideally during flexion and extension, the patella glides up and down on the groove like a train on a track. In a pathological situation, this ability is lost and the patella shifts out of track creating friction on the undersurface of the patella causing retropatellar pain. The pain is most profound with eccentric loading as in squatting, going up and downstairs. The reason being, in a knee bent position the congruency of the patella is challenged as it is being pulled by the soft tissue above and below. The following are reasons for possible lateral tracking of the patella (Fig. 27.1).

As the foot pronates abnormally beyond 4 to 6° and beyond 25% of the stance phase, the tibia is carried into excessive and prolonged internal rotation. This causes the femur to migrate into external rotation. The result is an increase in the Q-angle which is the quadriceps angle of pull in line with the femur superiorly relative to the pull of the patellar tendon inferiorly at the tibial tuberosity. When the Q-angle increases, there is a relative increase in the genu valgum angle and the patella is pulled laterally, resulting in lateral patellar tracking and patellofemoral pain. The situation is made worse if the vastus medialis obliquus (VMO) is weak and the laterally placed iliotibial band and lateral retinaculum is tight. The VMO works to pull the patella medially and when weak, the tight iliotibial band can favor lateral tracking. Congenitally, if the trochlear surface is flat, which normally has a groove, then it encourages excessive patella mobility. A superiorly placed patella as in patella alta is also a predisposing factor.

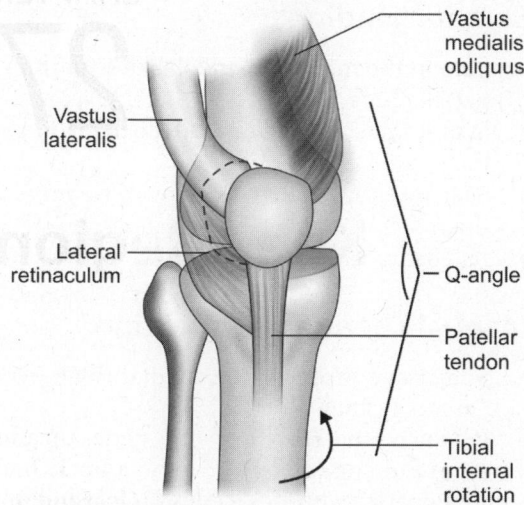

Fig. 27.1: Causes for lateral patella tracking.

Somatic Findings

- Clicking in the patellar area on flexion and extension of the knee
- Pain on squatting and going up- and downstairs
- Tenderness over the lateral retinaculum and the inferomedial aspect of the patellafemoral joint
- Swelling over the superolateral aspect of the patella
- Pain on medial tilt of the patella to stretch the retinaculum
- Superolateral patella
- Weak vastus medialis obliquus
- Tight iliotibial band
- Foot pronation
- Tibial internal rotation.

Manual Therapy Intervention

- Soft tissue mobilization, superolateral patella
- Patella medial tilt
- Patella inferior glide
- Ankle and foot mobilization for pronation (see next section)
- Frictions to VMO bulk.

PATELLAR TENDINITIS

Patella tendinitis is another condition causing anterior knee pain at the inferior pole of the patella.[1] It is also called a jumpers knee as it is more seen with activities related to repetitive jumping. The vulnerability is higher when the patella is in a high position called patella alta. When the length of the patella tendon is measured from the inferior pole of the patella to the tibial tubercle it should be equal to the length of the patella measured from the superior to the inferior pole. A ratio of 1:1, however, varying degrees of change in this ratio is considered to be a patella alta especially if the distance between the inferior pole of the patella to the tibial tubercle is higher than the length of the patella.

Somatic Findings

- Pain located in the patellar tendon between patella and the tibial tubercle
- Pain with running and jumping
- Pain in going up- and downstairs

Manual Therapy Intervention

- Soft tissue mobilization, superolateral and superomedial patella
- Patella medial tilt
- Patella inferior glide
- Frictions to patella tendon.

MEDIAL KNEE PAIN

MEDIAL LIGAMENT STRAIN

The medial collateral ligament (MCL) runs from the medial surfaces of the femur and the tibia and has two parts, a deep band that attaches to the cartilage, meniscus and joint margins, and a superficial band that attaches from medial aspect of the upper femoral condyle to the superior and medial surface of the tibia. It functions to prevent valgus stress and hence injured by excessive valgus moments.

Somatic Findings

Foot pronation with valgus and internal rotation.

Manual Therapy Intervention

Manual therapy for foot pronation with orthotics (see next section).

SAPHENOUS NERVE IRRITATION

The saphenous nerve is a pure sensory nerve that arises from the L3 and L4 spinal segments. It offers sensory supply to the medial lower thigh and knee. This nerve can be entrapped in the Hunter's canal in the medial aspect of the thigh, by dynamic muscle contractions of the VMO and adductors (Fig. 27.2). Often, contusions to the medial thigh or medial knee surgeries also cause dysfunction.[2]

Patients present with pain in the thigh, knee pain about the infrapatellar region, and possibly paresthesias in the leg and foot. Deep palpation over the medial aspect of the thigh and over the vastus medialis reproduces symptoms.

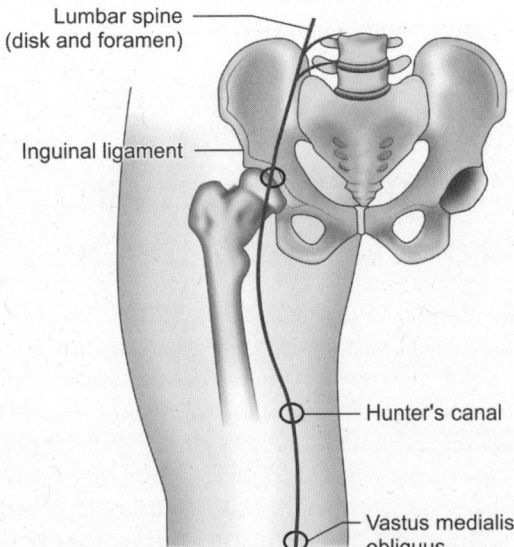

Fig. 27.2: Sites of saphenous nerve irritation.

Somatic Findings

- Pain in the mid thigh, medial knee or infrapatellar area
- Symptom reproduction on deep palpation of the medial thigh or VMO
- Scarring or palpable cords over the medial thigh
- Patella tracking dysfunction.

Manual Therapy Intervention

- Soft tissue mobilization medial thigh over Hunter's canal
- Patella medial tilt
- Patella inferior glide
- Ankle and foot mobilization for pronation (see next section)
- Frictions to VMO bulk.

PES ANSERINE BURSITIS

This condition is seen in inferomedial knee pain where the tendinous insertion of the gracilis, sartorius and semitendinosis are padded by this bursa. Prolonged internal rotation of the tibia can cause a hyperirritability of these muscles as they rotate the tibia inwards, subsequently irritating the bursa beneath it.[3] Tightness of the medial hamstrings can predispose to a similar condition.

Somatic Findings

- Tenderness over the pes anserine area on the superomedial aspect of the tibia
- Foot pronation with tibial internal rotation.

VASTUS MEDIALIS OBLIQUUS STRAIN

A source of medial knee pain is the vastus medialis obliquus. It tends to work in excess due to faulty patellar tracking or lack of terminal extension at the knee predisposing to excessive cross bridging and pain. Prolonged internal roation of the tibia as seen in a pronated foot may irritate the tendons of the sartorius, gracilis and semitendinosus predisposing to pain in these structures.

Somatic Findings

- Local tenderness
- Extension lag or patellofemoral syndrome
- Foot pronation with tibial internal rotation
- Tenderness over the medial sartorius bulk.

Manual Therapy Intervention for Pes Anserine Bursitis and Vastus Medialis Obliquus Strain

- Same as patellar tracking dysfunction, saphenous nerve irritation at the VMO, and foot pronation.
- Add frictions to the sartorius bulk at the knee for pes anserine bursitis.

LATERAL KNEE PAIN

PATELLA COMPRESSION (LATERAL)

See anterior knee pain.

ILIOTIBIAL BAND DYSFUNCTION

The tensor fascia latae (TFL) acts through the iliotibial tract by pulling it superiorly and anteriorly. It assists in flexion, medial rotation and abduction of the hip and extension of the knee joint. The TFL arises from the anterior part of the outer lip of the iliac crest, lateral aspect of the anterior superior iliac spine and the upper part of the anterior border of the iliac wing. The iliotibial band (ITB) also attaches into the posterior gluteus maximus muscle in the back. Distally it inserts on the patella, tibia, and biceps femoris tendon. When the TFL and gluteal muscles contract, they increase tension on the band. Often, one muscle dominates the movement pattern causing an imbalance to occur which may lead to injury. The common imbalance being weakness of the gluteal muscles and overactivity of the TFL. This situation is further aggravated in the presence of hip flexor tightness as the glutei work best in extension. Intrisic situations that favor femoral external rotation accompanied by the tibial internal rotation can cause the lateral condyle of the femur and the Gerdy's tubercle of the tibia to become more prominent. As the ITB crosses over these structures, repetitive flexion activity of the knee can create friction between the ITB and lateral condyle creating symptoms.[3]

Somatic Findings

Tightness in the TFL and ITB. This encourages external rotation of the femur and weakness of gluteals. Ober's test may be positive.
- A capsular pattern of restriction at the hip which favors femoral external rotation and hip flexion which will increase tension on the band.
- Weakness of hip abductors.
- Weakness of knee extension as the ITB has to excessively amplify knee extension.
- Excessively flat feet or pronation which causes tibial internal rotation and subsequent femoral external rotation.
- Leg length inequality.
- Overuse in flexion as in cycling or repeated stair climbing.

Manual Therapy Intervention

- IT band stretching with care
- Hip distraction and internal rotation stretch
- Tibia anteriomedial glide
- Manual treatment for foot pronation (see next section).

COMMON PERONEAL NERVE ENTRAPMENT

This nerve is superficial at the head of the fibula and can be irritated due to various causes. Varus stress that opens the lateral aspect of the knee joint, as described above can stress the superior tibiofibular articulation resulting in nerve irritation.[2]

The peroneus longus, however, is a more common cause. This muscle works to plantarflex the first ray for foot propulsion. However, during excessive or prolonged foot supination, the first ray plantarflexes excessively to get the forefoot flat on the ground for propulsion. Hence, it may be restricted in a plantarflexed position. This results in contracted and hyperactive states of the peroneus longus and irritation of the nerve as it passes through this muscle (Fig. 27.3).[4]

A supination of the foot can cause an external tibial rotation. This in turn can displace the fibula head laterally due to a varus stress and can cause an irritation of this nerve.

RETINACULAR NERVE ENTRAPMENT

Lateral patellar tracking dysfunction can cause tightness of the lateral retinaculum and result in what is described as a lateral patellar hyperpressure syndrome. The retinacular nerve that is in close proximity can be irritated and is a source of lateral knee pain. This condition is also seen in following lateral retinacular release, which is the procedure done for lateral patellar tracking dysfunction.[5]

Somatic Findings

- Tightness of the superior tibiofibular joint
- Tenderness over the peroneus longus located just below the fibular head
- Genu varum
- Foot supination with tibial external rotation
- Decreased medial tilt.

Manual Therapy Intervention

- Patella medial tilt
- Anterior posterior (AP) glide, superior tibiofibular joint
- IT band stretching
- Tibia posteriomedial glide
- Manual treatment for foot supination (see next section).

SUPERIOR TIBIOFIBULAR JOINT/ PERONEAL DYSFUNCTION

The tibia and fibula articulate at their proximal and distal ends and are called proximal and distal tibiofibular joints, respectively. The proximal tibiofibular joint is a plane type of synovial joint between the head of the fibula and lateral condyle of the tibia. Movement occurs at the superior tibiofibular joint during dorsiflexion and plantar flexion of the ankle joint. Restriction of the superior tibiofibular articulation is seen in chronic supination or pronation which diminish the gliding ability of the fibula. Inability of the fibula head to glide anteriorly is the most common restriction seen. The peroneus longus and soleus are attached to the head of the fibula at the superior tibiofibular joint. Dysfunction of the fibula head can predispose to irritability of the peroneus longus and subsequently the peroneal nerve.[4] Additionally, dysfunction of the

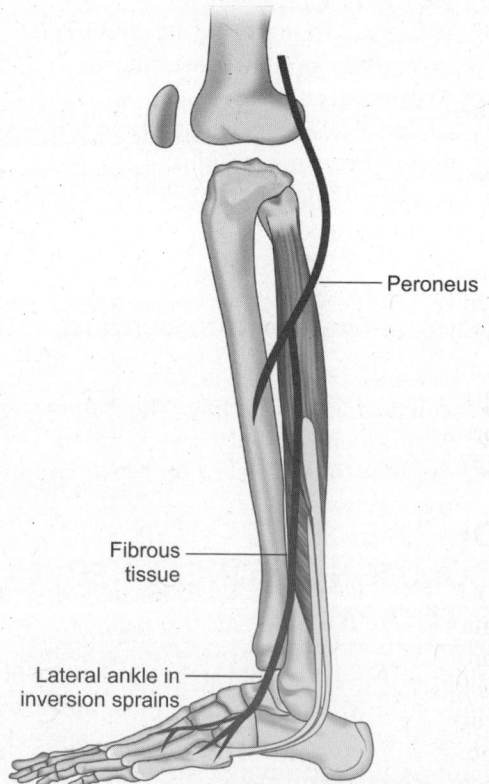

Fig. 27.3: Sites of common peroneal nerve entrapment.

fibula head can also predispose to dysfunctions of the lateral collateral ligament and iliotibial band causing lateral knee pain. It is also seen as a collateral in tibiofemoral osteoarthritis.[4]

What to Look For

- Tightness of the superior tibiofibular joint
- Tenderness over the peroneus longus located just below the fibular head
- Genu varum
- Foot supination with tibial external rotation
- Varus stress test may be positive.

Manual Therapy Intervention

- Patella medial tilt
- AP glide and superior tibiofibular joint
- IT band stretching
- Tibia posteromedial glide
- Manual treatment for foot supination (see next section).

LATERAL LIGAMENT STRAIN

The lateral collateral ligament (LCL) is part of a complex of structures collectively named posterolateral corner or arcuate complex. The structures in the arcuate complex include LCL, popliteal ligament, arcuate ligament, and posterolateral joint capsule. The LCL is separated from the lateral meniscus by a fat pad. It functions to prevent varus stresses and hence injured by varus stresses.

Somatic Findings

Foot supination with varus and external rotation.

Manual Therapy Intervention

Manual therapy for foot supination (see next section).

POSTERIOR KNEE PAIN

POPLITEUS INJURY

The popliteus muscle runs from the lateral femoral condyle distally to the posterior aspect tibia in a diagonal fashion. It assists in stabilizing the posterolateral corner of the knee and prevents anterior translation of the tibia. Its function is especially important in eccentric loading as in downhill running. It is also an internal rotator of the tibia. The tendon or muscle belly may be vulnerable to injury secondary to overuse or prolonged internal rotation of the tibia as in foot pronation or sudden violent external rotation.[6]

Somatic Findings

- Local tenderness over the posterior and posterolateral aspect of the knee
- Pronation tibial internal rotation.

Manual Therapy Intervention

- Soft tissue mobilization over the popliteus
- Manual treatment for foot pronation and tibial internal rotation (see next section).

ARTHRITIS

The term arthritis is generic and should be used with caution especially when you are labeling a patient as having 'arthritis'. The most common is just plain wear and tear which is universal. Technically, then, anybody over age 25 has some type of arthritis. The plain wear and tear type is what is known as osteoarthritis. There are, however, other types of arthritis which may require other forms of investigation and diagnosis and subsequently have a different prognosis.[7,8] The most common are described as follows:

DEGENERATIVE

Osteoarthritis of the knee occurs when the interposing articular cartilage which acts as a protective cushion between the tibia and femur, is subject to wear and tear. As the articular cartilage is lost, the joint space between the bones narrows. This is an early symptom of osteoarthritis of the knee and is visible on X-rays. Symptoms of knee pain on loading, stiffness and resting pain can develop. As the condition progresses, the cartilage thins, becoming grooved and fragmented. The underlying bone, called sub-chondral bone is subject to microfracture and react by becoming thicker and harder. They grow outward and form spurs. The synovium becomes inflamed and thickened and causes additional swelling. As the problem continues, the cartilage is completely worn and the bone makes contact over the bone which makes the condition very painful. This when it is considered bone-on-bone and warrants a replacement of the joint surfaces. This description of the knee applies to all joints in the human body including spine.

Several causative factors for developing osteoarthritis are:

Heredity: There is some evidence that genetic mutations may make an individual more likely to develop osteoarthritis.

Age and weight: Weight increases pressure on joints such as knee.

Gender: Women who are older than 50 years of age are more likely to develop osteoarthritis of the knee than men as their pelvic obliquity and knee angulation make them vulnerable.

Trauma, impact loading and repetitive stress: Previous injury to the joint including sports injuries, and a history of overuse can lead to osteoarthritis.

Metabolic: Repeated episodes of gout or septic arthritis, metabolic disorders can increase the risk of developing osteoarthritis.

Intrinsic: More recently the awareness of diet factors leading to wear and tear is offering new insight. Certain foods are pro-inflammatory's as in processed meats, enriched flour, refined sugars. These are claimed to increase the rate of wear and tear in the body. Other factors are lack of vitamins C and D, poor posture or bone alignment, poor aerobic fitness, and muscle weakness.

Manual Therapy Intervention

- Patella medial tilt
- Patella inferior glide
- AP glide superior tibiofibular joint
- IT band stretching
- Tibia distraction
- Tibia glides
- Manual treatment for foot pronation and tibial internal rotation (see next section)
- The goal is to distribute stresses within the joint, hence, the cartilage is not excessively loaded in one area.

REFERENCES

1. Waryasz GR, McDermott AY. Patellofemoral pain syndrome (PFPS): a systematic review of anatomy and potential risk factors. Dyn Med. 2008;7-9.
2. Saidoff DC, McDonough AL. Critical pathways in therapeutic intervention: extremities and spine, 2002, St. Louis Mosby.
3. O'Keeffe SA, Hogan BA, Eustace SJ, et al. Overuse injuries of the knee. Magn Reson Imaging Clin N Am. 2009;17:725-39.
4. Ozcan O, Boya H, Oztekin HH. Clinical evaluation of the proximal tibiofibular joint in knees with severe tibiofemoral primary osteoarthritis. Knee. 2009;16:248-50.
5. Fulkerson JP, Tennant R, Jaivin JS, et al. Histologic evidence of retinacular nerve injury associated with patellofemoral malalignment. Clin Orthop Relat Res. 1985;(197):196-205.
6. Geissler WB, Corso SR, Caspari RB. Isolated rupture of the popliteus with posterior tibial nerve palsy. J Bone Joint Surg Br. 1992;74:811-3.
7. Koopman WJ, Moreland LW. Arthritis and allied conditions: A textbook of rheumatology, 15th edn, 2005, Lippincott Williams and Wilkins, Philadelphia.
8. Poiraudeau S, Berenbaum F, Corvol M. [Cartilage degradation and articular inflammation]. Rev Prat. 1996;46:2180-5.

CHAPTER 28

Ankle and Foot Region

PLANTAR/MEDIAL ANKLE AND FOOT PAIN

Note: Many of the conditions described under this section require adequate manual intervention, however, the most effective maintenance of objectives achieved by manual intervention is good orthotic prescription. Hence the value of orthotic prescription cannot be undermined.

PLANTAR FASCITIS AND HEEL SPUR

The plantar fascia is a strong layer of white fibrous tissue with a thick central part and thinner lateral portions. The central portion arises from the calcaneal tubercle and projects distally as five divisions. They hold the flexor tendons and attach to the base of the proximal phalanx of all the toes. They provide stability of the first metatarsaphalangeal joint and medial arch through what is called the windlass mechanism. This mechanism has the effect of shortening the distance between the hallux and heel. By this process it raises the arch. This has the effect of making the foot a rigid and stable structure when the propulsive forces from above are applied. The foot hence supinates in preparation for push off. This mechanism is assisted by the tibialis posterior and gastrosoleus. Plantar fasciitis[1] occurs when the plantar fascia develops tears in the tissue resulting in pain and inflammation. The pain of plantar fasciitis is usually located close to where the fascia attaches to the calcaneus. During the normal gait cycle, following initial contact, the ankle and foot pronate to absorb the shock of weight bearing. This is the phase when the plantar fascia is maximally stretched. Following midstance, the foot reverses into supination to provide a rigid lever for push off. This is where the windlass mechanism is required. However, in situations where the foot is chronically pronated, the reversal does not occur and push off may occur in a pronated position resulting in excessive stretching of the plantar fascia. When this continues with prolonged weight (Fig. 28.1) bearing, running, etc. the fascia is subjected to repeated stretching resulting in tears and inflammation. Plantar fasciitis is the result. Treating the fascia would result in a very symptomatic

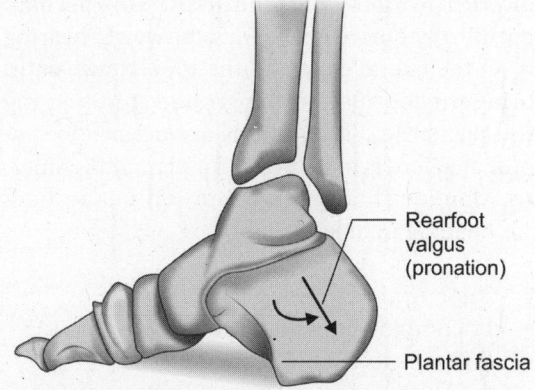

Fig. 28.1: Effect of pronation on plantar fascia.

approach, whereas correcting the causes for prolonged pronation will address the cause.

Somatic Findings

The patient complains of pain on the inside of the heel with local tenderness over the medial and anterior border of the heel pad. Observation reveals a typically pronated foot with rearfoot valgus and a flattened arch. The patient reports that after a period of rest the first few steps hurt the most with a gradual reduction on continued weight bearing. However, if the weight bearing is further prolonged the pain returns. This is most apparent on waking in the morning.

Subtalar neutral: The patient is lying prone and the clinician faces the patient from the leg side. The clinician then grasps the lateral metatarsals with one hand, while the other hand palpates both sides of the subtalar joint. The clinician alternately inverts and everts the foot and palpates both sides of the subtalar joint to look for symmetry in compression. When this is felt, the position of the heel in relation to the tibia is observed and maintained as neutral as possible. Now the position of the first ray in relationship to the fifth ray is observed. If the first ray is higher than the fifth ray, then it is a forefoot varus. On weight bearing when the forefoot is flat on the ground and a compensatory rearfoot valgus occurs. The result is a *pronated* foot.

Conversely, if the position of the heel is inverted (rearfoot varus) and first ray is higher than the fifth ray. On weight bearing the weight bearing is on the lateral aspect of the foot. However, to bring the foot flat on the ground, the first ray will plantarflex. The result is a *supinated* foot. A pronated foot is more prone for plantar fasciitis.

- Manual Therapy Intervention has to be a heading in block letters
- Talocrural distraction
- Talocrural posterior glide
- Friction to abductor hallucis
- Frictions to medial plantar fascia

PLANTAR NERVE ENTRAPMENT

The medial plantar nerve is a branch of the tibial nerve and it passes beneath the spring ligament on the medial side of the foot.[2] Excessive pronation can stretch this ligament and compress the medial plantar nerve below it. It is often termed as 'jogger's foot'.

Excessive pronation can also stress and compress the lateral plantar nerve as it passes between the deep fascia of the abductor hallucis and flexor accessories muscles. In a more neutral foot the long flexors of the great toe complete push off on gait, however, in pronation, the more medial position of the foot entails the abductors to work namely abductor hallucis (Fig. 28.2). The bulk of the abductor hallucis is place on the medial aspect of the heel, thereby causing medial heel pain secondary to overuse. In addition, the plantar nerve that passes through the muscle bulk also gets entrapped causing pain and dysfunction.

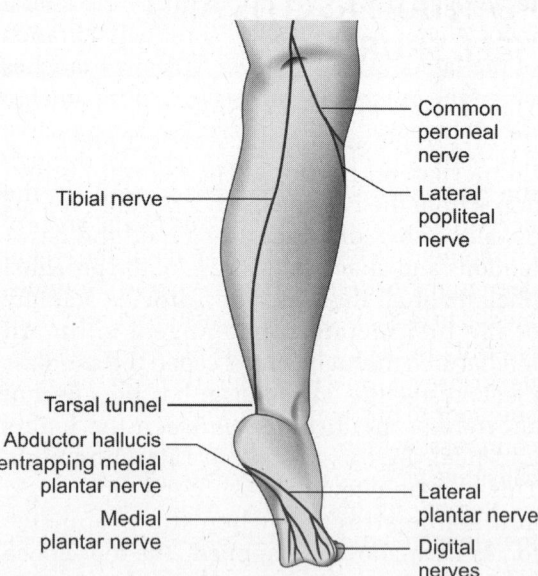

Fig. 28.2: Representation of tibial and plantar nerves.

Somatic Findings

- Foot pronation with tibial internal rotation
- Adverse neural tension of the tibial and plantar nerve may be possible
- Tinnel's sign may be positive at the medial ankle or medial heel
- Local tenderness over the abductor hallucis
- Symptom reproduction on pressure over the abductor hallucis or resisted great toe abduction.

Manual Therapy Intervention

- Talocrural distraction
- Talocrural posterior glide
- Friction to abductor hallucis
- Neural mobilization of the plantar nerve.

BAXTER'S NERVE ENTRAPMENT

Baxter's nerve entrapment refers to an entrapment of the calcaneal branch of the posterior tibial nerve.[3] Although it seems very similar to a 'jogger's foot', the difference is the lateral involvement. Baxter's nerve, or the first branch of the lateral plantar nerve, typically branches off, of the lateral plantar nerve just proximal to the abductor hallucis muscle. As Baxter's nerve descends deeper into the foot, it passes through the porta pedis. This is one location for the nerve to become entrapped. Additional areas of entrapment for Baxter's nerve include the region deep to the plantar fascia. The nerve continues medial to the calcaneal tuberosity and continues laterally between the quadratus plantae and flexor brevis muscles to its insertion into the abductor digiti minimi muscle. Pronation with compression of the porta pedis is considered the causative factor of this condition.

Somatic findings and management is similar to management of plantar nerve entrapment.

TARSAL TUNNEL SYNDROME

This condition refers to an entrapment of the posterior tibial nerve and artery as they pass through a fibrous osseous tunnel located posteromedial to the medial malleolus. The roof of the tunnel consists of the lanciate ligament and the floor by underlying bony structures (Fig. 28.3). The diameter of this tunnel can be reduced due to excessive pronation as this stretches the lanciate ligament. This results in pain and radicular symptoms in the distribution of the tibial nerve and medial and lateral plantar nerves as these are branches of the tibial nerve.[4]

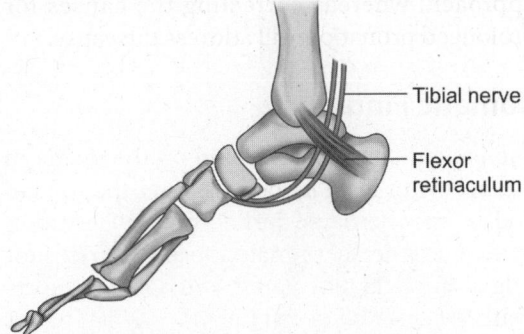

Fig. 28.3: Tarsal tunnel.

Somatic Findings

- Foot pronation with tibial internal rotation
- Adverse neural tension of the tibial and plantar nerve may be possible
- Tinnel's sign may be positive at the medial ankle
- Local tenderness below the medial malleolus.

Manual Therapy Intervention

- Talocrural distraction
- Talocrural posterior glide
- Friction to tibialis posterior and abductor hallucis
- Neural mobilization of the plantar nerve.

FLEXOR HALLUCIS LONGUS TENDINITIS

It arises from the inferior two-third of the posterior surface of the body of the fibula, and is inserted into the base of the last phalanx of the great toe. It traverses through the tarsal tunnel. (Fig. 28.4). It acts as a flexor of the great toe, elevates the arch, and assists with plantar flexion

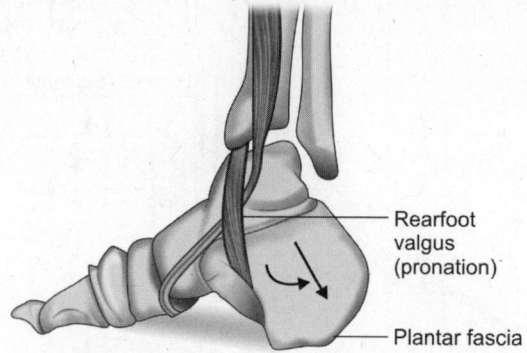

Fig. 28.4: Flexor hallucis longus tendon.

of the ankle. Patients with flexor hallucis longus (FHL) tenosynovitis usually present with pain in the tarsal tunnel. The pain improves with rest and increases in activities requiring repeated push off and extended running. The tendon can get irritable at three sites, the entrance of the fibro-osseous tunnel between medial and lateral talar tubercles, the tarsal tunnel, and between the sesamoids of the great toe.[5]

Somatic Findings

- Pain and weakness are noted with resistance to plantar flexion of the first metatarsophalangeal (MTP) joint.
- Pain and local tenderness in the tarsal tunnel.

Manual Therapy Intervention

Same as for tarsal tunnel syndrome.

TIBIALIS POSTERIOR TENDINITIS

The tibialis posterior originates on the inner posterior borders of the tibia and fibula. It is also attached to the interosseous membrane which attaches to the tibia and fibula. The tendon of tibialis posterior descends posterior to the medial malleolus and to the plantar surface of the foot where it inserts on to the tuberosity of the navicular, first and third cuneiforms, cuboid and second, third, and fourth metatarsals. This muscle inverts and plantarflexes the foot, however, its most important function is to decelerate pronation from initial contact to midstance. When there is chronic pronation of the foot, the muscle by virtue of its position gets overstretched and loses its decceleration ability. This predisposes to pain and dysfunction.[6]

Somatic Findings

- Medial ankle, medial lower leg pain
- Local tenderness medial to the medial malleolus and over the navicular
- Pain on resisted plantarflexion and inversion
- Foot pronation with tibial internal rotation.

Manual Therapy Intervention

- Talocrural distraction
- Talocrural posterior glide
- Friction to tibilialis posterior and abductor hallucis.

LATERAL ANKLE AND FOOT PAIN

LATERAL LIGAMENT STRAIN

Lateral sprains are most common and is usually secondary to faulty alignment of the rearfoot. A posterolateral dysfunction of the talus is usually a causative factor. This inverts the calcaneus and results in a rearfoot varus. Since the rearfoot is in varus, the forefoot pronates excessively to bring the foot flat on to the ground. This increases the height of the arch and overall renders the foot with faulty alignment and a tendency to buckle inwards especially when landing on one leg (as in running or jumping) (Fig. 28.5). When this occurs, the lateral ligament is prone to be injured.[7,8] The reverse can occur if the reverse mechanics is present which can eventually stress the medial ligamentous structures, although less common.

Somatic Findings

- Rearfoot varus with foot supination and tibial external rotation
- Tenderness over the anterior talofibular ligament and/or the middle calcaneofibular ligament

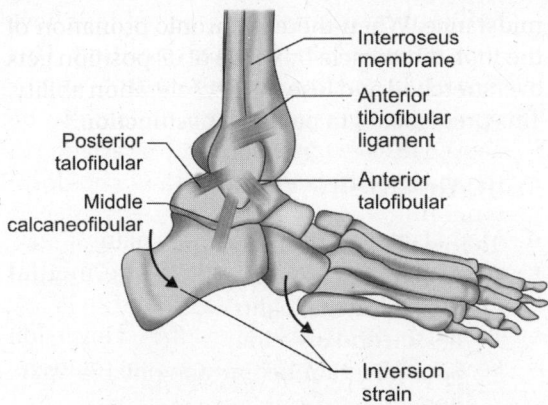

Fig. 28.5: Lateral ligament of ankle.

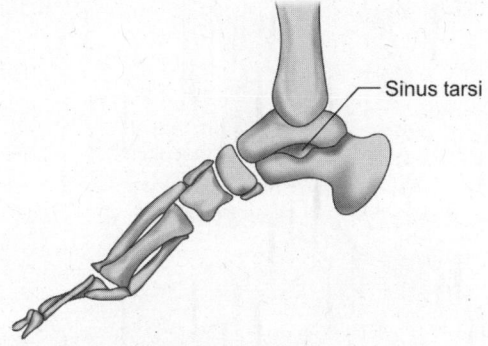

Fig. 28.6: Sinus tarsi.

- Symptom reproduction on plantar flexion and inversion for the anterior talofibular ligament and neutral inversion for the middle calcaneofibular ligament
- Weakness of the peroneal muscles as in resisted eversion.

Manual Therapy Intervention

- Talocrural distraction
- Talocrural anterior glide
- Frictions to anterior talofibular ligament
- Soft tissue mobilization of the peronei over the lateral aspect of the lower leg
- Cuboid manipulation in internal rotation
- Navicular anterior posterior AP glide
- Cuneiform depression manipulation.

LATERAL IMPINGEMENT SYNDROME

See impingement under dorsal foot pain.

SINUS TARSI SYNDROME

The sinus tarsi[9] is a small osseous canal which runs into the ankle under the talus. It is formed by the sulcus tali and sulcus calcanei (Fig. 28.6). Damage to the sinus tarsi can be caused from overuse in conjunction with over pronation. Inversion ankle sprains are also causative factors. The sinus tarsi contains synovial fluid and soft tissue which is vulnerable and can become inflamed. It may also occur with inflammatory conditions such as gout or osteoarthritis. Inversion sprains can cause overstretching to the area, whereas pronation causes a compression at the sinus tarsi.

What to Look For

See impingement under dorsal foot pain.

PERONEAL TENDON INJURY AND DYSFUNCTION

The peroneus longus originates from the upper two-third of the lateral surface of fibula and after crossing the plantar surface of the foot deep to intrinsic muscles, it inserts on medial cuneiform and base of 1st metatarsal. The peroneus brevis originates from the lower one-third of the lateral surface of the fibula tuberosity and inserts into the base of 5th metatarsal (Fig. 28.7). The peroneus tertius originates from the distal part of anterior surface of the fibula and inserts into the dorsum of shaft of the 5th metatarsal bone. The main function of the peroneal tendons are to stabilize the foot and ankle and protect them from inversion moments.[10]

Types of Peroneal Tendon Injuries

1. *Tendinitis:* It is an inflammation of the peroneal tendons. The inflammation is caused by the activities involving repetitive use of the tendon. Repetitive overuse can occur if there are repeated inversion strains. A supinated

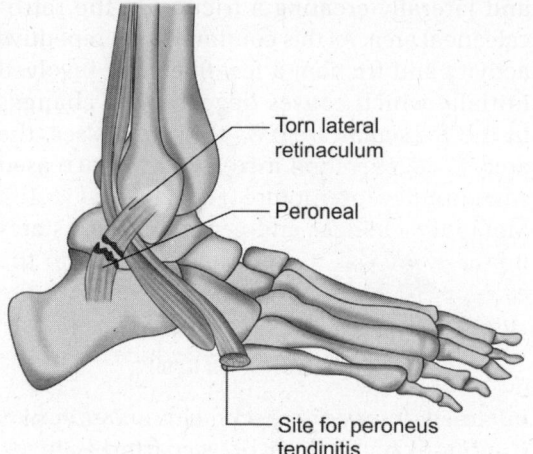

Fig. 28.7: Sites for peroneal dysfunction.

foot with a rearfoot varus can render more stress on the laterally placed peroneal tendons.
Symptoms of tendonitis include:
- Pain
- Swelling
- Warmth to the touch.

2. *Peroneal tears:* They are caused by repetitive activity or trauma. The factors mentioned above in the section on tendinitis may be precedents for a tear. The differentiation is that the ankle is now unstable.
Symptoms of acute tears include:
- Pain
- Swelling
- Weakness or instability of the foot and ankle.

3. *Degeneration:* It is the next cause for peroneal dysfunction. Again the above factors should be considered. As the repetitive stress progresses with possible added metabolic factors, the tendon may wear thin and has a potential to rupture. The clinician should watch for:
- Sporadic pain on and off on the outside of the ankle
- Weakness or instability in the ankle.

4. *Subluxation:* The peroneal tendons or the conjoint tendon of the longus and brevis pass under the lateral malleolus and are held in place by the peroneal retinaculum. Subluxation occurs when the tendons have slipped out of their normal position. This is seen in trauma secondary to heavy or repetitive inversion sprains. It can also be caused in a person is born with a variation in the shape of the lateral malleolus or peroneal tendon.
The symptoms of subluxation may include:
- A snapping feeling of the tendon around the lateral malleolus especially on dorsiflexion and eversion.
- Sporadic pain behind the outside ankle bone.
- Ankle instability.

Manual Therapy Intervention (Tendinitis Only)

- Talocrural distraction
- Talocrural anterior glide
- Calcaneal eversion
- Soft tissue mobilization of the peronei on the lateral aspect of the lower leg
- Superior tibiofibular joint AP glide
- Cuboid manipulation in internal rotation
- Navicular AP glide
- Cuneiform depression manipulation.

CUBOID SUBLUXATION

Inversion sprain is one of the most traumatic injuries to the ankle. Besides the ligament, tendon and retinaculum, a less recognized condition which is often a sequalae of an inversion stress at the ankle is injury to the joints and ligaments around the tarsal cuboid, resulting in cuboid subluxation. This condition is called cuboid syndrome.[11] A common cause for cuboid syndrome is pointe work as in ballet or repetitive jumping.

What to Look For

- Tenderness over the cuboid on plantar to dorsal pressure
- Lateral foot pain
- Weakness on push off
- Decreased midtarsal internal rotation.

Manual Therapy Intervention

- Talocrural distraction
- Talocrural anterior glide
- Calcaneal eversion
- Cuboid manipulation in internal rotation
- Navicular AP glide
- Cuneiform depression manipulation.

POSTERIOR ANKLE AND FOOT PAIN

Achilles Tendinitis/Tendon Calcification and Degeneration/ Retrocalcaneal Bursitis

Achilles tendinitis, although implying inflammatory as in tendinitis, is now being referred to as a tendinopathy.[10,12] A similar situation has come up with lateral epicondylitis. This is because it is no longer thought to be an inflammatory condition, as the main finding is usually degenerated tissue with a loss of normal fiber structure. The tendoachilles is a tendon formed by three muscles in the lower leg, gastrocnemius, soleus, and plantaris. It is the thickest and strongest tendon in the body. It is an extension of the muscle bulk which is inserted into the middle part of the posterior surface of the calcaneus. A bursa lies interposed between the tendon and retrocalcaneal area (Fig. 28.8). The lower end which is about 3 or 4 cm above the heel is called 'watershed zone' as it is relatively avascular. During gait, as the foot pronates and supinates, the tendon whips medially and laterally creating a friction in the retrocalcaneal area. As this continues with repetitive activity and friction, a few fibers are involved initially which causes degenerative changes in the avascular area. As this progresses, the area of degeneration increases with increased susceptibility to a rupture (Figs. 28.9 and 28.10). Metabolic changes and certain disease states increase the risk. Certain medications in the category of fluoroquinilones also increase the vulnerability.

To summarize the causes which is mostly overuse:

- Increase in activity in distance, speed or hills
- Less recovery time between activities
- Change of footwear or training surface
- Weak calf muscles
- Decreased range of motion at the ankle joint, usually cause by tight calf muscles.
- Overpronation or supination.

What to Look For

- Initial symptoms of achilles tendonitis
- Gradual onset of pain over a period of days
- Pain at the onset of exercise which fades as the exercise progresses, but resumes if exercise is prolonged
- Pain eases with rest
- Tenderness on palpation.

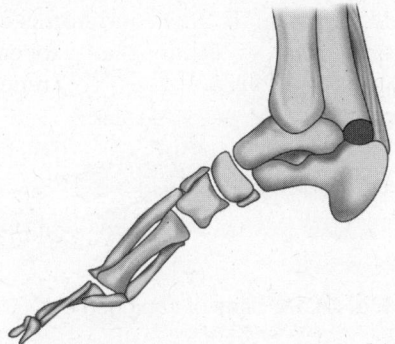

Fig. 28.8: Retrocalcaneal bursitis.

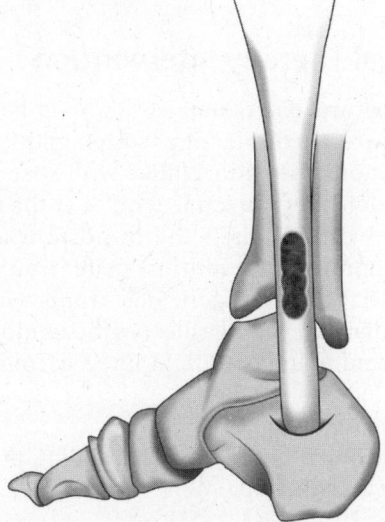

Fig. 28.9: Tendoachilles tendon degeneration.

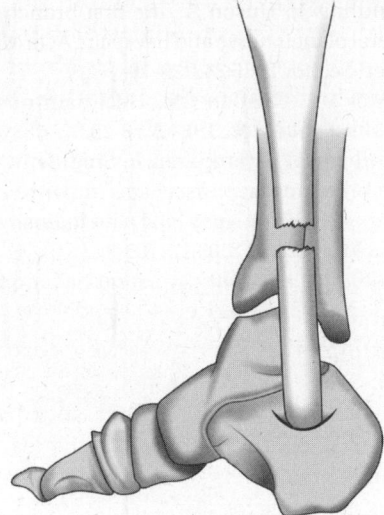

Fig. 28.10: Tendoachilles tear.

Chronic Symptoms

- Pain with all exercise which is constant throughout
- Pain in the tendon when walking especially up hill or upstairs
- Pain and stiffness in the achilles tendon especially in the morning or after rest
- There may be tender nodules or lumps in the achilles tendon, more so on the medial side of the watershed zone.

Manual Therapy Intervention

- Talocrural distraction
- Talocrural anterior or posterior glide
- Frictions to tendoachilles with scar mobilization over the tendoachilles at the watershed zone. This is the important aspect of manual intervention to rearrange the haphazard collagen. It is done over the medial and lateral aspect of the tendon
- Cuboid manipulation in internal rotation if the foot is supinated
- Navicular AP glide
- Cuneiform depression manipulation if the foot is supinated.

DORSAL ANKLE AND FOOT PAIN

Impingement and Deep Peroneal Nerve Entrapment

On reviewing mechanics dorsiflexion at the ankle is accompanied by a posterior glide of the talus and plantar flexion by an anterior glide. Chronic pronation is accompanied by a plantar flexed talus (a relative anterior talar glide). Due to its inability to freely glide posterioly, activities that challenge dorsiflexion as in climbing, walking downstairs, walking uphill, tend to impinge the soft tissue structures in the anterior aspect of the ankle mortise creating pain. The extensor retinaculum and the capsule can be the pain sources secondary to impingement. Occasionally the dorsally placed deep peroneal nerve can get entrapped under the extensor retinaculum causing dorsal foot pain. A similar impingement can also occur on the lateral aspect of the ankle mortise secondary to chronic pronation causing an anterolateral impingement syndrome (Fig. 28.11).[13]

Somatic Findings

- Pain and tenderness over the anterolateral aspect of the ankle joint/sinus tarsi area
- Pronation with rearfoot valgus
- Pain reproduced on single leg squat

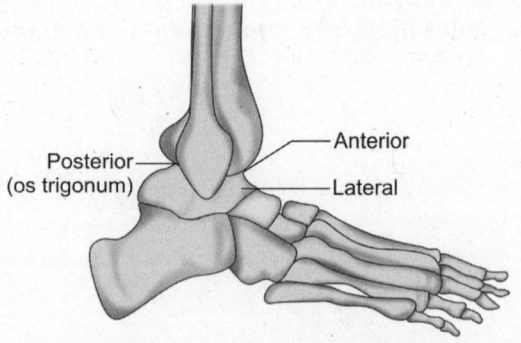

Fig. 28.11: Sites of Impingement.

Manual Therapy Intervention

- Talocrural distraction
- Talocrural posterior glide
- Frictions to the extensor retinaculum.

LUMBAR RADICULOPATHY

The lumbar roots emerging from the foramina of the respective vertebrae are vulnerable to compression. Intervertebral disk herniation and degeneration are the most common sources of compressive radiculopathy. Degeneration causes the intervertebral disk spaces to narrow, thereby narrowing the foramen and subsequently impinging the nerve root. Alternatively, a posterolateral disk herniation can also encroach the foramen causing radicular pain. Pain can radiate along the posterior thigh and the posterolateral aspect of the leg due to an L5 or S1 radiculopathy. An S1 irritation may radiate pain to the lateral aspect of the foot causing lateral foot pain. An L5 radiculopathy may radiate pain to the dorsum of the foot and to the large toe causing dorsal foot pain.

What to Look For

See lumbopelvic section for neurologic examination includes dermatomes, myotomes, reflexes and adverse neural tension testing.

REFERENCES

1. Furey JG. Plantar fasciitis. The painful heel syndrome. J Bone Joint Surg Am. 1975;57:672-3.
2. Rondhuis JJ, Huson A. The first branch of the lateral plantar nerve and heel pain. Acta Morphol Neerl Scand. 1986;24:269-79.
3. Baxter DE, Thigpen CM. Heel pain-operative results. Foot Ankle. 1984;5:16-25.
4. Gondring WH, Trepman E, Shields B. Tarsal tunnel syndrome: assessment of treatment outcome with an anatomic pain intensity scale. Foot Ankle Surg. 2009;15:133-8.
5. Schulhofer SD, Oloff LM. Flexor hallucis longus dysfunction: an overview. Clin Podiatr Med Surg. 2002;19:411-8.
6. Smerdelj M, Madjarevic CM, Oremus K. [Overuse injury syndromes of the calf and foot]. Arh Hig Rada Toksikol. 2001;52:451-64.
7. Lin CF, Gross ML, Weinhold P. Ankle syndesmosis injuries: anatomy, biomechanics, mechanism of injury, and clinical guidelines for diagnosis and intervention. J Orthop Sports Phys Ther. 2006; 36:372-84.
8. Fong DT, Chan YY, Mok KM, et al. Understanding acute ankle ligamentous sprain injury in sports. Sports Med Arthrosc Rehabil Ther Technol. 2009;1-14.
9. Herrmann M, Pieper KS. Sinus tarsi syndrome: what hurts? Unfallchirurg. 2008;111:132-6.
10. Simpson MR, Howard TM. Tendinopathies of the foot and ankle. Am Fam Physician. 2009;80:1107-14.
11. Adams E, Madden C. Cuboid subluxation: a case study and review of the literature. Curr Sports Med Rep. 2009;8:300-7.
12. Arya S, Kulig K. Tendinopathy alters mechanical and material properties of the achilles tendon. J Appl Physiol.2010;108:670-5.
13. Linklater J. MR imaging of ankle impingement lesions. Magn Reson Imaging Clin N Am. 2009; 17:775-800.

CHAPTER 29

Shoulder Region

SUPERIOR SHOULDER PAIN

FIRST RIB DYSFUNCTION

(See thoracic section under Thoracic Outlet Syndrome)

TRAPEZIUS STRAIN

The upper trapezius[1] arises from the external occipital protuberance, nuchal ligament, superior nuchal line, and the spinous processes of C7-T12 and from the corresponding portion of the supraspinous ligament. It inserts into the lateral third of the clavicle, acromion process, and into the spine of the scapula. It assists in shrugging the shoulders, positioning the glenoid when bringing the arm up and sidebending and rotating the head. It most importantly helps with the upward rotation of the scapula. This muscle can be injured or affected by a sudden abrupt displacement of the head/neck as in a whiplash injury, poor posture, and poor ergonomics. As it is inervated by a cranial nerve (spinal accessory) it is high strung.

LEVATOR SCAPULA STRAIN

The levator scapula[1] originates from the transverse processes of the atlas, axis and from the transverse processes of the third and fourth cervical vertebrae. It is inserted into the superomedial vertebral border of the scapula. It helps with ispilateral head rotation, and with the trapezius, the shrugging movement. It obviously hence works in all upright postures and is vulnerable during static postures of the neck. However, it has a tendency for pain and dysfunction when there is the presence of a subcranial dysfunction especially restrictions of the atlanto-occipital and atlantoaxial joints. Pain presentation is usually at the shoulder girdle area with temporary relief on stretching the muscle by contralateral rotation or sidebending.

Somatic Findings (Trapezius and Levator scapula)

- Forward head posture with upper thoracic kyphosis
- Somatic subcranial and midcervical dysfunction
- Restriction of active cervical rotation and sidebending which increases in the shoulder shrug position
- Restriction of passive rotation and sidebending to the opposite side (levator scapula) and sidebending opposite/rotation to the same side (trapezius), in the absence of subcranial and midcervical joint restriction
- Local tenderness over the upper/middle trapezius and levator scapula trigger points
- Positive somatic scapula dysfunctions.

Manual Therapy Intervention

- Suboccipital release
- Osteoarthritis OA forward nod
- Atlantoaxial AA rotation

- Midcervical opening/closing or side glides
- Levator stretch
- Upper trapezius stretch
- Scapula retraction
- Scapula upward rotation.

IMPINGEMENT

(See Impingement Section)

ANTERIOR SHOULDER PAIN

IMPINGEMENT

(See Impingement Section)

COSTOCLAVICULAR SYNDROME

(See Thoracic Section under Thoracic Outlet Syndrome)

BICIPITAL TENDINITIS

The biceps tendon (Fig. 29.1) is also a vulnerable structure for impingement and usually occurs secondary to a rotator cuff pathology.[2] The biceps tendon passes between the supraspinatus and subscapularis. Its intimate association with the cuff has extended its partnership to assist in humeral head depression which is one of the important functions of the cuff. The missing downward force of the cuff during dysfunctional states results in a further upward displacement of the humeral head causing an impingement of the coracoacromial arch on the biceps tendon. The other cause for bicipital tendinitis is due to humeral internal rotation is a primary bicipital tendinitis and is less common than a secondary bicipital tendinitis that accompanies a rotator cuff pathology.

Somatic Findings

- History of anterior shoulder pain

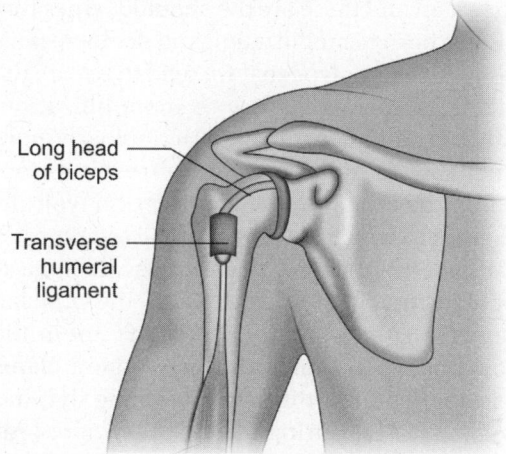

Fig. 29.1: Course of long head of biceps.

- Local tenderness over the bicipital groove
- Associated presence of rotator cuff pathology
- Anterior and medially rotated humerus
- Scapula downward rotation
- Scapula protraction.

Manual Therapy Intervention

- Levator stretch
- Upper trapezius stretch
- Scapula retraction
- Scapula upward rotation
- Distraction humerus
- Posterior glide humerus
- External rotation humerus.

CAPSULITIS

Adhesive capsulitis, otherwise known as frozen shoulder, is a condition characterized by inflammation of the shoulder joint capsule with stiffness and pain in the shoulder joint. Signs and symptoms begin gradually, worsen over time and then resolve usually within a two year period. The causes are varied. More recently a classification was published,[3] however, for purpose of description in a simplified manner, the causes could be primary or secondary. If one happens to see there are patients who wake up one morning with a stiff shoulder for no reason and these are the shoulder types that are stubborn to mobilization and do not resolve easily. The other type that we tend to see are the stiff shoulders postinjury or immobilization. These type of capsular restrictions are more amenable to mobilization and resolve more readily than the primary type. Flexion typically improves first, followed by external rotation and lastly internal rotation. There is an overemphasis for abduction in the frontal plane. The clinician must remember that the glenoid is not in the frontal plane but rather in the scaption plane. It is abduction in the scaption plane that has to be assessed during the treatment process. The causes for the primary type are usually connective tissue disorders, gout, diabetes, etc. These patients tend to contract their capsule as an insidious mechanism. When trauma or surgery or pain warrants immobilization the capsule contracts secondary to lack of mobility and results in a capsulitis of an adhesive nature.

Somatic Findings

- History of sudden onset of shoulder pain or preceding history of shoulder trauma and immobilization
- Classical capsular pattern of restriction of shoulder external rotation, abduction, internal rotation and flexion
- Associated scapular dysfunction.

Manual Therapy Intervention

- Levator stretch
- Upper trapezius stretch
- Scapula retraction
- Scapula upward rotation
- Distraction humerus
- Posterior glide humerus
- External rotation humerus
- Stretch inferior capsule
- Stretch posterior capsule
- Anterior glide humerus
- Stretch anterior capsule.

PECTORALIS MINOR STRAIN

The pectoralis minor originates from the upper margins and outer surfaces of the third, fourth, and fifth ribs, pass upward and laterally and converge to form a flat tendon which inserts into the coracoid process of the scapula. It draws the scapula downward and medially toward thorax, and throwing the inferior angle backward. Hence when tight it has a tendency to protract and tip the scapula.[1] The pectoralis minor in dysfunctional states tends to cause the following conditions:

- The tipping and protraction tends to compress the acromioclavicular joint causing pain and dysfunction
- It causes the 'hyperabduction syndrome', a subset of 'thoracic outlet syndrome' secondary to a tight pectoralis minor entrapping the lower trunk of the brachial plexus during repetitive abduction.
- It causes an anterior rib dysfunction where the rib is displaced anteriorly secondary to a tightness of the muscle.
- It is an entrapment interface of the median nerve.
- It tends to be an aggravating factor for cervical dysfunction as it adds to the upper thoracic kyphosis.
- It tends to aggravate a shoulder impingement syndrome as the tipping displaces the acromion closer to the tendon with the protraction which further adds to persistent internal rotation of the humerus. The consequence of a persistent internal rotation of the humerus is described under the section on somatic diagnosis.

Somatic Findings

All of the above and positive pectoralis minor tightness in supine lying.

Manual Therapy Intervention

- Scapula retraction
- Scapula upward rotation

- Distraction humerus
- Posterior glide humerus
- External rotation humerus
- Pectoralis minor stretch.

MUSCULOCUTANEOUS NERVE ENTRAPMENT

The musculocutaneous nerve arises from the lateral cord of the brachial plexus from the fifth, sixth, and seventh cervical nerves. It passes through the coracobrachialis (Fig. 29.2) and between the biceps and brachialis, supplying these three muscles. This nerve is vulnerable for entrapment by all three muscles it supplies. Sensory loss over the lateral aspect of the forearm and weakness are the key clinical features. However, pain can be a symptom if the sensory aspect, the lateral antebrachial cutaneous nerve is involved in isolation. The pain sensation can be at the insertion of the biceps and paraesthesias over the lateral aspect of the forearm.[4]

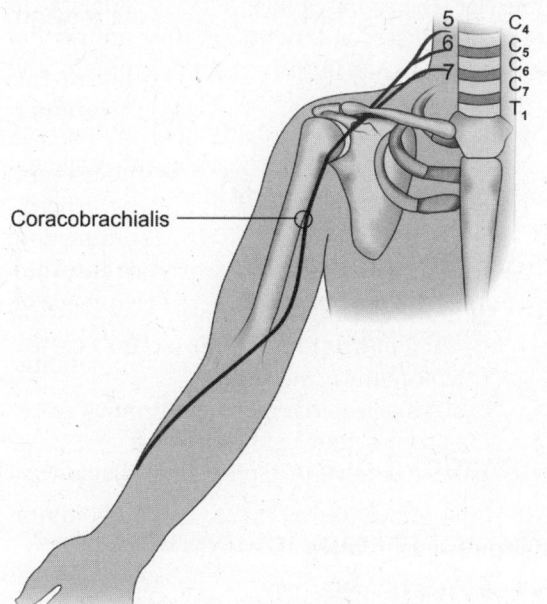

Fig. 29.2: Musculocutaneous nerve entrapment at coracobrachialis.

Somatic Findings

- History of anterior shoulder pain
- C6 like symptoms with negative findings on neurological examination (myotomes, dermatomes and reflexes).
- Local tenderness over the coracobrachialis.

Manual Therapy Intervention

- Scapula retraction
- Scapula upward rotation
- Distraction humerus
- Posterior glide humerus
- External rotation humerus
- Frictions over coracobrachialis.

LATERAL SHOULDER PAIN

RADIAL NERVE ENTRAPMENT

(see Triangular Interval Syndrome)

C5 RADICULOPATHY

The C5 nerve root compressed at the cervical spine may present as shoulder pain. Classically compression reproduces the pain and sensory testing may reveal diminished sensation at the tip of the lateral aspect of the shoulder and lateral forearm.

Somatic Findings

- Positive clinical prediction rule for cervical radiculopathy
- Diminished sensation over the tip of the shoulder and lateral forearm
- Possible weakness in abduction and internal rotation
- Possible presence of a decreased biceps reflex.

Manual Therapy Intervention

As in cervical nerve root irritation.

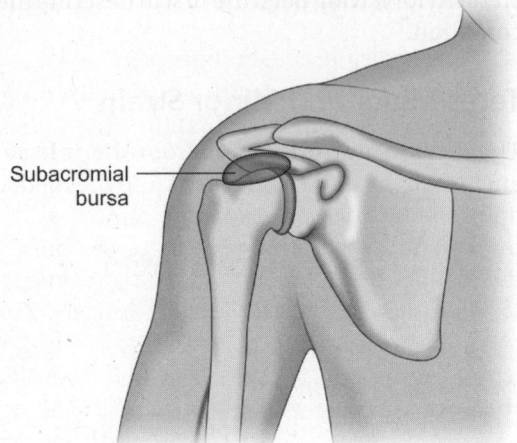

Fig. 29.3: Location of subacromial bursa.

SUBACROMIAL BURSITIS

The subacromial bursa is the intervening structure between the acromion and supraspinatus and is one of the first structure to be compromised in the impingement scenario (Fig. 29.3). See impingement section for a description.

Rotator Cuff Syndrome (See Impingement Section)

POSTERIOR SHOULDER PAIN

IMPINGEMENT

(See Impingement Section)

SUPRASCAPULAR NERVE ENTRAPMENT

(Spinoglenoid/transverse scapular)
The suprascapular nerve arises from the fifth and sixth cervical nerves. It runs laterally and enters the supraspinatous fossa through the suprascapular notch below the transverse scapular ligament. It then passes beneath the supraspinatus, and curves around the lateral border of the spine of the scapula under the spinoglenoid ligament to enter

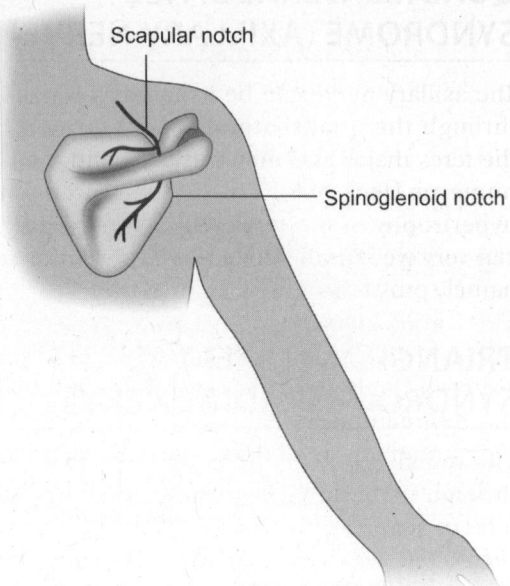

Fig. 29.4: Suprascapular nerve entrapment sites.

the infraspinous fossa (Fig. 29.4). It innervates the supraspinatus muscles and infraspinatus muscles. The suprascapular nerve is vunerable to entrapment[5] secondary to excessive protraction of the scapula or fibrosis and thickening of the spinoglenoid and transverse scapular ligament. Symptoms mimic a rotator cuff pathology, however, classically, impingement is negative with weakness in abduction and external rotation.

Somatic Findings

- All findings of C5 nerve root compression but the clinical prediction rule for cervical radiculopathy is negative
- No signs of impingement syndrome
- No capsular pattern of restriction
- Tenderness over the spinoglenoid ligament.

Manual Therapy Intervention

- Levator stretch
- Upper trapezius stretch
- Scapula retraction
- Scapula upward rotation
- Frictions to spinoglenoid ligament (supero-lateral border of scapula).

QUADRILATERAL SPACE SYNDROME (AXILLARY NERVE)

The axillary nerve can be irritated as it passes through the quadrilateral space[6] formed by the teres major and minor, triceps and medial humerus (Fig. 29.5). This is seen often with hypertrophy of the teres minor muscle but it can very well occur with scapular dysfunctions namely protraction.

TRIANGULAR INTERVAL SYNDROME (RADIAL NERVE)

The radial nerve can be irritated as it passes through the triangular interval formed by the teres major and minor, triceps (Fig. 29.5). This is seen often with hypertrophy of the triceps and teres major muscle but it can very well occur with scapular dysfunction, namely protraction. Prolonged faulty postures of scapular protraction and humeral internal rotation, or punching in the air as seen in martial arts are some causes. The pain presentation may be over the posterolateral aspect of the scapula or the lateral aspect of the humerus at the radial groove. The author is credited for having been the first to describe this condition.[7]

Teres Major and Minor Strain

The teres major originates from the inferior angle of the scapula, and inserts into the medial lip of the bicipital groove of the humerus. The teres minor originates from the upper part of the axillary border of the scapula and inserts on the greater tubercle of the humerus. The teres major internally rotates the shoulder, while the teres minor externally rotates the shoulder. Both muscles assist in stabilizing the head of the humerus in the glenoid. The two muscles form the boundaries to two vulnerable spaces, quadrilateral and triangular causing entrapment syndromes of the axillary and radial nerve, respectively. Hypertrophic bands have been described in these muscles as seen in cadavers for reasons unknown. The prolonged internal rotation (resting/functional) positions of the arm may render the teres major shortened and potentially dysfunctional. They are often palpated as tender and fibrous bands over the lateral border of the scapula and are a source of posterolateral shoulder pain.

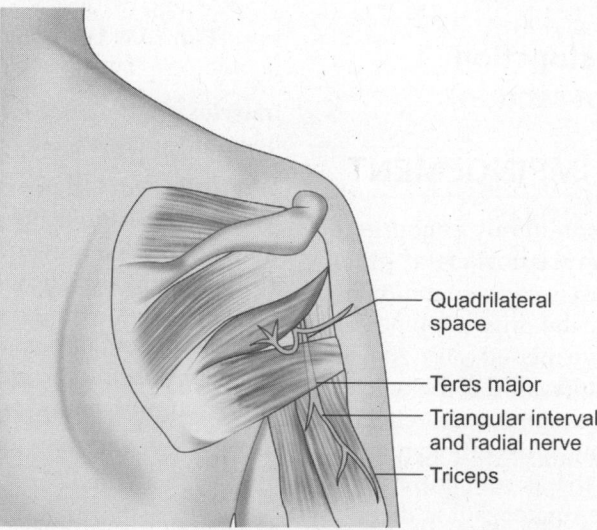

Fig. 29.5: Quadrilateral space and triangular interval.

Somatic Findings for Quadrilateral, Triangular Interval Syndrome and Teres Major and Minor Strain

- History of posterior-lateral shoulder pain
- History of radicular pain in the right upper extremity with negative findings on application of clinical prediction rule for cervical radiculopathy
- Local tenderness over the superolateral aspect of the scapula on passive retraction
- Passive retraction with compression over the superolateral aspect of the scapula reproduces symptoms down the arm and locally.
- Positive adverse neural tension of the radial nerve for triangular interval syndrome.

Manual Therapy Intervention

- Levator stretch
- Upper trapezius stretch
- Scapula retraction
- Scapula upward rotation
- Neural interface mobilization of the radial and axillary nerve by frictions over the teres major and minor and superior aspect of triceps
- Neural mobilization of the radial nerve.

Subscapularis Dysfunction (See Impingement section)

ROTATOR CUFF IMPINGEMENT

The rotator cuff is a commonly encountered terminology for the musculoskeletal practitioner. With varying levels of presentation and confusing terminology the different types and levels of involvement are missed (Figs. 29.6 and 29.7). An accurate identification of the type and presentation makes treatment more effective. We aim to simplify rotator cuff pathology and its subtypes in a manner that is contemporary yet clinically relevant. The rotator cuff is made up of four muscles that connect the scapula to the humerus and are known as the scapulohumeral

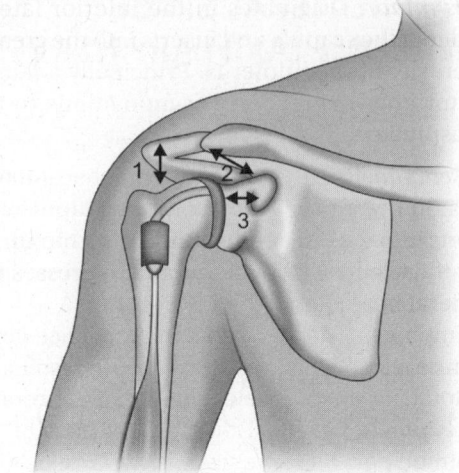

Fig. 29.6: Sites of impingement: 1. Subacromial, 2. Coracoacromial, 3. Subcoracoid.

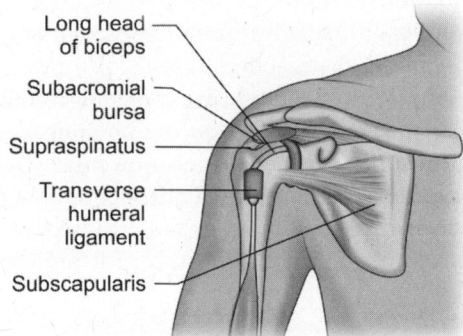

Fig. 29.7: Location of structures in the impingement complex.

muscles.[7-9] The anatomy is enumerated in the beginning of this section, and to review.

Supraspinatus: Originates in the supraspinous fossa of the scapula and inserts into the greater tuberosity of the humerus. This muscle initiates abduction at the shoulder and is one of the primary external rotators of the shoulder. Acting with the deltoid, it helps to contain the head of the humerus into the glenoid cavity during the entire range of motion at the shoulder.

Infraspinatus: Originates in the infraspinous fossa of the scapula and inserts into the greater tuberosity of the humerus. Function is to laterally rotate the shoulder and depress the humeral head.

Teres minor: Originates in the inferior lateral border of the scapula and inserts into the greater tuberosity of the humerus. Principally a lateral rotator and its function is synonymous to the infraspinatus.

Subscapularis: Originates in the subscapularis fossa on the anterior aspect of the scapula and inserts into the lesser tuberosity of the humerus. This muscle medially rotates and depresses the humeral head.

Impingement[9] is a subacromial space compromise resulting in irritation of the supraspinatus tendon. The supraspinatus tendon of the rotator cuff is pinched against the undersurface of the acromion portion of the scapula during elevation of the arm. The types are:

Primary Impingement

Primary impingement typically occurs in the subacromial space on the superior bursal side. The most common etiology of a primary impingement is degeneration and spurring, hence a radiological examination is strongly recommended. This commonly seen in the industrial population and more due to mechanical factors. The supraspinatus, infraspinatus and the long head of the biceps may be involved. The shape of the acromion also has a big part to play. A description of the acromion types and incidence of impingement is listed below:

Acromial Morphology

Type I: Flat acromion, low incidence of impingement

Type II: Curved acromion, higher incidence of impingement

Type III: Beaked acromion, very high incidence of impingement.

What to Look For

- Aging
- Mechanical narrowing of the subacromial space (see somatic diagnosis section)
- AC joint degeneration
- Subacromial type 2 and 3
- Rotator cuff/scapular weakness (see somatic diagnosis section)
- Increased thoracic kyphosis.

Manual Therapy Intervention

- Scapula upward rotation
- Scapula retraction
- Humerus distraction
- Humerus inferior glide
- Humerus posterior glide
- Humerus external rotation
- Frictions over supraspinatus
- Frictions over levator scapula
- Soft tissue mobilization of the trapezius and erector spinae in the interscapular area
- Midthoracic closing manipulation
- Stretch posterior capsule.

Secondary Impingement

Secondary impingement indicates an unstable situation of the humeral head in the glenoid fossa. Causes are weakness of the rotator cuff called functional instability in combination with the glenohumeral joint capsule and ligaments that are loose known as microinstability. The main cause for impingement is the anterior translation of the humeral head. The site of compromise is the coracoacromial space as opposed to the subacromial space seen in the primary impingement. Functional instability usually precedes microinstability. The supraspinatus and the long head of biceps may be involved.

What to Look For

- Pain is located in the anterior or anterolateral aspect of the shoulder.
- The symptoms are usually reproduced by the overhead activity.
- Neer impingement is positive
- Presence of instability.

Manual Therapy Intervention

When instability is present manual therapy for the joints is contraindicated, however, soft tissue mobilization for structures in the complex may be indicated. This conditions warrants strengthening exercises.

Subcoracoid Impingement

The subcoracoid space is the interval between the tip of the coracoid and humeral head and is called coracohumeral interval. The space measures 8 to 11 mm, however, stenotic situations occur when this area is less than 6 mm. Subcoracoid impingement is an impingement of the coracoid process against the lesser tuberosity of the humerus when the humerus is flexed, adducted and internally rotated. The susbscapularis that is in between these structures is vulnerable for tears.

What to Look For

- Patients present with anterior shoulder pain with coracoid tenderness especially on flexion, adduction and internal rotation
- Hawkins Impingement sign is positive
- Crossover sign may be positive
- Instability signs are usually absent
- Thoracic kyphosis.

Manual Therapy Intervention

- Scapula upward rotation
- Scapula retraction
- Humerus distraction
- Humerus inferior glide
- Humerus posterior glide
- Humerus external rotation
- Frictions over supraspinatus
- Frictions over levator scapula
- Soft tissue mobilization of the trapezius and erector spinae in the interscapular area
- Midthoracic closing manipulation
- Stretch posterior capsule.

Anterior Internal Impingement

This is a more recently described entity and occurs in stable shoulders. The suggested impingement is said to occur between the anterosuperior labrum and rotator cuff tendon. The prevalence is considered to be more in the swimming population.

What to Look For

Internal rotation resisted strength test may be positive.

Posterior superior Glenoid Impingement (PSGI)

Posterior superior glenoid impingement (PSGI) is considered the most common cause of posterior shoulder pain in the throwing or overhead athlete. It is caused by the impingement of the posterior edge of the supraspinatus and anterior edge of the infraspinatus (Fig. 29.8) against the posterior superior glenoid and glenoid labrum. This pathological situation can occur in athletes that repetitively throw using the extension, abduction, external rotation sequence. It is also prevalent in the industrial population involving repetitive overhead activity in the same fashion. It is also seen in individuals lifting weights, incorporating poor lifting techniques.

The other cause for posterior impingement of the shoulder is instability. Functional stability as we know it is provided by the rotator cuff complex. Throwing individuals may present with excessive external rotation and decreased internal rotation. Retroversion of the humeral head may also be present as an underlying

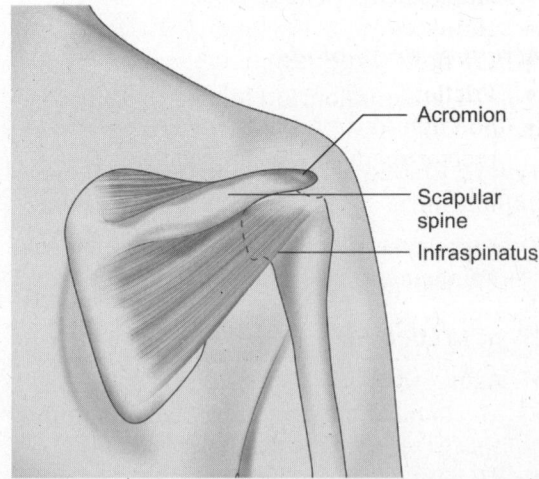

Fig. 29.8: Infraspinatus tendon and relationship to acromion and posterior glenoid.

etiology to reduced Internal rotation. Excessive external rotation will requires the antagonist internal rotator to work harder in an eccentric fashion to reduce momentum. This structure is the subscapularis, working harder in an eccentric fashion. This renders the muscle lax and encourages anterior instability. This may further aggravate symptoms in the throwing athlete or overhead worker.

What to Look For

- Pain is primarily associated with the athletic or overhead activity
- Slow onset, no history of trauma
- Posterior shoulder pain in the throwing shoulder during the cocking phase
- Posterior shoulder pain during the cocking phase that worsens during early acceleration
- Eccentric subscapularis weakness
- Scapular dyskinesia
- Increased external rotation with decreased internal rotation
- Relocation test is positive
- Neer test is positive.

Manual Therapy Intervention

- Scapula upward rotation
- Scapula retraction
- Humerus distraction
- Humerus posterior glide in excess avoided
- Humerus external rotation in excess avoided
- Frictions over supraspinatus
- Frictions over levator scapula
- Soft tissue mobilization of the trapezius and erector spinae in the interscapular area
- Midthoracic closing manipulation
- Stretch posterior capsule.

REFERENCES

1. Gazielly DF. Sports injuries of the shoulder. Baillieres Clin Rheumatol. 1989;3:627-49.
2. Churgay CA. Diagnosis and treatment of biceps tendinitis and tendinosis. Am Fam Physician. 2009;80:470-6.
3. Kelley MJ, McClure PW, Leggin BG. Frozen shoulder: evidence and a proposed model guiding rehabilitation. J Orthop Sports Phys Ther. 2009;39:135-48.
4. Ma H, Van Heest A, Glisson C, Patel S. Musculocutaneous nerve entrapment: an unusual complication after biceps tenodesis. Am J Sports Med. 2009;37:2467-9.
5. Ligh CA, Schulman BL, Safran MR. Case reports: unusual cause of shoulder pain in a collegiate baseball player. Clin Orthop Relat Res. 2009;467:2744-8.
6. Drez DJ Jr. Surgical decompression of the quadrilateral space in overhead athletes. Am J Sports Med. 2008;36:E8.
7. Sebastian D. Triangular interval syndrome: a differential diagnosis for upper extremity radicular pain. Physiother Theory Pract. 2010;26:113-9.
8. Burbank KM, Stevenson JH, Czarnecki GR, et al. Chronic shoulder pain: part I. Evaluation and diagnosis. Am Fam Physician. 2008;77:453-60.
9. Sahrmann S. Diagnosis and treatment of movement impairment syndromes, 2001. St Louis, Mosby.
10. Buss DD, Freehill MQ, Marra G. Typical and atypical shoulder impingement syndrome: diagnosis, treatment, and pitfalls. Instr Course Lect. 2009;58:447-57.

CHAPTER 30

Elbow, Wrist and Hand Region

MEDIAL ELBOW, WRIST AND HAND PAIN

MEDIAL EPICONDYLITIS (GOLFER'S ELBOW)

This is an overuse syndrome of the common flexor origin of the elbow (Fig. 30.1). Although the throwing mechanism is one of the causative factors, it is more so repetitive, wrist flexion and ulnar deviation that causes this condition. This condition, although originally considered an inflammatory condition is now being replaced by a degenerative sequelae. Angiofibroblastic tendinosis is the newly coined term to describe the syndrome and the tendons described to be most involved are the pronator teres and flexor carpi radialis.[1]

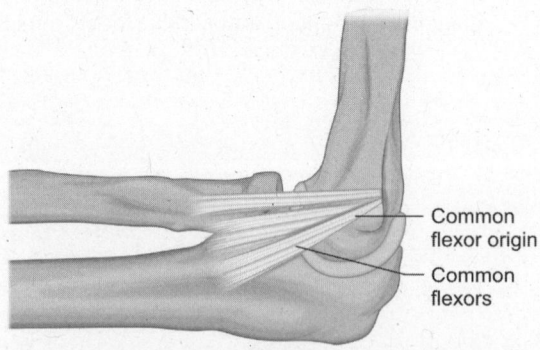

Fig. 30.1: Location of irritation in Golfer's elbow.

Somatic Findings
- Pain on resistance with wrist flexion and ulnar deviation
- Palpate the medial epicondyle with the arm in elbow flexion, forearm supination and wrist extension. Pain is reproduced as the elbow is extended.

Manual Therapy Intervention
- Deep frictions to the common flexor origin
- Distraction radiocarpal
- Volar glide radiocarpal
- Dorsal glide radiocarpal.

MEDIAL COLLATERAL LIGAMENT STRAIN

This ligament arises from the medial epicondyle of the humerus. It has three bands, anterior, posterior and intermediate. The anterior band attaches to the coronoid process of ulna and the posterior band attaches to the olecranon process (Fig. 30.2). These two ligaments are joined together by the intermediate fibers. Throwing involves a starting position of shoulder extension with abduction and external rotation, while the elbow is flexed. Then the motion consists of the trunk and shoulder moving rapidly forward, while leaving the arm behind. This causes an extension moment at the elbow which is rapid and jerky. This will cause the radius to glide

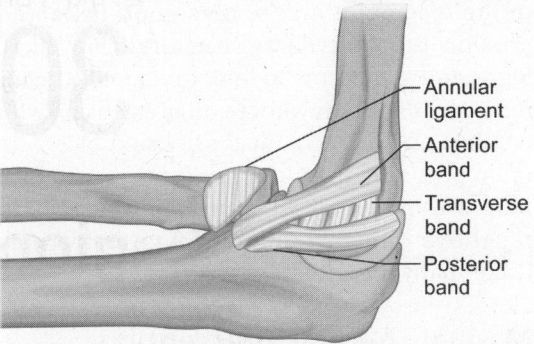

Fig. 30.2: Medial collateral ligament of elbow.

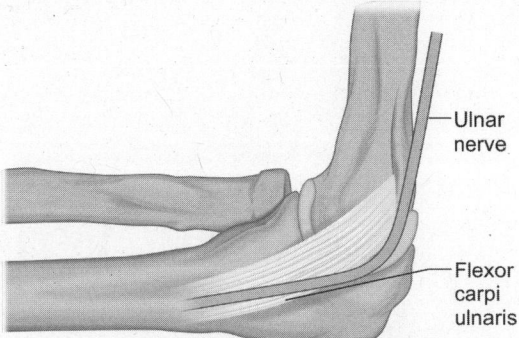

Fig. 30.3: Cubital tunnel.

inferiorly with the radial head gliding posterior. This causes a valgus stress at the medial aspect of the elbow and increased the tensile forces. However, if the arthrokinematic radial inferior glide is restricted it increases compressive forces on the lateral side which further increases the tensile forces on the medial side of the elbow. The medial collateral ligament is most vulnerable. In addition, it causes overuse injury of the musculature, capsular injury, ulnar traction spurs and medial epicondylitis.[2]

Somatic Findings

- Local tenderness
- Pain on valgus stress
- Postive ulnar variance.

Manual Therapy Intervention

- Inferior glide radial head
- AP glide, inferior radioulnar joint
- Manual intervention to improve shoulder external rotation
- Distraction radiocarpal
- Volar glide radiocarpal
- Dorsal glide radiocarpal.

CUBITAL TUNNEL SYNDROME

Cubital tunnel syndrome[3] describes an ulnar nerve compressive neuropathy at the elbow. Compression of the ulnar nerve at the elbow often has a component of extrinsic compression and may be static or dynamic. The dynamic cause maybe of greater relevance to the physical therapist and may be summarized as follows. With flexion of the elbow, the aponeurosis covering the cubital tunnel stretches changing the cross-sectional geometry of the cubital tunnel from smooth and round to flattened and triangular. This both decreases the volume of the tunnel by half and significantly increases the intraneural pressure, therefore putting the nerve at risk of compression. This pressure can further increase significantly with shoulder abduction, elbow flexion, and wrist extension, as in the throwing motion. Additionally, contraction of the flexor carpi ulnaris may further increase the pressure on the ulnar nerve (Fig. 30.3). This includes repeated flexion at the elbow and ulnar deviation of the wrist. Systemic diseases such as diabetes, chronic alcoholism, renal failure, and malnutrition may also predispose the patient to compressive neuropathy. Other causes include spurs, triceps and anconeus epitrochlearis, and space occupying lesions.

Somatic Findings

- Local tenderness over the medial aspect of the olecrenon (spur)
- Positive ulnar variance
- Tinel's sign at the elbow

Principles of Manual Therapy

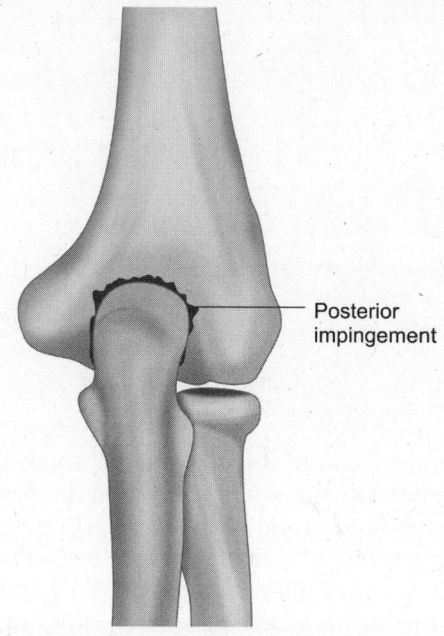

Fig. 30.4: Site for posterior impingement elbow.

- Positive adverse neural tension for the ulnar nerve
- Pain on resisted wrist flexion and ulnar deviation
- Possible history of repetitive throwing.

Manual Therapy Intervention

- Inferior glide radial head
- AP glide and inferior radioulnar joint
- Frictions over flexor carpi ulnaris
- Neural mobilization of the ulnar nerve
- Distraction radiocarpal
- Volar glide radiocarpal
- Dorsal glide radiocarpal
- Shoulder external rotation to be addressed if ligamentous valgus instability in the elbow is present.

POSTERIOR ELBOW PAIN OLECRANON IMPINGEMENT

Throwing activity of a repetitive nature is the cause for this condition. It is an impingement of the olecranon on the olecranon fossa and possibly the intervening structures (Fig. 30.4). Signs and symptoms to look for are clicking or locking of the elbow with terminal extension with crepitus and a mechanical extension block are often present. Elbow extension may reproduce pain with possible valgus instability as seen in repetitive throwing. Radial compression may accompany the situation.[4]

Manual Therapy Intervention

- Ulna distraction
- Medial and lateral glide of the olecranon over olecranon fossa
- Low load long duration anterior capsule stretch (caution: Risk of myositis ossificans).

LATERAL ELBOW, WRIST AND HAND PAIN

LATERAL EPICONDYLITIS (TENNIS ELBOW)

This is an overuse syndrome of the common extensor origin of the elbow (Fig. 30.5). Although the gripping mechanism is one of the causative factors, it is more so repetitive, wrist extension

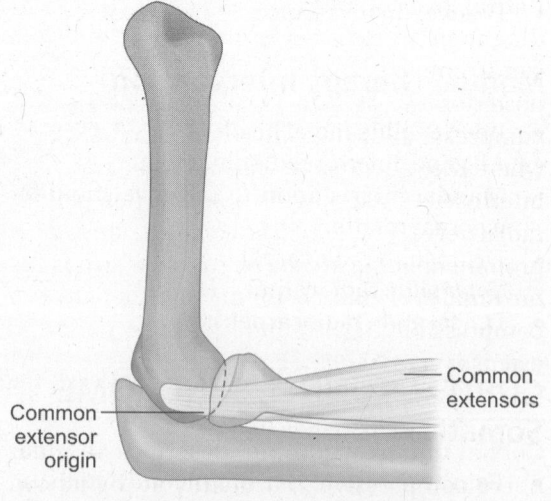

Fig. 30.5: Common extensor origin.

and radial deviation that causes this condition. This condition, although originally considered an inflammatory condition is now being replaced by a degenerative sequelae. Angiofibroblastic tendinosis is the newly coined term to describe the syndrome and the tendons described to be most involved are the extensor digitorum communis and extensor carpi radialis brevis.[5]

Somatic Findings

- Pain on resistance with wrist extension and radial deviation (cozen's test)
- Pain on resistance of the middle finger (maudsley's test)
- Positive ulnar variance
- Restriction of terminal extension of the wrist.

Manual Therapy Intervention

- AP glide and radial head
- AP glide and inferior radioulnar joint
- Inferior glide and radial head
- Frictions over extensor carpi radialis brevis (ECRB), and brachioradialis
- Distraction radiocarpal
- Volar glide radiocarpal.

RADIAL TUNNEL SYNDROME

Radial tunnel syndrome[6] is a differential diagnosis for lateral epicondalgia and is a syndrome arising from compression of the posterior interosseous nerve at the elbow. This compression occurs in the proximal forearm where the radial nerve splits into the posterior interroseus nerve and the sensory branch of the radial nerve (Fig. 30.6). The compression is most prominent at the arcade of Frohse which is the proximal border of the supinator. Other areas of compression include radiocapitellar joint and extensor carpi radialis brevis.

Somatic Findings

- Pain resembling lateral epicondylagia and radiating into the forearm

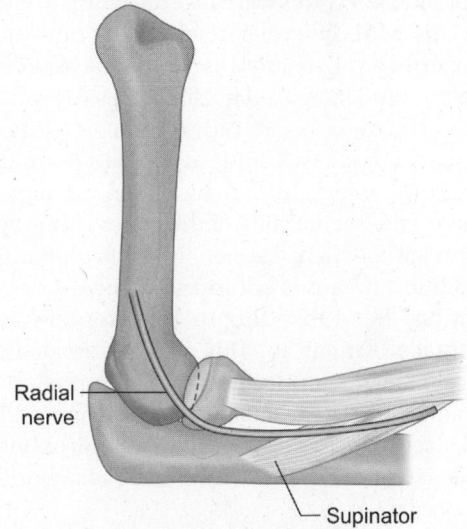

Fig. 30.6: Radial tunnel.

- Tenderness over the bulk of the supinator which lies under the bulk of the brachioradialis
- Positive adverse neural tension of the radial nerve
- Terminal restriction of wrist extension
- Possible positive ulnar variance.

Manual Therapy Intervention

- AP glide and radial head
- AP glide and inferior radioulnar joint
- Inferior glide and radial head
- Frictions over ECRB, and brachioradialis
- Neural mobilization of the radial nerve
- Distraction radiocarpal
- Volar glide radiocarpal.

RADIAL HEAD COMPRESSION/ FIBRILLATION/RADIOCAPITELLAR CHONDROMALACIA

Throwing involves a starting position of shoulder extension with abduction and external rotation, while the elbow is flexed. Then the motion consists of the trunk and shoulder moving rapidly forward while leaving the arm behind. This causes an extension moment at the elbow which is rapid and jerky. This will cause the radius to glide inferiorly with the radial head gliding posterior. This causes a valgus stress at the medial aspect of the elbow and increased tensile forces. However, if the arthrokinematic radial inferior glide is restricted it increases compressive forces on the lateral side, which further increases the tensile forces on the medial side of the elbow. Although the medial collateral ligament is most vulnerable, in addition it causes compressive stresses over the radial head resulting in compression and eventually fibrillation. This condition is called radiocapitellar chondromalacia. Compression of the radiocapitellar articulation sometimes results in damage to the radial head, capitellum, or both. Frank osteochondral fracture and loose bodies may occur.[7]

Somatic Findings

- Positive ulnar variance
- The typical presenting symptoms are catching, locking and lateral elbow pain with active use of the elbow. Swelling and localized tenderness are noted at the affected site.
- An axial load applied with passive supination and pronation often provokes pain and can be helpful in differentiating radiocapitellar chondromalacia from lateral tennis elbow.
- Radiographs may show a loss of joint space, marginal osteophytes, and possibly loose bodies.

Manual Therapy Intervention

- AP glide and radial head
- AP glide and inferior radioulnar joint
- Inferior glide and radial head
- Frictions over ECRB, and brachioradialis
- Neural mobilization of the radial nerve
- Distraction radiocarpal
- Volar glide radiocarpal.

MUSCLES AND TENDONS

Overuse strains are seen in several of small muscles of the hand and forearm, the most commonly involved are the interossei, flexor digitorum profundus and superficialis. As mentioned earlier these may occur secondary to faulty arthrokinematics as well. Similarly the extensor tendons and tendon sheaths are also prone to injury secondary to overuse. It is also important to address the normal arthrokinematics of extension and radial deviation.

Manual Therapy Intervention

- Distraction radiocarpal
- Volar glide radiocarpal
- Frictions to the interossei, flexor digitorum profundus and superficialis.

ANTERIOR/VOLAR ELBOW, WRIST AND HAND PAIN

PRONATOR SYNDROME/ ANTERIOR INTEROSSEOUS NERVE SYNDROME

This is a condition characterized by an entrapment of the median nerve distal to the elbow.[66] The muscular interface is the pronator teres (Fig. 30.7). It often occurs in individuals presenting with anterior elbow pain after participating in racquet or throwing sports. Anterior pain and distal paresthesias are characteristic symptoms secondary to an entrapment of the anterior interroseus nerve.

Somatic Findings

- Pronator compression at the anterior aspect of the elbow, an inch below the elbow crease reproduces symptoms
- Hypertrophied pronator muscle distal to the antecubital fossa.
- The pain worsens when pronation is performed against resistance.
- Tingling or paresthesias in the distribution of the median nerve often with a positive Tinel's sign.

Elbow, Wrist and Hand Region

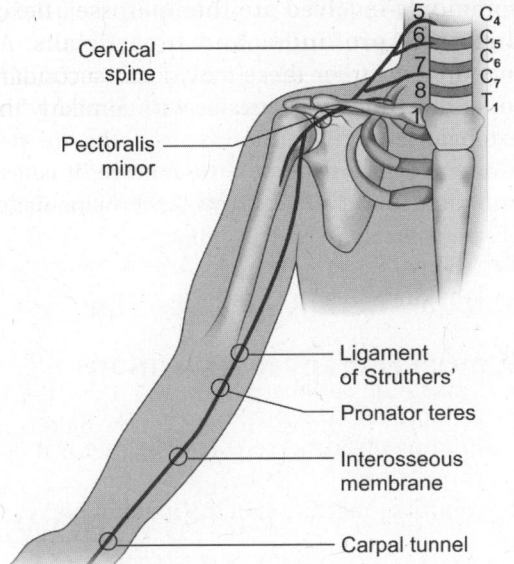

Fig. 30.7: Median nerve entrapment sites.

Manual Therapy Intervention

- AP glide and inferior radioulnar joint
- Frictions pronator teres
- Neural mobilization of the medial nerve.

GUYON'S CANAL SYNDROME

This condition describes an irritation of the ulnar nerve characterized by a stretching of the nerve secondary to a faulty combination of hyperextension and ulnar deviation of the wrist. It is seen commonly in cyclists. The nerve then gets irritated between the pisiform and hook of the hamate (Fig. 30.8). Faulty arthrokinematics during extension of the wrist may also be a causative factor. The pisohamate ligament is essentially two fibrous bands, the pisohamate and pisometacarpal ligaments that run from the pisiform and hamate and the pisiform and fifth metacarpal. These are in reality extensions of the flexor carpi ulnaris muscle and are susceptible to dysfunction with prolonged and repetitive flexion movements of the wrist. This is seen in occupational situations and in sports like volleyball, cricket and golf. Hence faulty arthrokinematics of wrist flexion and ulnar deviation are the causative factors as well.[6]

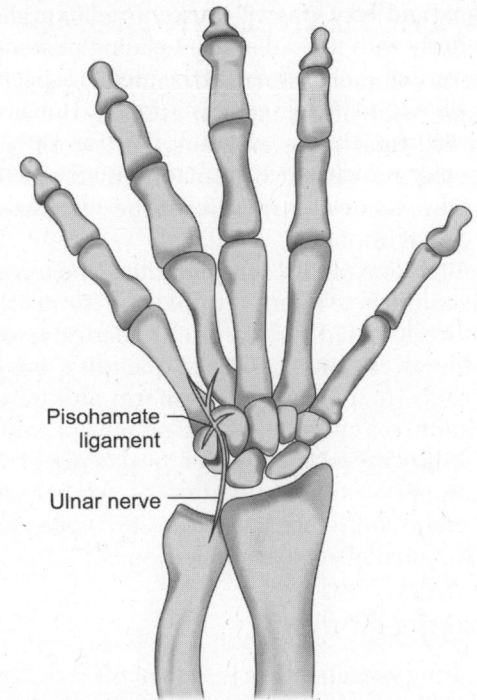

Fig. 30.8: Guyon's canal.

Somatic Findings

- History of repetititve hyperextension and ulnar deviation of the wrist or in some cases flexion and ulnar deviation of the wrist
- Possible history of cycling
- Pain and paraesthesia over the ulnar side of the hand and little finger, possibly the lateral half of the ring finger
- Local tenderness over the Guyon's canal and symptom reproduction on pressure.

Manual Therapy Intervention

- Frictions over pisohammate ligament
- Neural mobilization of the ulnar nerve.

CARPAL TUNNEL SYNDROME

This is a commonly described condition involving compression of the median nerve at the wrist (Fig. 30.9) and has several causative factors.[6] The ones that are relevant to the manual therapist are:
- Fibrosis or contracture of the transverse carpal ligament
- Alteration of the bony margins of the tunnel secondary to injury, arthrokinematic restriction and faulty alignment secondary to fractures (colles). The carpals that are of concern are hammate/pisiform and trapezium/scaphoid. A tight ligament or faulty arthrokinematics can alter the patency of the tunnel resulting in symptoms. An anterior subluxation of the lunate can also predispose to a medial nerve compression.

Somatic Findings

- History of repetititve flexion of the wrist and gripping
- Possible history of prolonged periods of typing, keyboard work
- Pain and paraesthesia over the radial side of the hand and the lateral three and a half fingers
- Local tenderness over the transverse carpal ligament and symptom reproduction on pressure
- Positive Phalen's test
- Weakness of grip.

Manual Therapy Intervention

- Carpal mobilization
- Frictions transverse carpal ligament if not very acute
- Neural mobilization of the median nerve.

CARPOMETACARPAL ARTHROSIS

This is an obvious arthrokinematic restriction that occurs in the carpometacarpal (CMC) joint of the thumb as it is most vulnerable for osteoarthritis. It is seen during chronic overuse involving gripping or racquet sports. The restriction is usually in the direction of abduction. Since it restricts thumb mobility, it can significantly affect function including the sharp pain that it is associated with. Local tenderness over the first CMC joint is characteristic.

Somatic Findings

- Pain in the first CMC joint increased with gripping
- Restriction of mobility.

Manual Therapy Intervention

- Distraction first CMC
- Dorsal and volar glides, first CMC.

REFERENCES

1. Bayes MC, Wadsworth LT. Upper extremity injuries in golf. Phys Sportsmed. 2009;37:92-6.
2. Hayter CL, Giuffre BM. Overuse and traumatic injuries of the elbow. Magn Reson Imaging Clin N Am. 2009;17:617-38.

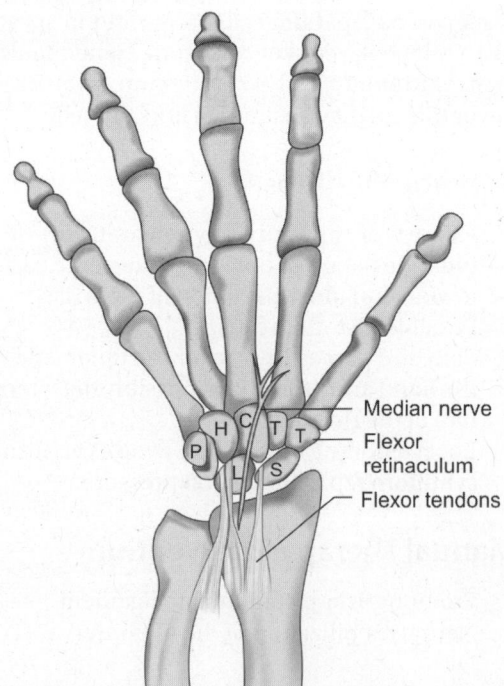

Fig. 30.9: Carpal tunnel.

3. Palmer BA, Hughes TB. Cubital tunnel syndrome. J Hand Surg Am. 2010;35:153-63.
4. Damert HG, Altmann S, Schneider W. Soft-tissue defects following olecranon bursitis. Treatment options for closure. Chirurg. 2009;80:448, 450-4.
5. Walz DM, Newman JS, Konin GP, et al. Epicondylitis: pathogenesis, imaging, and treatment. Radiographics. 2010;30:167-84.
6. Neal S, Fields KB. Peripheral nerve entrapment and injury in the upper extremity. Am Fam Physician. 2010;81:147-55.
7. Antuna SA, O'Driscoll SW. Snapping plicae associated with radiocapitellar chondromalacia. Arthroscopy. 2001;17:491-5.

PART 4

The Critical and Neglected Zones of the Upper and Lower Quarter in the Management of Regional Conditions

Chapter 31: The Upper Quarter
Chapter 32: The Lower Quarter

INTRODUCTION

The musculoskeletal system working as chains and links, is a well understood concept in contemporary practice. Manual practitioners incorporate this principle as a routine in the management of musculoskeletal dysfunction. There is currently a clearer understanding of the relationship and need in treating adjacent joints to accomplish desired outcomes in a region,[1] for example, the need to address foot pathomechanics while managing knee dysfunction. While some areas are more obvious, others tend to be subtle and indirect, nevertheless relevant. This chapter aims to address these areas with a larger emphasis on clinical relevance to regional conditions more than just mobility, as their treatment on a more individual basis is described in the previous chapters.

CHAPTER 31

The Upper Quarter

SCAPULA

The scapula has steadily gained importance in the management of mechanical dysfunction of the shoulder. While this is imperative, the clinician must also understand that addressing mechanical dysfunction of the scapula is critical to the management of not just the shoulder but of all upper quarter dysfunction.[1] This includes cranial pain and headaches, cervical dysfunction and thoracic dysfunction.

Anatomy

The scapulae are a pair of flat, symmetrical bones on either side of the upper thoracic region. They lie 2–3 inches lateral to the thoracic vertebrae and extend approximately between T2-T8. To contour to the rib cage, it is slightly protracted, forward tipped and upward rotated. It attaches to the axial skeleton to form the scapulo-thoracic joint and is not a true anatomic joint as it has none of the usual joint characteristics (union by fibrous, cartilaginous, or synovial tissues). Its true bony integrity is derived by its attachment to the clavicle via the acromioclavicular (AC) joint and the corresponding ligaments that attach the scapula to the clavicle.

The soft tissue integrity of the scapula is worth describing. A clinician with good examination skills can identify imbalances and subsequently balance these tissues for a very desired outcome while treating most upper quarter dysfunction. The scapula and its attachments to the thorax is synonymous to a mountain climber scaling a peak. He or she uses the concept of anchoring; utilizing hooks and ropes to anchor and scale a peak. The scapula is literally hanging on the posterior wall of the thorax and anchoring itself via ligamentous and muscular attachments to the thorax, clavicle and humerus, and serving as an intermediary to most upper quarter function.

The superior and inferior acromioclavicular ligaments strengthen the attachment of the scapula to the lateral end of the clavicle. The coracoclavicular ligament runs from the lateral end of the clavicle to the coracoid process. It consists of two parts, conoid ligament which resists forward movement of the scapula, and trapezoid ligament which is stronger and restricts backward movement of the scapula.

The muscles acting on the shoulder complex are as follows:
1. Muscles connecting the scapula to the spine
2. Muscles connecting the scapula to the humerus.

Their function is described below:

Muscles connecting the scapula to the spine:
- *Trapezius:* The upper fibers adduct, elevate and upwardly rotate the scapula and glenoid. The middle fibers adduct the scapula and glenoid and the lower fibers adduct depress and upwardly rotate the scapula and glenoid.
- *Levator scapula:* This muscle adducts, elevates and downwardly rotates the scapula and glenoid. Acting unilaterally it rotates

and side bends the cervical spine to the same side. Acting bilaterally, it extends the cervical spine.

- *Rhomboids:* They adduct, elevate and downwardly rotate the scapula and glenoid.
- *Serratus anterior:* This muscle abducts and upwardly rotates the scapula. It also holds the scapula to prevent it from winging from the rib cage on the medial side.
- *Pectoralis minor:* This muscle tilts the scapula anteriorly and downwardly rotates the scapula.

Muscles connecting the scapula to the humerus:
- *Deltoid:* The anterior fibers flex and medially rotate the shoulder. The middle fibers abduct the shoulder and the posterior fibers extend and laterally rotate the same.
- *Supraspinatus:* This muscle initiates abduction at the shoulder and is one of the primary external rotators of the shoulder. Acting with the deltoid, it helps to contain the head of the humerus into the glenoid cavity during the entire range of motion at the shoulder.
- *Infraspinatus:* Functions to laterally rotate the shoulder and depress the humeral head.
- *Teres minor:* Principally a lateral rotator and it's function is synonymous to the infraspinatus.
- *Subscapularis:* This muscle medially rotates and depresses the humeral head. Another important function of this muscle is to provide anterior stability and prevent anterior migration of the humeral head.
- *Teres major:* It functions to medially rotate, adduct and extend the shoulder.
- *Biceps brachii:* This muscle flexes the elbow and with the elbow in extension, it assists to flex the shoulder. It is also a powerful supinator of the forearm and assists in adduction of the shoulder with the humerus in external rotation.
- *Lattismus dorsi:* This versatile muscle medially rotates, adducts, extends and depresses the shoulder. Acting bilaterally, it extends the spine and tilts the pelvis anteriorly.

Dysfunctional States of the Scapula Previously Described[2]

Winging

Winging is a pathomechanical situation where the medial border of the scapula excessively elevates off the rib cage during arm movements. It can occur due to weakness of the serratus anterior and is obvious on shoulder flexion and on push up. However, winging can also occur during return from flexion back to midline. This obviously is not due to weakness of the serratus but due to a timing problem. The possible cause is that the scapulohumeral muscles do not relax as rapidly as the axioscapular muscles.

Scapular winging can compromise the subacromial space and predispose to compression at the acromioclavicular joint.

Adducted/Downward Rotation

This is implied as stated where the scapula along with the scapular spine and acromion moves excessively in a downward direction during arm elevation. Thus, the scapula rotates downward during the initial phase of shoulder abduction, instead of the normal upward rotation after the initial setting phase. The possible causes for this dysfunction are:
- Tightness of levator scapulae.
- Insufficient activity of the lower trapezius.

Again, during the last phases of humeral elevation, the scapula fails to rotate upward. The causes for this dysfunction are as above but also due to tightness of the levator scapula and pectoralis minor.

A downward rotation of the scapula can compromise the subacromial space predisposing to impingement. A dysfunction of the levator scapula and upper fibers of the trapezius can predispose to myogenic headaches.

Abducted/Protraction

In this dysfunction, the scapula protracts excessively during shoulder flexion. The possible causes for this dysfunction are:

- Tightness of the pectoralis minor, pectoralis major, teres major and serratus anterior.
- Weakness of the scapular retractors.

A protracted scapula predisposes to a forward head posture and rounded shoulders. This primarily compromises the subacromial space causing impingement and also increases compression at the acromioclavicular joint. It can also predispose to irritability of the rhomboids and by virtue of their attachment to the thoracic spine causes thoracic dysfunctions. Protraction can also cause tightness of the pectoralis minor causing a compromise of the thoracic outlet. A protracted scapula can also cause traction on the suprascapular nerve causing symptoms. It can also compromise the quadrilateral space and triangular interval causing an irritation of the axillary and radial nerves, respectively.

Primary Dysfunction

Excessive Scapula Forward Tipping (A Combination of Downward Rotation, Protraction and Winging)

Normally, the scapula rests at a position we term the scaption plane. It rests on the posterior thorax where it is internally rotated 30° to 45° from the coronal plane, is tipped anteriorly approximately 10° to 20° from vertical, and is upwardly rotated 10° to 20° from vertical. While all is well in this position, the risk is rendered when the proximal and lateral anchors of the scapula shorten. The anchors are as follows:

- Coracoclavicular ligaments (trapezoid and conoid)
- Pectoralis minor
- Teres major

When these structures shorten, the scapula is tilted anteriorly.[3] However, owing to the superior and lateral placement of these structures, in the forward tipped position, the scapula is in a position of downward rotation, protraction and medial border elevation predisposing to winging (Fig. 31.1).

The dynamic challenges to the muscles in this position are as follows:

- A greater challenge for the trapezius to upwardly rotate the scapula (downward rotation)
- A greater challenge for the serratus anterior to flatten the medial border of the scapula to the medial thoracic wall (winging)
- A greater challenge for the trapezius and rhomboids to hold the medial border of the scapula in the midline (protraction).

Clinical Relevance of Excessive Scapula Forward Tipping to most Upper Quarter Dysfunction

The clinical relevance of the excessively anteriorly tipped position (with its concurrent downward rotation, protraction and winging) to shoulder dysfunction is obvious and is described in detail in the shoulder chapter. Its relevance to neck[1,4] and thoracic dysfunction requires explanation, thus making the scapula a needed treatment destination to address 'all' upper quarter dysfunction.

Relevance to Neck Dysfunction and Headaches

The direct attachments of the scapula to the cervical spine and the cranium are via the following structures:

- Trapezius (spine of scapula to external occipital protuberance, nuchal line, all cervical spinous processes)

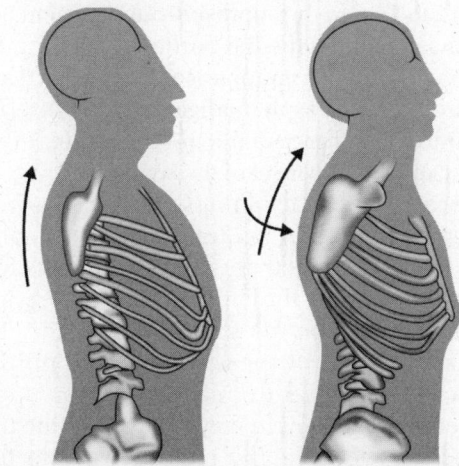

Fig. 31.1: Neutral and forward tipped scapula.

- Levator scapula (superior medial border of scapula to transverse processes of C1-C4 vertebrae)

Scapula forward tipping (with its concurrent downward rotation, protraction and winging) can cause hyperactivity of the trapezius and levator scapula owing the change in length tension causing a drag on the cervical vertebrae and occipital region. The constant stress of these muscles combined with wear and tear from activity can result in cervical spondylosis, facet joint degeneration leading to foraminal narrowing and nerve root irritation/cervical radiculopathy. A larger emphasis on the upper cervical attachments can contribute to cervicogenic headaches. Additionally, in combination with other relevant factors, it can contribute to occipital headaches. As the pectoralis minor remains tight, repetitive overhead activity can entrap the lower trunk of the brachial plexus causing thoracic outlet syndrome.

Relevance to Thoracic Dysfunction

The direct attachments of the scapula to the thoracic spine are via the following structures:
- *Trapezius:* The middle fibers attach to C7, T1, T2, T3. The lower fibers attach to T4–T12. They collectively insert over the superior aspect of the spine of scapula.
- *Rhomboids:* The rhomboid major arises from T2 to T5 and the supraspinous ligament and inserts on the medial border of the scapula. The rhomboid minor arises from C7, T1, and from the supraspinous ligament. It is inserted into a small area of the medial border of the scapula at the level of the scapular spine.

Scapula forward tipping (with its concurrent downward rotation, protraction and winging) can cause hyperactivity of the trapezius and rhomboids owing the change in length tension, causing a drag on the thoracic vertebrae. The constant stress of these muscles combined with wear and tear from activity of the upper extremity can result in mechanical dysfunction of the thoracic region. The prolonged contraction of these hyperactive muscles can result in persistent actin and myosin cross-bridging of the rhomboids, trapezius and serratus anterior, resulting in mid-thoracic, interscapular and rib pain.

Point to Note

The reverse is also true as in treatment of a forward head, cervical dysfunction and thoracic dysfunction is also needed to manage scapula and shoulder dysfunction.

Examination of Presence

Scapula backward tipping test (SBTT): The procedure consists of having the individual lay on the stomach in a neutral head position with palms in the anatomical position. The clinician places one hand on the inferior angle of the scapula and the fingers of the other hand hooked the under surface of the coracoid process. With a firm inferiorly directed stabilizing force on the inferior angle of the scapula, a gentle pull is imparted in an upward direction (Fig. 31.2) to sense tightness and to observe movement of the acromion up to the tragus of the ear. Care must be taken to not hook the fingers under the clavicle as this would place a stretch on the acromioclavicular joint and not the pectoralis minor. The author is credited to have first described this test.[3]

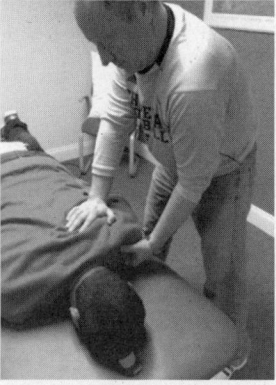

Fig. 31.2: Hand positioning for SBTT.
[Scapula backward tipping test (SBTT)]

Management of Excessive Scapula Forward Tipping

The primary intervention in managing an excessive forward tipping of the scapula is to stretch the pectoralis minor and teres major. The procedure to stretch the pectoralis minor is like performing the SBTT. It consists of having the individual lay on the stomach in a neutral head position with palms in the anatomical position. The clinician places one hand on the inferior angle of the scapula and the fingers of the other hand hooked the under surface of the coracoid process. With a firm inferiorly directed stabilizing force on the inferior angle of the scapula, a gentle pull is imparted in an upward direction (Fig. 31.2) to stretch the pectoralis minor. Care must be taken to not hook the fingers under the clavicle as this would place a stretch on the acromioclavicular joint and not the pectoralis minor.

The teres major is stretched using the following method. The patient is lying prone. The thumbs of the clinician stabilize the spine of the scapula and hook on to the superior medial border of the scapula. The other fingers of both hands are taken over the scapula and hooked on the lateral border of the scapula. The clinician then imparts an upward and inward stretch over the lateral border of the scapula (Fig. 31.3).

Strengthening the Serratus Anterior and Lower Trapezius

The patient is either standing or supine lying. The arms are in the 90° shoulder flexion position with the elbows fully extended. A resistance band is used as shown in the figure and is wrapped around the scapular area and held by the hands. In the lying position, a pair of dumbbells are used. In this position, the patient protracts both scapula as if to reach forward in standing, or reach for the ceiling in supine lying. The protraction is kept to a minimum the elbow, as a mandate, does not flex throughout the procedure (Fig. 31.4).

A safe and nonimpingement position to strengthen the lower fibers of the trapezius is achieved in standing with a resistance band. The band is pulled to achieve adequate tension but the elbow does not move past the trunk. At any point, the elbow is not pulled past the trunk and is maintained static. Now with the resistance maintained, the scapula is drawn back and down (Figs. 31.5 and 31.6).

GLENOHUMERAL CAPSULE TIGHTNESS

The joint capsule is the enclosing structure of an articular joint and is a highly sensitive structure.

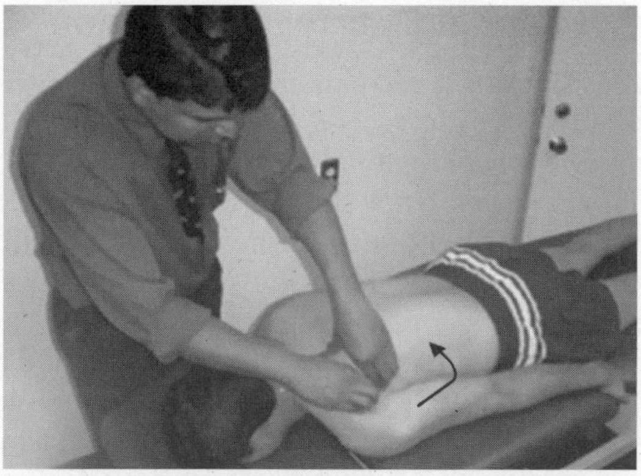

Fig. 31.3: Manual technique to stretch the teres major.

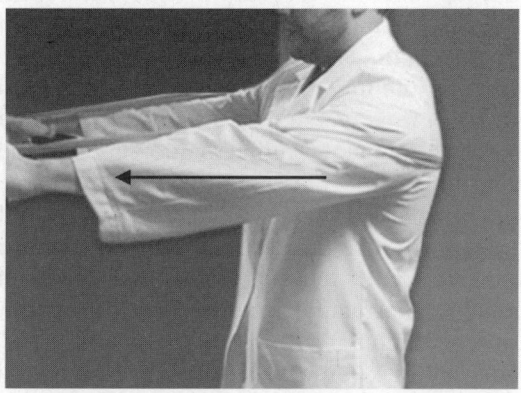

Fig. 31.4: Serratus anterior strengthening.

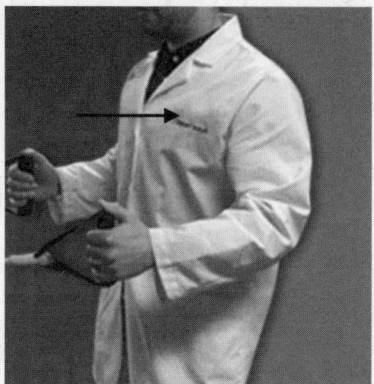

Fig. 31.5: Lower trapezius strengthening.

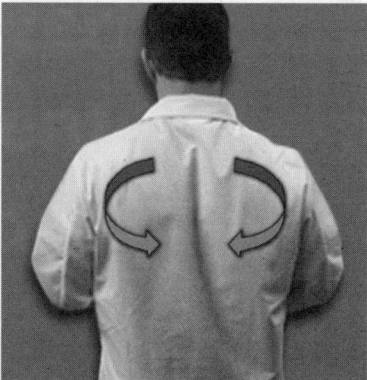

Fig. 31.6: Direction of scapula in lower trapezius strengthening.

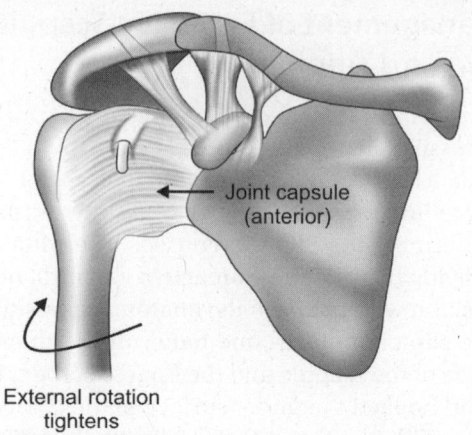

Fig. 31.7: Depiction of glenohumeral capsule and humeral rotation.

It offers a sense of direction and proprioception. Musculoskeletal clinicians understand clearly that tightness or restricted mobility in a joint is primarily caused by tightness of the joint capsule. In the anatomical resting position, the joint capsule in the glenohumeral articulation runs in a transverse direction. As the image indicates, humeral external rotation tightens the anterior capsule, hence if the anterior capsule is contracted secondary to adhesions, external rotation may be limited (Fig. 31.7). A similar situation applies to the posterior capsule which limits internal rotation when tight and the inferior capsule which limits elevation when tight.

It is obvious in conditions like adhesive capsulitis/frozen shoulder, where limited and painful mobility are the result of an inflamed and tight capsule. While this should be considered, the clinician should be aware of the naturally occurring capsular tightness secondary to faulty postures, inactivity or faulty and repetitive activity. Sometimes the posterior capsule can be of greater concern creating an internal rotation deficit. This condition is called glenohumeral internal rotation deficit (GIRD).

In any case while the clinician is examining the shoulder, mid or end range restrictions of joint mobility are routinely assessed as a restriction in glenohumeral mobility challenge the entire upper quarter.

Clinical Relevance of Excessive Glenohumeral Capsule Tightness to most Upper Quarter Dysfunction

The clinician is recommended to examine the shoulder for mid or end range restrictions as a routine for all regional pain conditions of the upper quarter. When the glenohumeral capsule is rendered tight even in the terminal or end ranges, it vastly affects the scapulo-humeral rhythm. This in turn affects the mobility of the scapula and in many instances creating a hypermobility of the scapula. A hypermobile scapula has a directional preference of protraction, forward tipping, downward rotation and winging. The consequences of this to neck, shoulder and thoracic dysfunction have been already explained. Hence, investigating and addressing

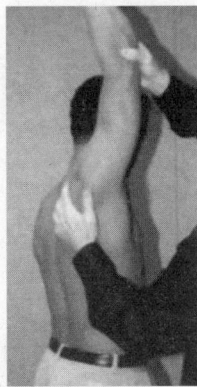

Fig. 31.8: Testing shoulder elevation.

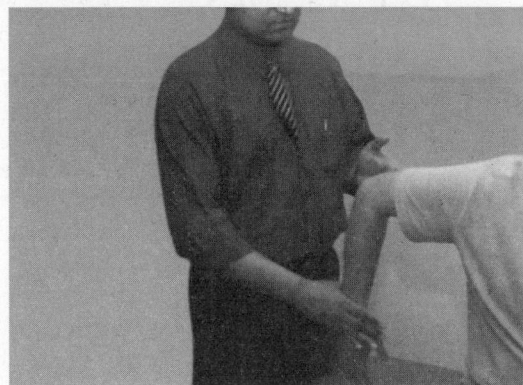

Fig. 31.10: Testing shoulder internal rotation arm by the side.

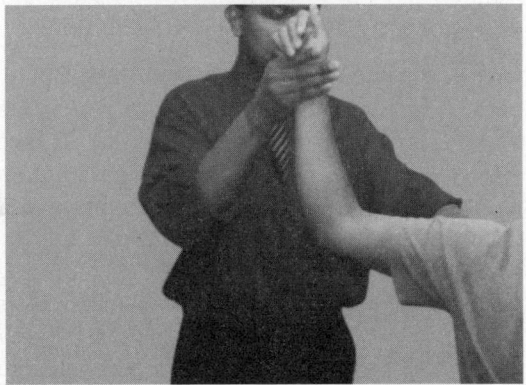

Fig. 31.9: Testing shoulder external rotation.

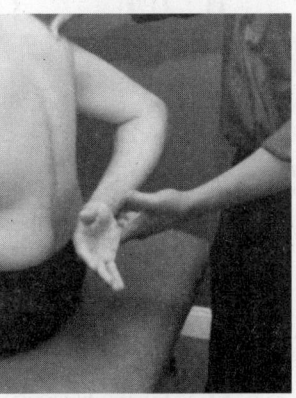

Fig. 31.11: Testing shoulder internal rotation arm behind the back.

glenohumeral capsule tightness is imperative for all upper quarter musculoskeletal dysfunction.[5,6]

When the capsule is overstretched secondary to overuse it is called hypermobility. Glenohumeral hypermobility is yet another cause for concern. While it causes shoulder dysfunction including secondary impingement, it can still affect scapula mechanics as described earlier. Hence, addressing glenohumeral micro-instability with the appropriate strengthening measures are highly recommended.

Examination of Presence of Excessive Glenohumeral Capsule Tightness

The examination to identify glenohumeral capsular tightness simply entails testing range of motion in the shoulder. Since frontal plane abduction is not functional, scaption and overhead elevation is assessed for available range (Fig. 31.8). Restricted mobility may suggest tightness of the inferior capsule.

External rotation is ideally assessed in slight or 90° of abduction to relieve tension off the coracohumeral ligament. Caution needs to be exercised in the presence of shoulder instability. Restricted mobility in external rotation may suggest tightness of the anterior capsule (Fig. 31.9).

Internal rotation may be assessed with the arm in abduction, however, full range internal rotation is assessed by visualizing the ability to reach behind the back (Figs. 31.10 and 31.11).

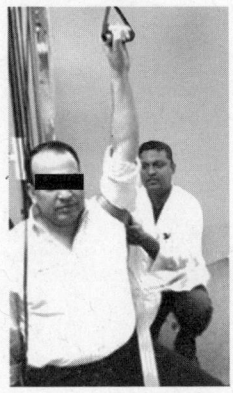

Fig. 31.12: End range flexion with inferior glide maintained with a mobilization strap and patient sustaining an end range stretch in elevation by using an overhead pulley.

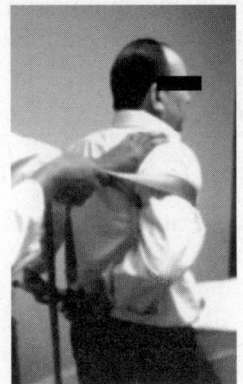

Fig. 31.14: End range internal rotation with posterior glide maintained manually by the clinician using a mobilization strap and patient sustaining an end range stretch in internal rotation using a cane.

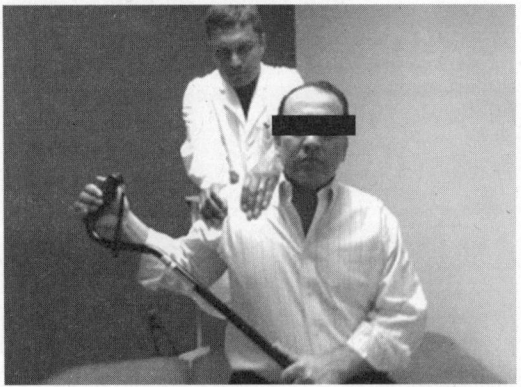

Fig. 31.13: End range external rotation with anterior glide maintained manually by clinician and patient sustaining an end range stretch in external rotation using a cane.

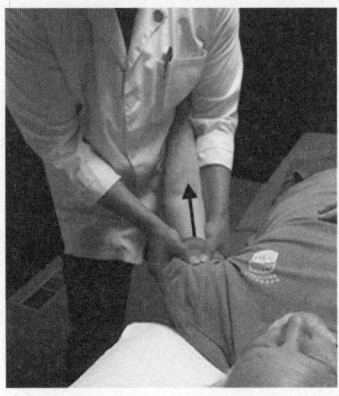

Fig. 31.15: Glenohumeral capsule long axis distraction.

Management of Excessive Glenohumeral Capsule Tightness

While joint mobilization is one of the most commonly used interventional procedures in a physical therapy practice, the most appropriate and effective method of delivery for the most optimal outcome has been routinely researched.[7] Currently, a stretch applied to the capsule utilizing a low load but extended over a period of time is considered most effective. More recent research has shown with the generalizability most appropriate for the glenohumeral capsule that end range glides combined with repetitive or a stretch of the desired motion was effective in improving joint range of motion in the shoulder joint[7] (Figs. 31.12 to 31.14).

Glenohumeral capsule long axis distraction is achieved with the patient in supine lying and the clinician facing the patient by the side. The clinician grips the upper end of the humerus with the thumbs over the anterior humeral head and fingers over posterior. A gentle yet firm distraction force is applied in the inferior direction (Fig. 31.15). (*Caution:* Do not attempt the above described shoulder techniques on patients with shoulder arthroplasty or recent fractures).

CRANIUM

Cranium and Cranial Sutures

Cranium or skull, although viewed as one rigid structure, like sacrum consists of the frontal, temporal, parietal and occipital surfaces. They are united by multiple synarthrosis called sutures. A synarthrosis is a type of fibrous joint which permits very little or no movement under normal conditions. Other examples include gomphosis, synostosis and synchondrosis. Sutures are bound together by Sharpey's fibers. Cranium is divided into two halves superiorly by the coronal suture. On the posteriorly placed occipital surface, the inverted v-shaped suture is called lambdoid suture. The frontal suture on the anterior aspect is perpendicular to the coronal suture. On the lateral aspect the squamous suture is in close relationship to the temporalis muscle. A tiny amount of movement is permitted in these sutures which contribute to the elasticity of the skull. The nature of whether these movements are active and palpable, or passive induced is subject to controversy [8,9]. Cranium is an ignored area as far as musculoskeletal dysfunction is concerned. Manual interventions described in this section, although not fully validated, may be of empirical value in the management of certain types of extracranial pain (headache) (Fig. 31.16).

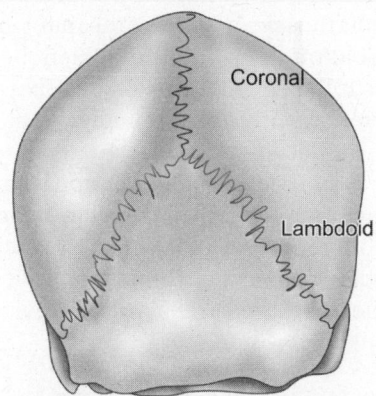

Fig. 31.16: Cranium and sutures.

Galea Aponeurotica (Epicranial Aponeurosis)

The galea aponeurotica or epicranial aponeurosis, is an intermediate tendon connecting the frontalis and occipitalis muscles. They collectively form the epicranius and resemble a close, tight-fitting, skull cap (Fig. 31.17).

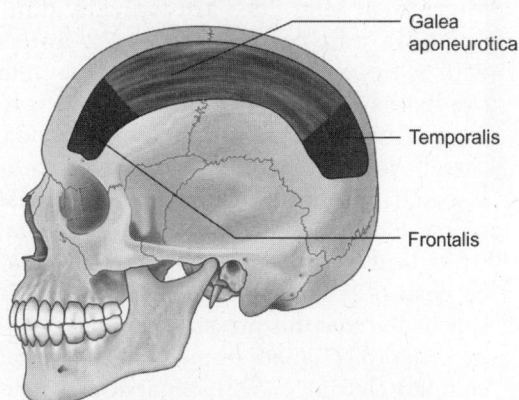

Fig. 31.17: Galea aponeurotica.

Mechanism of Pain and Dysfunction

The correlative anatomy described above support the hypothesis that the epicranial aponeurosis can cause an intrinsic tension tightness over the head and influence a compressive effect on the frontal, sagittal and lambdoid sutures. The cohort to this phenomenon is the more laterally placed

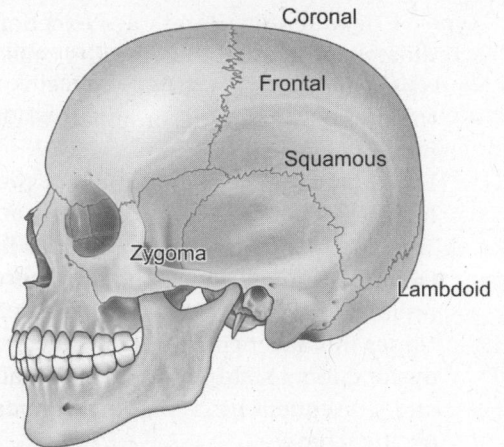

temporalis muscle. It is one of the main muscles of mastication and in habitual clenchers can cause a similar effect on the lateral aspect of the skull, temporal area. Additionally, it can cause the same impaction effect on the laterally placed squamous suture. This phenomenon is called an implosive compression or tension headaches and is different from that which occurs in the suboccipital region contributing to cervicogenic headaches. However, a tension and cervicogenic can occur side by side.

Examination of Presence

The (International Headache Society) IHS describes more than 300 type of headaches and are broadly classified as primary and secondary. The ones relevant to the musculoskeletal practitioner are listed below which are as follows [10]:

A. Primary Headaches

Primary headaches include migraines and tension-type.

- **Migraines:** Migraines are typically non-episodic and can last for 4-72 hours with 1-4 episodes a month and a female predisposition. They can have multiple triggers including bright lights, loud sounds, certain foods, smells and stress. Current research is beginning to point to intracranial pressure due to variations in cerebrospinal fluid and influence of the trigeminal cervical reflex in the cervical region. It is speculated that this pressure can be caused by structural changes in the cranio-cervical complex causing cerebrospinal flow related abnormalities. Manual therapy for this type of headache focuses on releasing impactions in the upper and mid-cervical spinal facets associated with myofascia and cranial sutures. Thus, freeing the patient from the internal and external pressure changes that causes migraines. Additionally, this can also help to re-establish the integrity of the trigeminal cervical reflex and the research supports this mechanism to be a reason for relief of migraine symptoms following manual intervention.

- **Tension-type headaches:** Tension headaches are the most common and is caused by tension in muscles found around the neck, head and face. The pain can be diffuse and bilateral and up to 30 episodes a month occurring equally in both males and females. They can be infrequent, frequent or chronic. The compressive phenomenon described in the section describing the galea aponeurotica clearly attests to this type of headache. While the research shows that manual therapy interventions to the sub-occipital and mid-cervical region are extremely effective, adding procedures to release impactions in the galea and cranial sutures have been found to have anecdotal clinical value, although lack validation. It is also important to note that migraine and tension type headaches can overlap presenting a mixed picture.

B. Secondary Headaches

Secondary headaches relevant to the musculoskeletal practitioner include cervicogenic, (temporomandibular joint) TMJ and vestibular related headaches.

- **Cervicogenic headaches:** They are common and often recur. This type of headache is caused by mechanical issues found in the neck. The pain is unilateral and typically begins occipital and radiates frontoparietal and orbital occurring equally in both males and females. Much like the tension type of headaches, the research shows that these type of headache sufferers are excellent candidates for manual therapy. The causes and clinical features are as follows:
    - Unilateral "ram's horn" or unilateral dominant headache
    - Exacerbated by neck movement or posture
    - Tenderness with restricted mobility in the OA and AA joints with a positive flexion rotation test (FRT)
    - Upper thoracic tightness that can cause dysfunctional states of the semispinalis and subsequent irritation of the greater occipital nerve

- Dysfunctional states of the suboccipital muscles and semispinalis with irritation of the greater occipital nerve
- Dysfunctional states of the scapulo-humeral and glenohumeral joints can be a contributor as well
- Association with neck and upper thoracic pain or dysfunction
- An associated history of whiplash injury
- Definitive diagnosis made through selective nerve blocking through injection of specific sites
- Compared to migraine headache and control groups, cervicogenic headache group patients tend to have increased tightness and trigger points in upper trapezius, levator scapulae, scales and suboccipital extensors
- Weakness in the deep neck flexors and thoracic and scapula retractors
- Increased activity in the superficial flexors particulary sternocleidomastoid (SCM)
- Atrophy in the suboccipital extensors and so the deep muscle sleeve which is important for active support of the cervical segments becomes impaired.
- **TMJ and Vestibular headache:** TMJ headaches are similar in nature to cervicogenic headaches in that they originate in one location (jaw) and send pain to another location. Vestibular headaches occur secondary to central or peripheral vestibular disorders. The reader is suggested to review relevant literature as this elaborate topic is beyond the scope of this chapter.

Management

A detail red flag examination as outlined in the cervical chapter should precede all manual interventions for headaches, this also includes a central neurological, vestibular, and TMJ evaluation. Some specific signs that may initiate a medical referral are:
- Sudden onset of severe headache called 'thunderclap'
- Headache with activity or exertion
- Vomiting relieves headache
- Increases with lying down and disturbs sleep
- Pulsating sensation in the head like heartbeat
- Headache associated with temporal tenderness, diplopia or seizures
- Associated neurological or symptoms affecting special senses.

Manual Therapy Intervention

The validation for manual therapy intervention is adequate suggesting favorable results for cervicogenic, tension and migraine headaches[11,12]. Understanding the mechanisms associated with these 3 types of headaches as outlined above can help with an appropriate order of intervention. The clinician must also understand that manual therapy is a component of a multimodal approach including pharmacological and psychological therapies (although manual therapy can be one of the main components of the multimodal approach). The order of manual intervention may be as follows:
- Address suboccipital, cranial, mid cervical and upper thoracic dysfunction followed by the scapulohumeral and glenohumeral regions
- Address soft tissue restriction prior to joint restriction.

Soft Tissue Mobilization: Suboccipital Stretch

In the supine lying position, the clinician's fingers are hooked on the nuchal line to offer a gentle long axis distraction (Fig. 31.18).

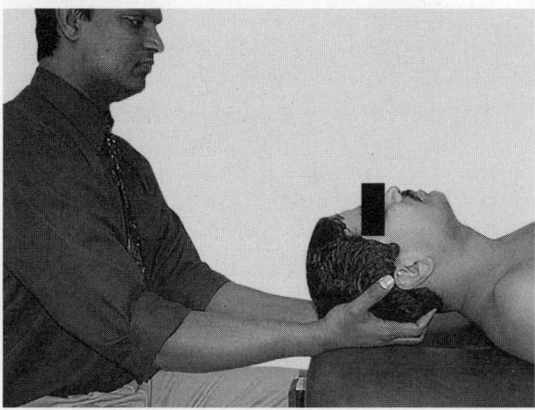

Fig. 31.18: Suboccipital stretch in supine lying position.

Splenius/Semispinalis Stretch

In the prone lying position one hand offers a counter on the external occipital protuberance and on nuchal line, while a stretch is imparted over the upper thoracic region (Fig. 31.19).

Occipitalis

In the prone lying position, the area between the external occipital protuberance and nuchal line is palpated. Using an index knobbler, or a light soft tissue mobilization tool with a rounded head, gentle kneading pressures are applied over the occipitalis (Fig. 31.20).

Frontalis

In the supine lying position, the clinician's thumbs are placed over the forehead and gentle kneading pressures are applied over the entire length of the forehead (Fig. 31.21).

Galea Aponerotica

In the supine lying position, the clinician's thumbs are placed over the vertex of the head and gentle kneading pressures are applied over the entire length of the head to mobilize the galea.

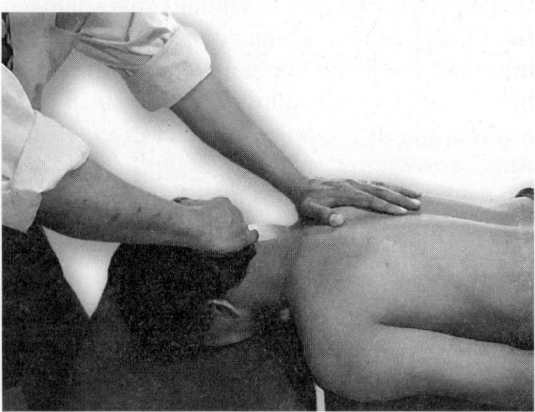

Fig. 31.19: Semispinalis Stretch.

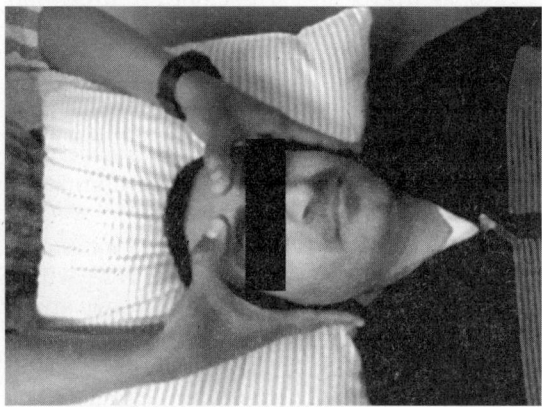

Fig. 31.21: Frontalis kneading.

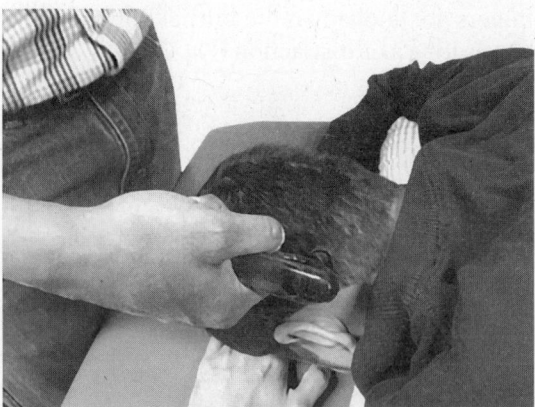

Fig. 31.20: Kneading pressure on occipitalis while using index knobbler.

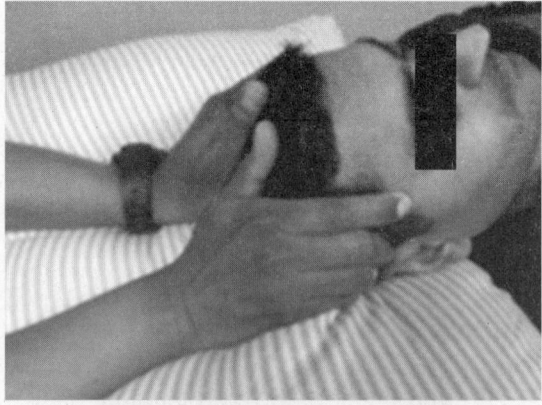

Fig. 31.22: Galea aponeurotica soft tissue mobilization.

Zygomatic Arch

In the supine lying position, the clinician's fingers are placed under the zygomatic arch and gentle kneading pressures are applied over the entire length to knead the masseter and pterygoid followed by a gentle upwardly directed distractive pressure (Fig. 31.23).

Articular/Joint Mobilization

Articular mobilization begins with addressing the OA/AA/C2/C3/Thoracic/scapula. Please refer to the cervical, thoracic and shoulder section for a detail description of techniques. Upon completion of manual work around the suboccipital region the following order of intervention may be incorporated in the extracranial region.

Squamous Suture Stretch

In the supine lying position, the clinician's fingers are placed under the squamous suture just over the ear where a dip is felt. The other side of the head is supported by the other hand and the fingers on the right side impart a gentle upwardly directed distractive pressure (Fig. 31.24).

Zygoma Depression and Frontal Suture Stretch

In the supine lying position, the clinician's fingers are placed over the zygoma. The other hand is placed over the frontal bone and imparts a gentle upwardly directed distractive pressure while a downward pressure is applied over the zygoma (Fig. 31.25).

Orbit Distraction

In the supine lying position, the clinician's fingers are placed over the superior orbit. To impart a gentle upwardly directed distractive pressure (Fig. 31.26).

Coronal Suture Stretch

In the prone lying position, the clinician's thumbs are placed centrally on the vertex of

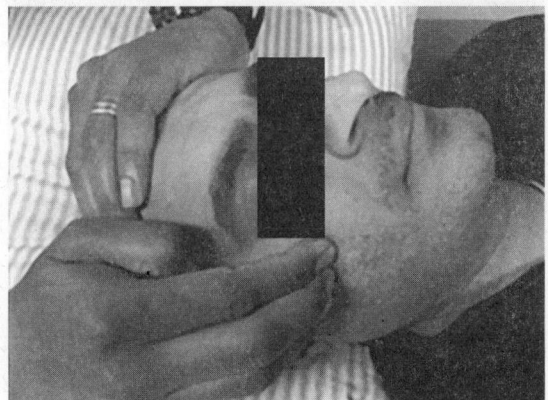

Fig. 31.23: Zygomatic arch soft tissue kneading.

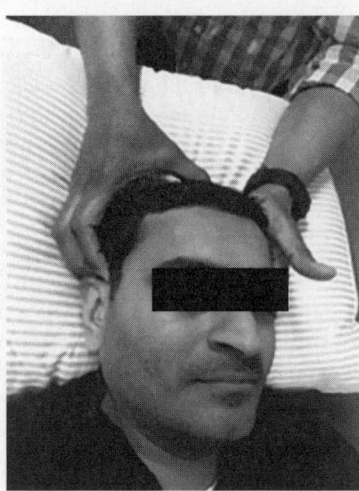

Fig. 31.24: Squamous suture stretch.

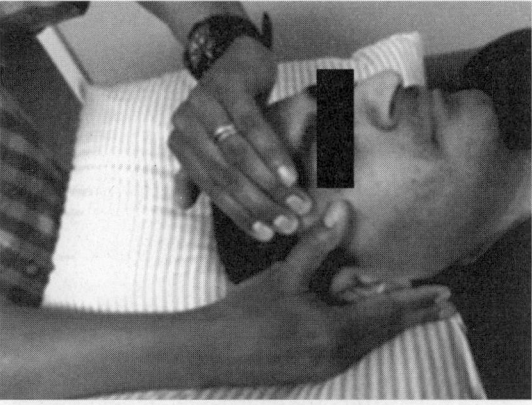

Fig. 31.25: Zygoma depression and frontal suture stretch

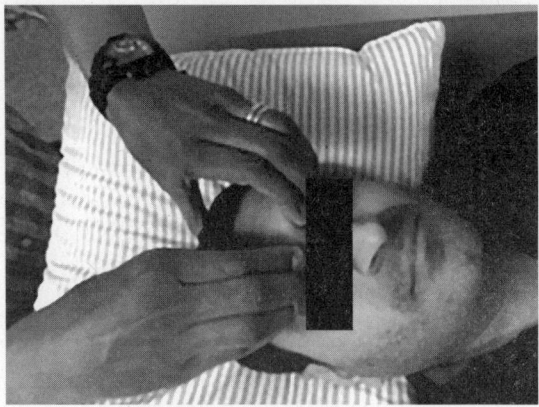

Fig. 31.26: Orbit distraction.

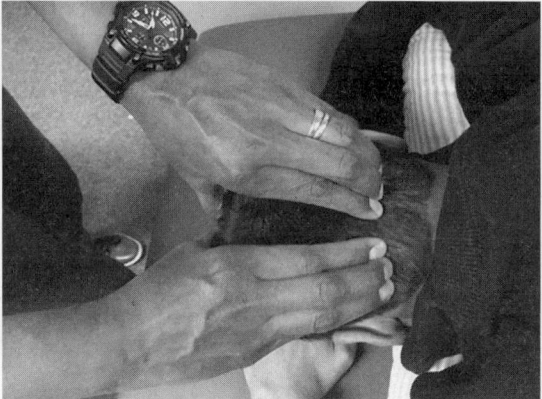

Fig. 31.28: Lambdoid suture strectch.

the head. and imparts a gentle downward and laterally directed distractive pressure (Fig. 31.27).

Lambdoid Suture Stretch

In the prone lying position, the clinician's fingers are placed about an inch over the nuchal line. and impart a gentle upwardly directed distractive pressure (Fig. 31.28).

Maxilla Distraction

In supine lying, one hand blocks the zygoma, while the other hand pinch grips the maxilla both intra-and extra-orally to impart an inferiorly directed stretch (Fig. 31.29).

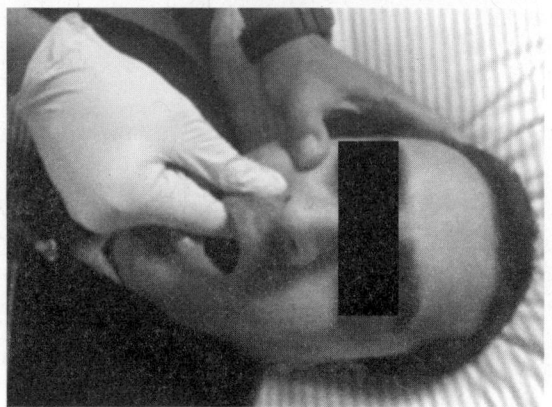

Fig. 31.29: Maxilla distraction.

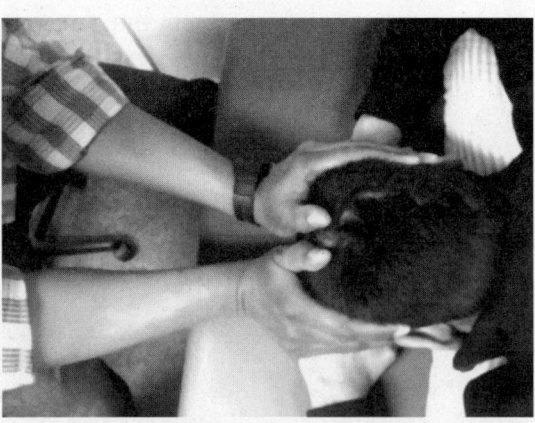

Fig. 31.27: Coronal suture stretch.

REFERENCES

1. Van Dillen LR, McDonnell MK, Susco TM, et al. The immediate effect of passive scapular elevation on symptoms with active neck rotation in patients with neck pain. Clin J Pain. 2007;23:641-7.
2. Sahrmann S. Diagnosis and treatment of movement impairment syndromes, 2001. St Louis, Mosby.
3. Sebastian D, Chovvath R, Malladi R. The scapula backward tipping test: an inter-rater reliability study. J Bodyw Mov Ther. 2017;21:69-73.
4. Kim SR, Kang MH, Bahng SY, et al. Correlation among scapular asymmetry, neck pain, and neck disability index (NDI) in young women with slight neck pain. J Phys Ther Sci. 2016;28:1508-10.

5. Pateder DB, Brems J, Lieberman I, et al. Masquerade: nonspinal musculoskeletal disorders that mimic spinal conditions. Cleve Clin J Med. 2008;75:50-6.
6. Valli J. Chiropractic management of a 46-year-old type 1 diabetic patient with upper crossed syndrome and adhesive capsulitis. J Chiropr Med. 2004;3:138-44.
7. Yang JL, Chang CW, Chen SY, et al. Mobilization techniques in subjects with frozen shoulder syndrome: randomized multiple treatment trial. Phys Ther. 2007;87:1307-15.
8. Parodi RZ et al. Cranial palpation pressures used by osteopathy students: Effects of standardized protocol training. The Journal of the American Osteopathic Association, 2009, 109, 79-85.
9. Downey PA, et al. Craniosacral therapy: the effects of cranial manipulation on intracranial pressure and cranial bone movement. J Orthop Sports Phys Ther. 2006;36:845-53.
10. Moore CS, Sibbritt DW, Adams J. A critical review of manual therapy use for headache disorders: prevalence, profiles, motivations, communication and self-reported effectiveness. BMC Neurol. 2017; 17: 61.
11. Chaibi A, Russell MB. Manual therapies for primary chronic headaches: a systematic review of randomized controlled trials. The Journal of Headache and Pain. 2014;15:67.
12. Schoensee SK, et al. The effect of mobilization on cervical headaches. J Orthop Sports Phys Ther. 1995; 21:184-96.

CHAPTER 32

The Lower Quarter

THE HIP CAPSULE AND FEMORAL ROTATION

In the anatomical resting position, the joint capsule in the coxofemoral (hip) articulation runs in an oblique direction. As the image indicates, femoral external rotation tightens the posterior capsule, hence if the posterior capsule is contracted secondary to adhesions or prolonged sitting postures with hip external rotation, internal rotation may be limited (Fig. 32.1). A similar situation applies to the anterior capsule which limits external rotation when tight (Fig. 32.2).

Owing to the nature of our lifestyles, we spend a major part of our day in a sitting position. When we visualize the typical sitting posture of a male, it is in a position of hip flexion, abduction and external rotation.

The female on the other hand predominates a flexion, adduction and internal rotation posture. Empirically, on examination, the male hence tends to shorten and tighten the posterior capsule. The female on the other hand tends to shorten and tighten the anterior capsule. Variations to the above hypothesis are bound to exist.

Rarely, on examination, internal rotation may be in excess with a typical external rotation tightness. This is seen in femoral neck anteversion and called a coxafemoral external rotation deficit (CERD).

In any case while the clinician is examining the hip, mid or end range restrictions of joint mobility are routinely assessed as a restriction in hip mobility challenge the entire lower quarter including lumbopelvic region.

Clinical Relevance of Excessive Coxofemoral (Hip) Capsule Tightness to Most Lower Quarter Dysfunction

The term 'hip at risk' can be used when the following are seen:
- Iliopsoas tightness

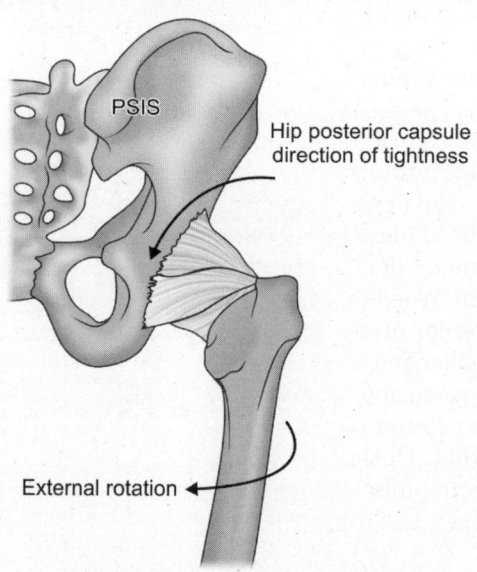

Fig. 32.1: Hip joint posterior view. (PSIS: posterior superior iliac spine)

The Lower Quarter

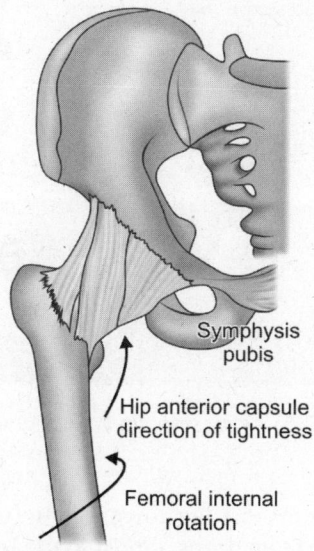

Fig. 32.2: Hip joint anterior view.

- Posterior capsule tightness causing restricted internal rotation
- Anterior capsule tightness causing restricted external rotation
- Gluteus maximus and medius weakness.

Of the above, the most common presentation is iliopsoas tightness with posterior capsule tightness causing restricted or lack of internal rotation, as posterior capsule tightness drags the femur into external rotation. Manual therapy intervention to address the above patho-mechanical presentation is imperative as its persistence can contribute to most lumbar, sacral, hip and knee dysfunction.[1,2-4]

Hip flexor tightness, as mentioned is a problem of lifestyle, as most spend a considerable amount of time during the day in a seated position. When the femur is dragged and fixated in a position of relative flexion, the gluteus maximus is challenged as it lacks the excursion of full range of extension. In a standing posture, this creates an anterior pelvic tilt with an excessive lordosis which closes the facets causing a foraminal compromise. This on persistence may lead to facet degeneration, lumbar radiculopathy, foraminal stenosis, stress on the par interarticularis and potential spondylolysis and listhesis. The progressive weakness of the gluteus maximus compromises the stability of the sacroiliac joint. The gluteus medius works optimally when abduction is done in a slightly extended position. Since extension is diminished the external rotators of the hip (primarily piriformis) and tensor fascia lata (TFL) compensate to perform the abduction moment required during stance. This causes TFL strain, buttock pain and potentially piriformis syndrome.

In the presence of concurrent posterior capsule tightness causing restricted internal rotation, the femoral head is in a position of relative external rotation in the acetabulum. When there are demands for internal rotation during the stance phase of gait, there is potential for the femoral head to be impinged over the acetabular rim, and when prolonged for a period, predisposes to osteoarthritis. The iliopsoas and trochanteric bursa (owing to the prominent greater trochanter combined with gluteal weakness) has the potential for being irritated causing bursitis and Iliotibial band friction and tension. Additionally, the tight capsule demands greater mobility of the ilia and sacrum, stressing the lumbar spine and sacroiliac joints. The cycle hence, vicious.

The femoral flexion and external rotation can result in involving the next joint in the lower extremity chain, knee. The resulting compensation being a relative internal rotation of the tibia. This can cause a relative knee flexion and a persistent lack of terminal knee extension. The consequence of this scenario is described in the next section.

In conclusion, the above description calls for functional mobility of the hip capsule, adequate length of the iliopsoas and functional strength of the gluteus maximus and medius for nearly 'all' mechanical pain syndromes of the lumbopelvichip-knee region.

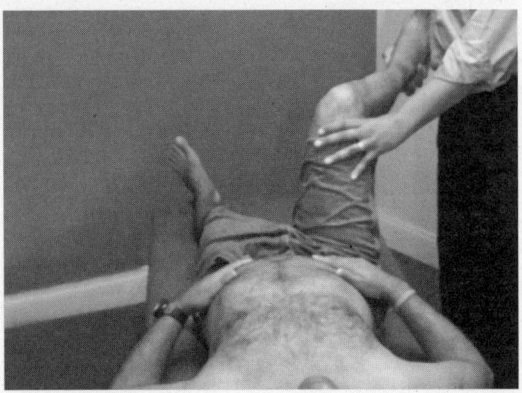

Fig. 32.3: Testing hip internal rotation (*Caution:* Do not attempt this maneuver on a hip replacement patient).

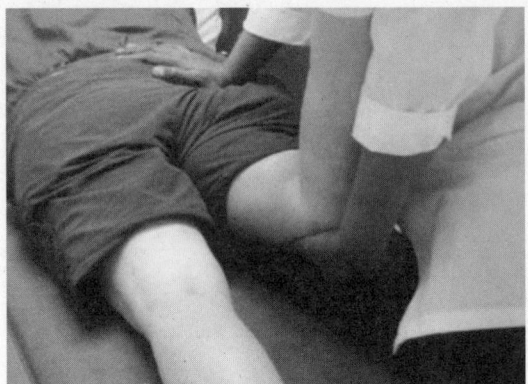

Fig. 32.5: Assessing hip flexor tightness.

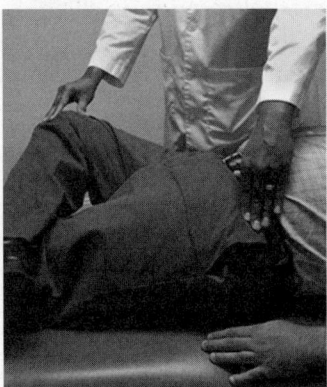

Fig. 32.4: Testing hip external rotation.

Examination of Presence of Excessive Coxofemoral (Hip) Capsule Tightness

Presence of Hip Capsular Pattern

The patient is lying supine and the examiner supports the ankle and knee of the patient. The ankle is moved outward maintaining 90° of flexion to test the internal rotation (Fig. 32.3).

To test the anterior capsule, the patient is lying supine. The patient's tested leg is placed in a "figure-4" position (Fig. 32.4) where the knee is flexed and ankle is placed on the opposite knee. The hip is placed in flexion, abduction, and external rotation (which is where the name FABER comes from). The examiner applies a posteriorly directed force against the medial knee of the bent leg towards the table top. Ideally the knee drops almost to the level of the ankle indicating an anterior capsule tightness, otherwise.

Prone Hip Flexor Tightness and Diminished Hip Extension

Patient is lying prone and the examiner holds the pelvis down to block lumbar extension. The knee is flexed and the other hand of the examiner supports the anterior aspect of the knee. The clinician then raises the knee off the table to assess range in hip extension and consequently the presence of hip flexor tightness (Fig. 32.5). The hip is blocked throughout the process to discourage lumbar extension which can mimic hip extension.

Assessing Gluteus Medius Strength

With patient in side lying, the leg is positioned in line with the trunk and not in slight flexion. The hip is rotated internally and resistance to abduction is applied (Fig. 32.6). Inability to maintain resistance indicates weakness.

Assessing Gluteus Maximus Strength

Patient is lying prone and the examiner holds the pelvis down to block lumbar extension. The knee is flexed to minimize hamstring activity and the patient is asked to raise the knee off the table (Fig. 32.7).

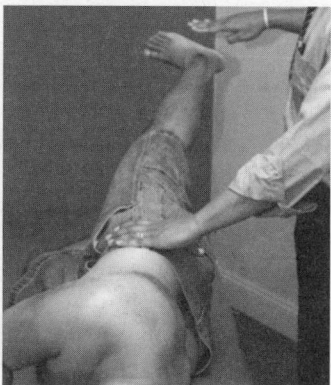

Fig. 32.6: Assessing gluteus medius strength.

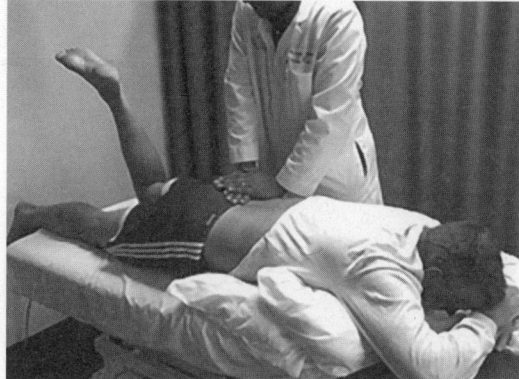

Fig. 32.7: Assessing gluteus maximus strength.

Management of Excessive Coxofemoral Capsule Tightness

The patient is lying prone with the knee flexed to 90° and a mobilization strap is used to maintain a lateral distraction at the hip. While distraction is maintained the ankle is moved outwards so as to stretch the posterior capsule into internal rotation (Figs. 32.8 and 32.9). (*Caution:* Do not attempt this maneuver on patient that has had a hip replacement or recent fracture).

The patient is lying supine with the knee flexed to 90° and ankle placed over the other knee, a mobilization strap is used to maintain a lateral distraction at the hip. While distraction is maintained the knee is moved outwards to stretch the anterior capsule into external rotation. Vice versa, the knee is moved inward to stretch the posterior capsule into internal rotation (Fig. 32.10). (*Caution:* Do not attempt this maneuver on patient that has had a hip replacement or recent fracture).

Stretching Iliopsoas

A localized stretch can be achieved by using the same maneuver as in testing. Patient is lying prone and the examiner holds the pelvis down at the level of the ischial tuberosity to block lumbar extension. Ideally it is held down by the clinicians' forearm. The knee is flexed and the other hand of the examiner supports the anterior

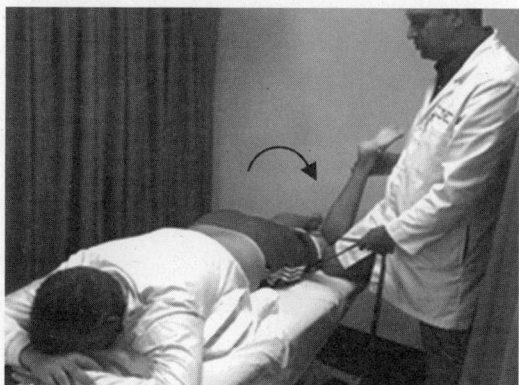

Fig. 32.8: Distraction mobilization technique for hip posterior capsule.

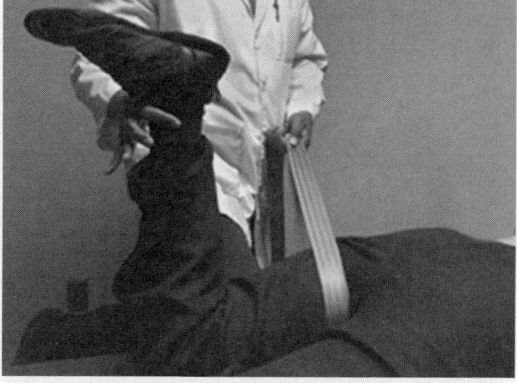

Fig. 32.9: Distraction mobilization technique for hip posterior capsule.

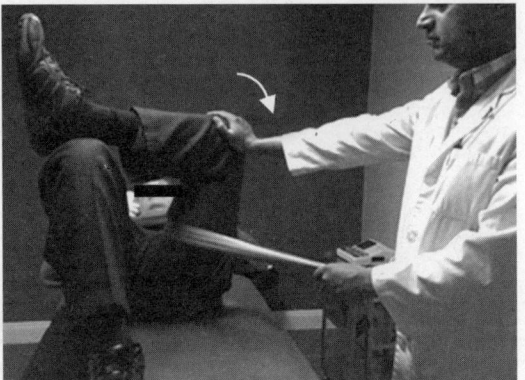

Fig. 32.10: Distraction mobilization technique for hip anterior capsule.

aspect of the knee. The clinician then raises the knee off the table into hip extension and sustains a stretch on the hip flexors. If the knee is fully flexed the rectus femoris may be engaged more effectively. The hip is blocked throughout the process to discourage lumbar extension which can mimic hip extension.

Strengthening Glutei

Gluteal strengthening is an elaborate topic and literature suggests several methods of engaging the glutei depending on the lesion diagnosis. The reader is suggested to review appropriate literature to employ best methods to strengthen the glutei.[9,10]

TIBIAL ROTATION/EXTENSION LAG AND SUPERIOR TIBIOFIBULAR JOINT

The knee is yet another joint to be considered in dysfunctions of the lower extremity chain. While trauma, flexion range of motion and instability are huge considerations in the knee, the 'neglected component' affects the lower extremity chain is lack of terminal knee extension and concurrent tibial internal rotation.

Lack of terminal extension and its consequences in the knee have been previously described. The terms flexion deformity or flexion contracture have been used and their occurrence has been mostly associated with postoperative knee surgery and osteoarthritis. Additional causes described are arthrogenic muscle inhibition (AMI) secondary to trauma to the knee, gastrocnemius, popliteus, hamstring tightness, and injury to the knee extensor mechanism. Terminal extension in the knee is a prerequisite for adequate stability and load distribution during the stance phase of gait and weight-bearing function. The lack of full extension at the knee results in a greater force of quadriceps activation and energy expenditure. It also results in slower walking velocity and abnormal gait mechanics, overloading the ipsilateral and contralateral joints resulting in pain and dysfunction. Residual knee flexion contractures have been associated with poorer functional scores and outcomes.

While some flexion contractures are obvious others can be subtle and missed. Additionally, it may not be a contracture but a diminished efficiency of the knee extensor mechanism. They may still result in a lack or lag of terminal knee extension with instability and consequences therein. This simply means that a lack in terminal knee extension may be an active or a passive restraint problem. It is active when the quadriceps extensor mechanism is deficient and passive when the posterior capsule of the knee is tight.

The posterior capsule of the knee is well depicted as a thick band like structure. Contractures of the posterior capsule which extends from the posterior femoral cortex to the posterior aspect of the tibia 1–2 cm below the level of the joint line may contribute to a passive knee extension lag. The intimate attachment of the semimembranosus, medial gastrocnemius head and popliteus may favor knee flexion and potentially contribute to a knee extension lag as these muscles flex the knee and internally rotate the tibia.

Knee flexion is brought about by the action of several muscles including hamstrings, gastrocnemius, sartorius, gracilis. While internal rotation of the tibia is considered a cohort of dynamic knee flexion popliteus muscle may also be inclusive. We can hence suggest that when the knee flexors lack full length a passive extension lag can result. Additionally, tightness in the hip flexors may also contribute to knee flexion during weight-bearing. Tight hip flexors contribute to an anterior pelvic tilt and a persistent hip flexion contracture is described to cause altered loading of the knee.[7]

Clinical Relevance of Terminal Knee Extension Lag to Most Lower Quarter Dysfunction

Tibial internal rotation associated with knee flexion and tibial external rotation with knee extension has been described. Persistent tibial internal rotation causes a myriad of dysfunctions in the knee. The medial condyle of the femur is larger than the lateral condyle. It rolls only for the first 10–15° of flexion, while the lateral condyle continues until 20° of flexion. This is the most stable range of the knee as the part of the femoral condyles involved in the articulation which is large. As the knee continues to flex beyond 20° this contact area decreases. This tends to result in the ligaments being more lax and subsequently favoring tibial internal rotation.

Besides the femur, this tibial rotation is greatly determined by the position of the foot on the ground and hip capsule flexibility. Pronation favors tibial internal rotation and supination, the opposite. Additionally, a tight hip posterior capsule rotates the femur externally, favoring tibial internal rotation. In conclusion, a persistent knee terminal extension lag, tight posterior hip capsule or abnormal pronation of the foot favor tibial internal rotation. Listed are some examples of the aftermath of prolonged internal tibial rotation:

Patellar Compression

Internal rotation of the tibia causes the lateral portion of the femoral trochlear groove to move anteromedially against the lateral patellar facet during weight-bearing. Chronic irritation of the lateral patellar facet can result in lateral patellar compression syndrome.

Patellar Tracking

As the foot pronates abnormally beyond 4 to 6° and beyond 25% of the stance phase, the tibia is carried into excessive and prolonged internal rotation. This causes the femur to migrate into external rotation. The result is an increase in the Q-angle which is the quadriceps angle of pull in line with the femur superiorly relative to the pull of the patellar tendon inferiorly at the tibial tuberosity. When the Q-angle increases, there is a relative increase in the genu valgum angle and the patella is pulled laterally resulting in lateral patellar tracking and patellofemoral pain.

Pes Anserine Bursitis

This condition is seen in inferomedial knee pain where the tendinous insertion of the gracilis, sartorius and semitendinosis are padded by this bursa. Prolonged internal rotation of the tibia can cause a hyperirritability of these muscles as they rotate the tibia inwards, subsequently irritating the bursa beneath it. Tightness of the medial hamstrings can predispose to a similar condition.

Iliotibial Band Friction Syndrome

The prolonged internal rotation that occurs secondary to abnormal foot pronation causes the femur to rotate externally and applies a tensile force to the attachment site of the iliotibial band at the Gerdy's tubercle on the lateral condyle of the femur. Since the band crosses the lateral femoral condyle, the external rotation of the femur makes this bony landmark more prominent, tethering the band that crosses over it. Repetitive flexion and extension at the knee can cause the inferior portion of the band to rub on the relatively prominent lateral femoral condyle resulting in an iliotibial band friction syndrome and lateral knee pain.

Medial Ligament and Medial Meniscus Strain

The effect of prolonged pronation and tibial internal rotation creates a genu valgum and opens the medial tibiofemoral joint space. This increases the tensile loading on the medial aspect of the knee resulting in stress on the medial ligament, medial meniscus and medial capsule. This factor should also be considered when rehabilitating a medial ligament strain that has already occurred or partial tears.

Anterior Cruciate Ligament

The anterior cruciate legament (ACL) functions to resist tibial movement in the anterior direction, however it has yet another function that is not frequently described. It also functions to resist tibial internal rotation and tibial valgum. Prolonged excessive tibial internal rotation and valgus of the tibia tends to cause a cumulative stress on the ligament increasing its vulnerability to injury. This should most definitely be considered when rehabilitating a reconstructed ligament or healing partial tears of the ACL.

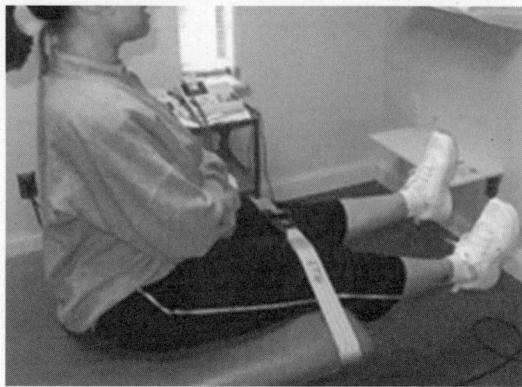

Fig. 32.11: Test position for 'active lag'.

Examination of Presence

Sitting active and prone passive lag test: An active lag is determined by the inability of the seated subject to actively extend the involved knee with the ankle in maximum dorsiflexion, to the same level as the normal knee held in a full extension position with the ankle dorsiflexed (Fig. 32.11). This is determined by the low position of the toes on the involved side (Fig. 32.12). A passive lag is determined by placing the subject prone with the knees just past the edge of the table (Fig. 32.13). With both legs fully extended and resting, the high position of the heel compared to the heel on the normal side determines the presence of a passive lag (Fig. 32.14). The differentiation between an active and a passive lag is mandatory as, when appropriately identified, the most appropriate management can be instituted. An active lag may indicate the need to address the contractile structures as in muscle strengthening, provided there are no passive restraints, while a passive lag may indicate the need to address tight restraints as in the posterior knee capsule, gastrocnemius, popliteus, hamstrings, iliopsoas and rectus femoris followed by the muscle strengthening. The author is credited to have first described this test.[7]

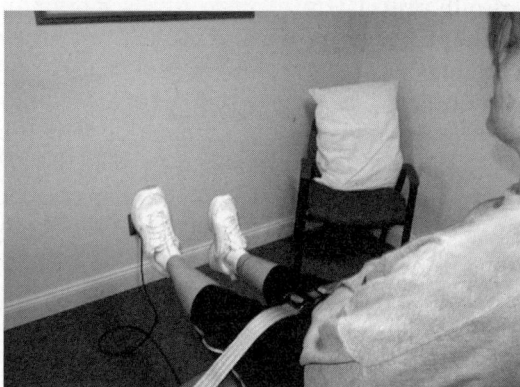

Fig. 32.12: A positive 'active lag' on the right.

SUPERIOR TIBIOFIBULAR JOINT AND TIBIAL ROTATION

The superior tibiofibular joint has received little or no attention while addressing pathology of knee and ankle. Tibial rotation, however, has received a wider importance in addressing knee and ankle dysfunction. While this is a

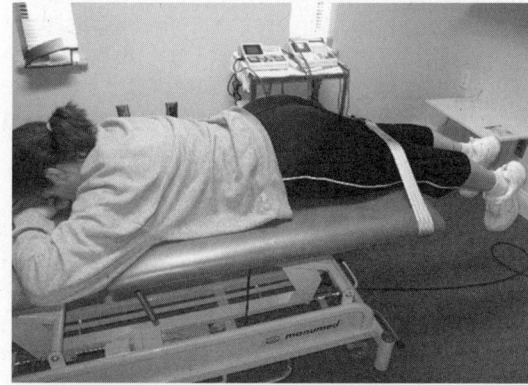

Fig. 32.13: Test position for 'passive lag'.

The Lower Quarter

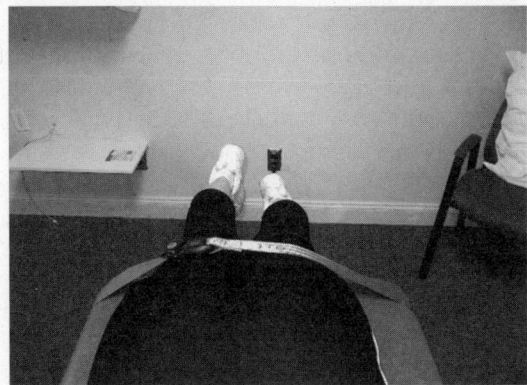

Fig. 32.14: A positive 'passive lag' on the right.

Clinical Relevance of Superior Tibiofibular Joint to Most Lower Quarter Dysfunction

Anterior and posterior translation of the fibular head relative to the tibia was consistently seen when external and internal rotation moments were applied to the tibia (Fig. 32.15). This can be explained from the functional anatomy of the joint. FCL transmits force to the head of the fibula. In external tibia rotation, this tensile force vector is oriented anteriorly causing anterior motion of the head of the fibula, and vice versa for internal rotation. There is still confusion as to the exact direction of restriction of fibula head gliding during internal and external rotation of the tibia. The common agreement however, is that when stiffness of the superior tibiofibular joint prevails, the ability of the tibia to rotate internally or externally is potentially inhibited. This may adversely affect knee and ankle mechanics thereby predisposing to dysfunctions of the lower quarter.

The effect of persistent internal rotation of the tibia has been described in the previous section. It also enumerates the clinical relevance of terminal knee extension lag to most lower quarter dysfunction.

It may be of value to note that with relevance to the superior tibiofibular joint, persistent

definite precedent in normalizing knee joint mechanics, it is of importance to understand that tibial rotation may largely require the integral functioning of the superior tibiofibular joint. The superior tibiofibular joint is a synovial membrane-lined, hyaline cartilage articulation. The joint capsule is comprised of a thick anterior capsule, anterior proximal tibiofibular ligament, and a thinner posterior capsule, posterior proximal tibiofibular ligament. The joint is the site of attachment of numerous structures which help to stabilize the tibiofemoral joint. These include the fibular collateral ligament (FCL), capsular arm of the short head of the biceps femoris, fabellofibular ligament, popliteofibular ligament and popliteus muscle.[5] In addition, the biceps femoris tendon and popliteus muscle insert onto the styloid process of the proximal fibula. This location collectively is called arcuate complex.

Studies have demonstrated obvious and substantial motion in the superior tibiofibular joint during weight-bearing.[5,6] They were largest in the anterior-posterior direction with translations of 1-3 mm observed during a range of physiological loading conditions. Additionally, applied internal-external rotation moment in the tibia had a significant effect on superior tibiofibular joint translation (Fig. 32.15). Preservation of proximal tibiofibular joint function and anatomical variations which affect this function, may need to be considered for normal mechanical functioning of the knee joint.

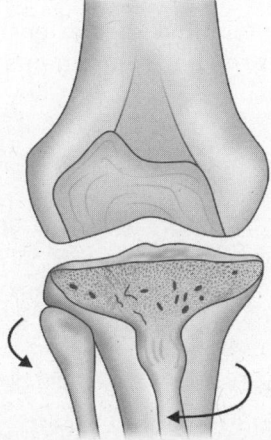

Fig. 32.15: Anterior translation of fibula with tibial external rotation.

tibial external rotation may also be a concern. Researchers[12] have quantified the force in the FCL and found it to be largest in the external rotation and varus loading suggesting that varus load should have an effect on superior tibiofibular joint motion as well (arcuate complex strain). Rearfoot supination during early to mid-stance may increase these varus stresses over the lateral aspect of the knee. When persistent this may predispose to painful lateral knee dysfunction including FCL strain, peroneus strain and peroneal nerve entrapment, stiffness of the superior tibiofibular joint and arcuate complex strain.

Examination of Presence

The patient is lying with the knees flexed to about 60 to 70°. The clinician palpates one fibular head at a time and grips it with the index, thumb and middle fingers and notes for asymmetry. A glide is applied in the anterior and posterior direction and the clinician senses for restriction and local tenderness (Fig. 32.16). Inability of the fibula head to glide anteriorly is the most common restriction seen.

Management of Knee Terminal Extension Lag and Superior Tibiofibular Dysfunction

Knee Extension Lag

To improve terminal knee extension, the soft tissue and articular components need to be addressed. The soft tissue components that require attention are the posterior capsule of the knee and the structures on the posteromedial aspect of the knee namely semimembranosus, medial gastrocnemius, popliteus and sartorius. Additionally, as tightness of the hip flexors contribute to knee flexion during weight-bearing, lengthening it may be of value.

The patient is lying prone and the medially placed tibial internal rotators are located over the posteromedial aspect of the knee. The medial hamstrings and medial gastrocnemius are posteromedial and above the knee joint line. The sartorius is central and medial and extends over the entire length of the medial aspect of the knee. The popliteus is also posteromedial but placed below the knee joint line. The clinician incorporates soft tissue mobilization as a direct technique over these structures in a horizontal direction to separate the individual fibers which run vertically (Fig. 32.17). The technique can be executed hands on or with a mobilization instrument. Techniques to stretch the hip flexors are described in the previous section.

The articular component of managing a knee extension lag involves gliding the medial condyle of the tibia anteriorly to facilitate tibial external rotation.

Tibia Anterior Glide Medial Condyle

The patient is lying prone and the knee is flexed to about 70°. The clinician faces the leg from the same side. One hand of the clinician supports

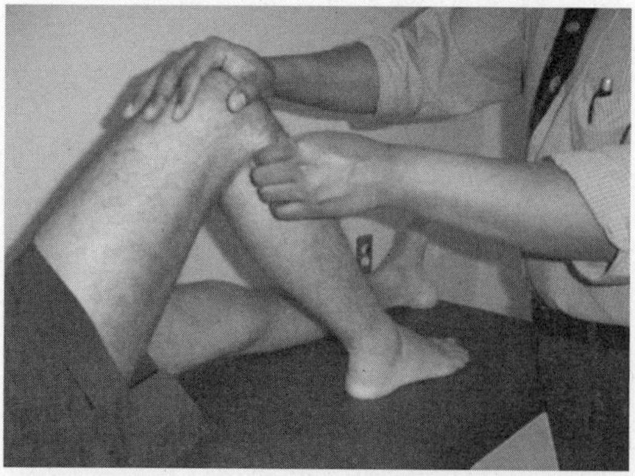

Fig. 32.16: Assessing superior tibiofibular joint mobility.

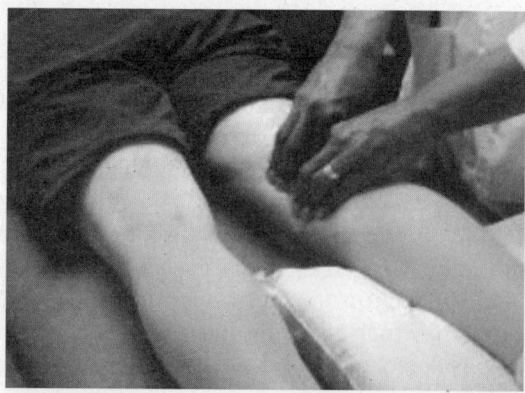

Fig. 32.17: Soft tissue mobilization to tibial internal rotators.

the ankle, while the thenar eminence of the other hand contacts the posterior aspect of the medial tibial condyle. A gentle mobilization force is imparted in an anterior direction (Fig. 32.18).

Stretching the Posterior Capsule of the Knee

Patient is lying prone with the leg past the edge of the treatment table at the level of the superior border of the patella. A heating pad may be used behind the knee to improve the viscoelasticity of the posterior capsule. Initially gravity may be used as the stretching force and based on tolerance a weight maybe added at the ankle level (Fig. 32.19). The literature suggests applying a low load over an extended period as optimal for tissue lengthening. Hence, the stretch position is maintained for a short period (5-10 minutes) based on tolerance for an optimal effect.[13] Caution is exercised while applying this technique especially following knee trauma or surgery.

Restricted Superior Tibiofibular Joint

For an anterior dysfunction, the patient is lying supine and the clinician faces the leg to be treated. The knee is flexed to about 70 to 80° and the tibia is rotated medially by placing the foot pointing inward. One hand of the clinician cups and supports the superior aspect of the knee. The base of the thumb and thenar eminence of the other hand contacts the head of the fibula. A gentle mobilizing force is imparted in a posterior direction (Fig. 32.20).

For a posterior dysfunction, the patient is lying prone and the knee is flexed to about 70°. The clinician faces the leg from the other side. One hand of the clinician supports the ankle, while the thenar eminence of the other hand contacts the posterior aspect of the fibular head. A gentle mobilization force is imparted in an anterior direction (Fig. 32.21).

Strengthening the Quadriceps

Quadriceps strengthening is an elaborate topic and literature suggests several methods of engaging the quadriceps depending on the legion diagnosis. The key however, is to emphasize the need for complete terminal extension and a hold to best address the active component of the extension lag. The reader is suggested to review appropriate literature to employ best methods to strengthen the quadriceps.[11]

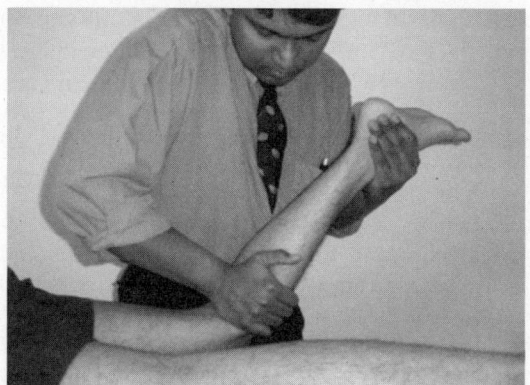

Fig. 32.18: Tibia anterior glide medial condyle.

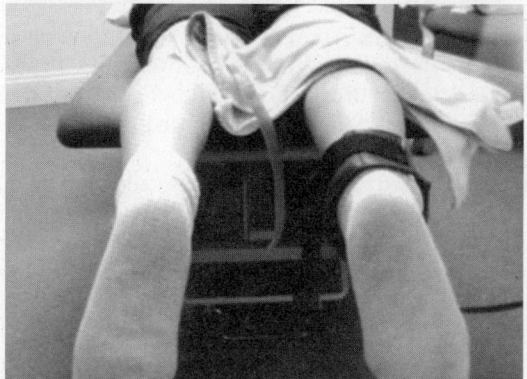

Fig. 32.19: Stretching the posterior capsule of the knee.

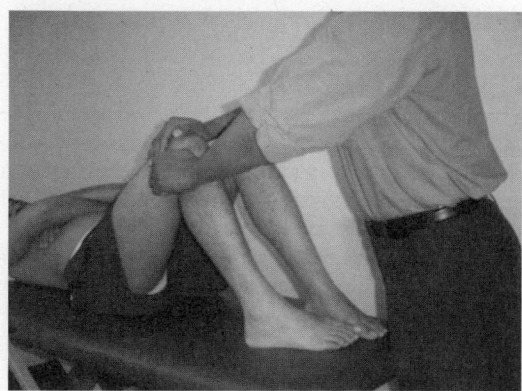

Fig. 32.20: Superior tibiofibular posterior glide.

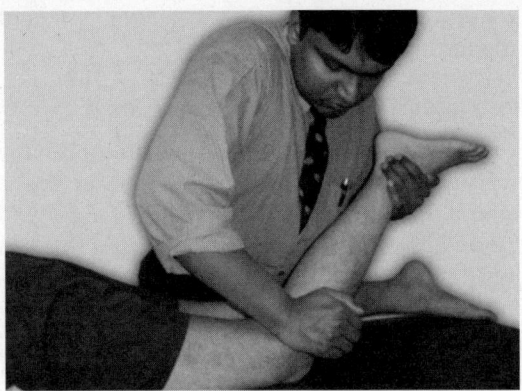

Fig. 32.21: Superior tibiofibular anterior glide.

Prior Correction of Hip Mechanics

Posterior capsule tightness at the hip favors femoral external rotation which in turn favors tibial internal rotation. Hence, addressing knee extension lag may be defeating the purpose in the presence of a persistent hip posterior capsule tightness. Addressing hip mechanics is hence recommended side by side.

Correction of Foot Mechanics

A pronated foot encourages tibial internal rotation, whereas a supinated foot favors tibial external rotation. Appropriate manual and strengthening intervention and orthotic measures are recommended to discourage prolongation of pronation and supination during the gait cycle. This may assist in minimize excessive loading in the patellofemoral,[8] tibiofemoral and superior tibiofibular joints.

REFERENCES

1. Steinberg N, Tenenbaum S, Hershkovitz I, et al. Lower extremity and spine characteristics in young dancers with and without patellofemoral pain. Res Sports Med. 2017;25:166-80.
2. McGregor AH, Hukins DW. Lower limb involvement in spinal function and low back pain. J Back Musculoskelet Rehabil. 2009;22:219-22.
3. Prather H, Cheng A, Steger-May K, et al. Hip and lumbar spine physical examination findings in people presenting with low back pain, with or without lower extremity pain. J Orthop Sports Phys Ther. 2017;47:163-72.
4. Mirzaie G, Kajbafvala M, Rahimi A, et al. Altered hip mechanics and patellofemoral pain. A review of literature. Ortop Traumatol Rehabil. 2016;18:215-21.
5. Jacob Scott, Ho Lee, Wael Barsoum, et al. The effect of tibiofemoral loading on proximal tibiofibular joint motion. J Anat. 2007;211:647-53.
6. Bellchamber TL, van den Bogert AJ. Contributions of proximal and distal moments to axial tibial rotation during walking and running. J Biomech. 2000;33:1397-403.
7. Sebastian D, Chovvath R, Malladi R. The sitting active and prone passive lag test: an inter-rater reliability study. J Bodyw Mov Ther. 2014;18:204-9.
8. Shih YF, Wen YK, Chen WY. Application of wedged foot orthosis effectively reduces pain in runners with pronated foot: a randomized clinical study. Clin Rehabil. 2011;25:913-23.
9. Stastny P, Tufano JJ, Golas A, et al. Strengthening the gluteus medius using various bodyweight and resistance exercises. Strength Cond J. 2016;38:91-101.
10. Boren K, Conrey C, Le Coguic J, et al. Electromyographic analysis of gluteus medius and gluteus maximus during rehabilitation exercises. Int J Sports Phys Ther. 2011;6:206-223.
11. Irish SE, Millward AJ, Wride J, et al. The effect of closed-kinetic chain exercises and open-kinetic chain exercise on the muscle activity of vastus medialis oblique and vastus lateralis. J Strength Cond Res. 2010;24:1256-62.
12. LaPrade RF, Tso A, Wentorf FA. Force measurements on the fibular collateral ligament, popliteofibular ligament, and popliteus tendon to applied loads. Am J Sports Med. 2004;32:1695-701.
13. Logerstedt D, Sennett BJ. Case series utilizing drop-out casting for the treatment of knee joint extension motion loss following anterior cruciate ligament reconstruction. J Orthop Sports Phys Ther. 2007;37:404-11.

Index

Page numbers followed by f refer to figure

A

Abduction 139, 152, 170, 171, 179, 180, 193
Abductor digiti minimi 228
Abductor hallucis 33, 298-300
    muscle 239, 299
Abductor pollicis
    brevis 212, 227
    longus 30, 199-201, 211, 212, 212f
Abducts carpometacarpal joint 199
Achilles tendinitis 303
Acromioclavicular inferior anterior glide 179, 180
Acromioclavicular joint 29, 167-169, 176, 327
    degeneration 172
Acromioclavicular mobility 176f
Acromioclavicular superior posterior glide 179, 180
Acromion 28
Adduction 139, 152, 170, 179, 193, 288
    horizontal 241, 242
Adductor 31, 160, 285
    local tenderness over 285
    magnus, tenderness of 286
    pollicis 212, 228
Adson's maneuver 80
Adverse neural tension 244-249
Alar ligament 55, 55f, 65
    atlantal part of 55
American Academy of Orthopedic Manual Physical Therapy 13
Ankle 131, 247
    and foot 32, 129
        complex 129
        region 297
    instability 302
    lateral 239, 247, 300
        ligament of 301f
    strain, recurrent 24
Annular ligament 186
Anterior sacrum, torsional positions of 113
Anterior shoulder pain, history of 307
Anterolateral impingement syndrome 133
Anticoagulant therapy 127
Arcade of Frohse 187, 189

Arch, lateral 131
Artery
    law of 9
    temporal 27, 56
Arthritis 295
Arthrokinematic 12, 47
    motion 17, 232
    radial inferior glide 317
Arthrosis, carpometacarpal 201, 322
Articular mobilization 339
Atlantoaxial joint 58
Atlantoaxial ligament 55
    anterior 55
    posterior 55
Atlantoaxial rotation mobilization 73f
Atlanto-occipital membrane 52
Atlas 54f
Axillary nerve 229f, 230, 311
    entrapment 173
Axonotmesis 215

B

Backward bending 35, 35f, 40f, 59, 62, 62f, 65, 73, 101f
Backward nodding restriction 71
Ball and socket joint 18f
Barbiturates 69
Basilar artery 56f
Battle sign 69
Baxter's nerve 299
    entrapment 299
Biceps
    brachii 169, 211, 328
        weakness of 174
    long head of 28, 307
    tendon 172, 307
Bicipital tendinitis 307
Bicycle test 277
Bladder bowel
    dysfunction 256, 272
    incontinence 50
Bone
    disease 50, 127

rotation 44
setting 9
translation 44
Boxer's muscle 267
Brachialis, myositis ossificans of 193
Brachioradialis 29, 212*f*, 319, 320
British Association of Manual Medicine 12
Bucket handle motion 89*f*
Bursa 45, 47, 161
Bursitis 159

C

Calcaneal eversion 302, 303
Calcaneocuboid ligament 130
Calcaneus
    eversion of 141, 142*f*
    inversion of 138, 141, 142*f*
Capsular pattern 138, 139, 152, 163, 179, 193, 284
Capsule tightness
    anterior 343
    posterior 343
Capsulitis 307
Carotid artery 27, 56
Carpal mobilization 322
Carpal tunnel syndrome 202, 322, 322*f*
Ceiling fan analogy 122
Central canal stenosis 274, 275
Cervical
    and thoracic flexion 238, 239
    area function, ligamentous apparatus of 52
    flexion 67
        release of 238, 240
    lateral flexion and depression, release of 241
    myelopathy 256
    nerve root irritation 309
    opening, left-mid 64*f*
    pathology 173
    radiculopathy 253
    region 253
    retractors 53
    rib, possible presence of 90
    side flexion away 241
    spine 27, 51, 167
    spinous processes 329
    spondylosis 60, 253, 269
    vertebra, typical 51*f*, 52
    vertebral bodies, superior surface of 52
Cervicis 54
Cervicothoracic complex 87
Cervicothoracic junction 85*f*
Cervicothoracic region 248
    faulty posture of 265

Cervicothoracic spine 169
Clay-Shoveler's fracture 69
Collateral ligament 198, 201
Compression 43
Condyloid joint 198
Connective tissue disorders 50, 127
Coracobrachialis 29, 309*f*
    hypertrophic 244
Coracoclavicular ligaments 329
Coracoid process 28
Coronal suture stretch 339, 340*f*
Costochondritis 90, 263
Costoclavicular space 244
Costoclavicular syndrome 90, 307
Coxafemoral external rotation deficit 342
Cranial nerves 217
Cranial sutures 335
Cranium 335, 335*f*
Cricoid 27
Cruciate ligament 55
    anterior 146, 147, 149, 348
    posterior 146, 147
Cubital tunnel syndrome 188, 317
Cuboid 32
    dorsal glide 138, 141, 141*f*
    dysfunctions of 132
    manipulation in internal rotation 301-304
    plantar glide 141*f*
    subluxation 302
Cuneiform
    depression manipulation 301-304
    elevated 135, 137
Cuneonavicular dorsal glide 138, 140, 141*f*
Cuneonavicular plantar glide 138, 141*f*
Cutaneous nerve
    lateral 248
    posterior 248
Cyriax' syndrome 92

D

De Quervain's disease 200
Deep peroneal nerve 226, 226*f*
    entrapment 304
Deltoid tuberosity 29
Dermatomes 237
Diarthrodial condyloid 139
Diarthrodial ginglymus 152
Diarthrodial hinge 138, 139, 193
Diarthrodial pivot 193
Diarthrosis 179
Digital nerve 225
Disk 232

degeneration 223
herniation 240, 242, 253, 255, 269, 270f, 271
pathology
    acute 50
    types of 254f
shearing 41f
Distal interphalangeal joint 143, 209
Distal radioulnar joint 197
Distraction 143, 164, 164f, 206
    calcaneus 138, 141, 141f
    humerus 307-309
    mobilization technique 345, 345f, 346f
    MTP joint 142f
    rotation 139, 142, 206, 208, 209
    talus 138, 139, 139f
Dorsal ankle 304
Dorsal glide 139, 142, 143, 206, 209, 210
Dorsal interrossei 212f
Dorsal root ganglion 217
Dorsal scapular nerve 79
Dorsal talonavicular ligament 130
Dorsiflexion 138
Down's syndrome 50, 66
Drop attacks 68
Dysarthria 68
Dysfunction 36, 38, 69
Dysfunctional segments 80
Dysphagia 68

E

Elbow 29, 186, 250, 316
    dysfunction
        anterior 188
        lateral 189
        posterior 188
    extension 242
    flexion 242
        release of 243
    joint 186, 189
    medial collateral ligament of 317f
    pain
        lateral 318
        posterior 188, 318
Elevated first rib 80, 83, 90, 92
Endoneurium 218
Epicondylalgia, lateral 189
Epicondylitis 188
    lateral 190, 318
Epicranial aponeurosis 335
Epineurium 218
Erector spinae 78, 107, 108, 123, 313-315
    muscle 238, 245

Excessive coxofemoral capsule tightness 333, 344
    management of 345
Excessive glenohumeral capsule tightness,
management of 334
Excessive scapula forward tipping, management of
331
Extended rotated side-bent 98, 100
    dysfunction 102
Extension 139, 152, 179, 193
    great toe 139
Extensor carpi radialis
    brevis 29, 44, 186, 187, 199, 211, 212f
    longus 44, 187, 199, 211, 212f
Extensor digitorum 211, 212f
    brevis 226
    communis 199
    longus 226
Extensor hallucis
    brevis 226
    longus 226, 272
Extensor origin 318f
Extensor pollicis
    brevis 30, 199-201, 211, 212
    longus 211, 212
Extensor retinaculum 305
External occipital protuberance 57f, 329
External rotation 170, 171
    end range 334f
    humerus 307-309
    of tibia 151f
Extraspinal interface entrapment 238, 240-243
Extremity joint dysfunction, management of 126

F

Facet
    capsule impingement 253-255, 269-271
    joint 35, 51, 97, 98
        degeneration 253-255, 269-271
    orientation of 51f
    restriction, consequences of 41f
    shearing 41f
    syndrome 223
Fascia 232
Fascial origin 243
Fascicles, superior longitudinal 55
Fatigue 155
Femoral head posterolateral direction 163f
Femoral nerve 221, 222f, 239, 246, 247
Femur
    lateral condyle of 31
    medial condyle of 31
Fibro-osseous tunnels 232

Fibrous bands 232
Fibrous capsule 55
Fibula
    anterior translation of 349f
    glide 154f
    head 31
        anterior glide of 151f
        posterior glide of 138
    mechanics 131
Fibular collateral ligament 349
Finger flexion 242
First rib
    depression 93f
        manipulation 84f
    dysfunction 306
    elevated 177
Flexed rotated side-bent 101
    dysfunction 102
Flexion 39, 139, 152, 169, 170, 179, 193
    rotation test 336
Flexor carpi
    radialis 227
    ulnaris 29, 187, 200, 211, 212, 212f, 250
        strain 189
Flexor digiti minimi 211
    brevis 228
Flexor digitorum
    longus 224
    profundus 199, 211, 227, 320
    sublimis 227
    superficialis 211
Flexor hallucis longus 224, 300
    tendinitis 299
    tendon 300f
Flexor pollicis
    brevis 227
    longus 227
Foot 131, 247
    dorsiflexion 238
    drop 215, 274
    mechanics, correction of 352
    pain 297, 300, 303, 304
        lateral 302
    pronation 150, 152, 291, 292
    supination 150, 152, 295
Foraminal stenosis 274
Forearm pronation 242
Forefoot 129
Forward bending 35, 35f, 39f, 59, 61, 65
Forward head posture 60, 60f, 90, 254-258, 260
Forward nodding 72
    restriction 71

Forward tipped scapula 329f
Fractures 50, 127
Frictions over
    coracobrachialis 309
    extensor carpi radialis brevis 319
    flexor carpi ulnaris 318
    levator scapula 313-315
    pisohammate ligament 321
    supraspinatus 313-315
Frictions pronator teres 321
Frictions transverse carpal ligament 322
Frontal suture stretch 339, 339f
Frontalis 338
    kneading 338f
Fryettes rules 35

G

Galea aponeurotica 335, 335f, 338, 338f
Gamekeepers thumb 201
Gastrocnemius 224
Genitofemoral nerve 220
Genu varum 295
Gerdy's tubercle 148, 293
Glenohumeral anterior glide 180, 183, 183f
Glenohumeral capsule 334
    depiction of 332f
    long axis distraction 334f
    tightness 331
Glenohumeral distraction 179, 180, 182, 182f, 183f
Glenohumeral inferior glide 180, 183, 183f
Glenohumeral internal rotation deficit 332
Glenohumeral joint 167-170
Glenohumeral posterior glide 180, 182, 183f
Glenoid impingement, posterior superior 314
Gluteus maximus 107, 123
    strength 344, 345f
Gluteus medius 31, 107, 108, 119f, 123, 270, 277, 284, 287, 288
    muscle 287
    soft tissue mobilization of 287
    strength 344, 345f
    tenderness 287
    weakness 287
Golfer's elbow 188, 316, 316f
Gracilis 31
Greater trochanter 31
Grip, weakness of 322
Groin pain, anteromedial 283
Gross neural mobilization 246, 247, 249, 250
Guyon's canal 243, 244, 250, 321f
    syndrome 202, 321

H

Hamate, hook of 30
Hamstring syndrome 224
Hand pain
　lateral 318
　medial 316
Hawkins impingement sign 314
Headache 329, 337
　cervicogenic 336
　muscular 79
　myogenic 24, 173, 259, 262
　primary 336
　secondary 336
　severe 337
　tension type 336
　vestibular 337
　vomiting relieves 337
Hemarthrosis 127
Hinge joints 198
Hip 30, 105, 131, 157
　abduction firing pattern 162, 162f, 163
　adductors 107, 109, 123
　anterior capsule 346f
　bursitis 160
　capsular pattern, presence of 344
　capsule and femoral rotation 342
　distraction 284, 286, 287
　extension of 239, 287, 344
　flexor 284, 288, 343
　　tightness 240, 344f
　impingement 159
　internal rotation 344f
　joint 157, 286
　　anterior view 343f
　　posterior view 342f
　　somatic diagnosis 161
　mechanics, prior correction of 352
　pain 157
　　anteromedial 283
　　lateral 286
　　mechanical 160
　　posterior 288
　posterior capsule 345, 345f
　region 283
　replacement 344f
　restriction, capsular 288
Human body, kinesiology of 12
Humeral head position 174f
Humeral rotation 174f
　depiction of 332f
Humerus 173

anterior
　glide of 308
　rotation of 184
distraction 313-315
external rotation 178f, 313-315
greater
　tubercle of 311
　tuberosity of 28
inferior glide 313, 314
medial rotation of 184
posterior glide 178f, 307-309, 313-315
superior 178, 184
　dysfunction of 175f
Hunter's canal 221, 292
Hyoid 27
Hyperabduction syndrome 308
Hyperextension 193
Hypertrophic teres 244
Hypertrophy 188, 242

I

Iliac crest 30, 115
Iliac spine
　anterior superior 30, 105, 160, 221, 287
　posterior superior 30, 105, 115, 342
Iliohypogastric nerve 220
Ilioinguinal nerve 220
Iliolumbar ligament 99, 106, 223f, 239, 246
Iliolumbar syndrome 223
Iliopsoas 107, 108, 123, 160, 270, 277, 285
　bursitis 159, 284
　functional length of 123
　stretching 345
　tightness 287, 342
Iliotibial band 31, 291, 293
　dysfunction 293
　friction syndrome 148, 347
Ilna styloid, posterior 191f, 203f
Inervertebral foramen 249
Inferior longitudinal fascicles 55
Inferior pubis 112, 120, 162
Inferior radioulnar joint 318-321
Inflammation, acute 127
Infraspinatus 168, 169, 229, 312, 328
　tendon 314f
　weakness of 174
Inguinal ligament 240, 246
　dysfunctional states of 160
Injury, consequences of 55f
Innominate dysfunctions 271
　diagnosis of 118
　manipulation of 284-288
　treatment of 121

Instability 50, 127, 171, 276
Intercarpal joints 208, 208f
Intercostal compression syndrome, anterior 91
Intercostal space stretching 94, 262
Intercostobrachial nerve 263
Intermetacarpal joints 208, 208f
Internal impingement, anterior 314
Internal rotation 170, 171
    end range 334f
    restricted 343
International Federation of Orthopedic Manual Therapy 12
International Headache Society 336
Interossei 198, 211
Interosseous nerve syndrome, anterior 188, 320
Interphalangeal joint, proximal 143, 209
Intersection syndrome 201, 212f
Interspinous ligament 99
Intertransverse ligament 99
Intervertebral disk 97
Intervertebral foramen 238, 240, 241, 243, 246, 248
Inverted calcaneus, correction of 136f
Irvin Korr's muscle spindle theory 11
Ischemia 234
Ischial spine 115
Ischial tuberosity 30

J

Jogger's foot 133, 298, 299
Joint
    atlanto-occipital 58, 65
    basics 138, 139, 152, 163, 179, 193
    carpometacarpal 42, 210
    disease 50, 127
    fusion, anomalous 50, 127
    interphalangeal 42, 198, 226
    line, medial 32
    Macconail's classification of 41, 42
    mobility 233
    mobilization 339
    play, restriction of 203
    replacement 127
    restriction 17, 18, 188
    subtalar 138, 141
    types of 138, 139, 152, 163, 179, 193

K

Kaltenborn concave-covex rule 43
Kneading pressure 338f
Knee 31, 131, 146, 246
    extension 152
        lag 238, 350
    flexion 118, 239, 346
    joint 146
        somatic diagnosis 149
    pain
        anterior 290
        lateral 293
        medial 291
        posterior 295
    region 290
    stretching posterior capsule of 351, 351f
    terminal extension lag, management of 350

L

Lambdoid suture stretch 340, 340f
Lateral collateral ligament 32, 147
Lateral femoral cutaneous nerve 221, 221f
Lateral impingement syndrome 301
Latissimus dorsi 79, 169, 328
Leg length 117
    discrepancy 271
Lesions 254f
Levator scapula 53, 74, 78, 79, 82, 168, 306, 327, 330
    strain 306
    stretch 74f
    syndrome 266
    tightness of 175
Levator stretch 307, 308, 310, 312
Ligament 45, 47, 232
    anterior longitudinal 52, 78, 98
    atlanto-occipital 55
    bifurcated 130
    insufficiency 50, 127
    lateral 55
    posterior
        longitudinal 52, 78, 98
        occipitoatlantal 55
    primary 146
    sacrospinous 106
    sacrotuberous 106
    strain 189, 201
        lateral 149, 295, 300
    supraspinous 52, 98
Ligamentum flavum 52, 99
Limb, lower 220, 237, 238
Long axis tissue stretch 101
Long plantar ligament 130
Longus cervicis 53
Longus colli 53, 54
Loose packed position 138, 139, 152, 163, 179, 193
Lower quarter dysfunction 342, 347, 349

Lower trapezius
    insufficient activity of 175
    strengthening 332*f*
Lumbar dysfunctions, manipulation of 287, 288
Lumbar herniated disk 223
Lumbar lordosis 270-276, 279-281
Lumbar paraspinals, strengthen 123
Lumbar radiculopathy 269, 305
Lumbar spine 30, 36, 96
    nonneutral dysfunctions of 108, 109
    somatic diagnosis 100
Lumbar spondylosis 223, 269, 270*f*
Lumbar stenosis 223
Lumbar vertebra, typical 97*f*
Lumbopelvic complex 122
Lumbopelvic hip 124*f*
    region 245
Lumbopelvic region 269
Lumbosacral junction 269
Lumbosacral ligament 223
Lunate 29
    anterior 203, 205, 208
    posterior glide 205*f*
Lymph nodes 27
    inguinal 31

M

Manipulation, types 14
Marfans syndrome 66
Maxilla distraction 340, 340*f*
Mechanical radicular pain, management of 245
Medial collateral ligament 147
    strain 188, 316
Medial cutaneous nerve 248
Medial elbow
    dysfunction 188
    pain 316
Medial epicondylitis 188, 316, 317
Medial intermuscular septum 242
Medial ligament strain 148, 291
Medial meniscus strain 347
Medial nerve
    neural mobilization of 321
    tension test 241*f*
Medial patellofemoral joint 32
Medial plantar
    fascia 298
    nerve 133, 225
Medial tibial condyle 31
    anterior glide of 153
    posterior glide of 153

Median nerve 227, 227*f*, 248, 250
    entrapment sites 321*f*
    neural mobilization of 322
    tension test 241*f*
Meralgia paresthetica 160, 287
Metacarpophalangeal
    distraction 208*f*
    dorsal glide 209*f*
    joints 42, 73, 198, 206, 208
    lateral glide 209*f*
    medial glide 209*f*
    rotation 208*f*
    volar glide 209*f*
Metatarsal arch 131
Metatarsal heads 33
Metatarsophalangeal joints 139, 142, 226, 300
Midcarpal
    dorsal glide 206, 207, 208*f*
    volar glide 205, 207, 207*f*
Midcervical
    closing 307
    dysfunctions 74
    opening 307
    side gliding 76*f*
    spine 36, 61, 73, 177
        osseous anatomy 51
        somatic diagnosis 63
Midfoot 129, 130
    internal rotation restriction 137*f*
Midthoracic closing manipulation 313-315
Mid-thoracic spine 83
    closing restriction of 86
    opening restriction of 85*f*, 86*f*
Migraines 336
Minimally supports test 6
Moderately supports test 6
Motion, planes of 18*f*
MTP joint
    lateral glide of 143
    medial glide of 143
Multifidus 53, 107, 109
Multisegmental ligaments 98
Muscles 45, 161, 200, 232, 243, 320
    action, inversion of 285
    attaching thoracic spine 78
    connecting scapula
        to humerus 328
        to spine 327
    energy technique 11, 14, 16
    inhibition, arthrogenic 346
    length imbalances 131
    of cervical area 53

of elbow 186
of forearm 211
pathologies 258, 265, 272
strain 132
  intercostal 91
suboccipital 53, 260f
weakness 19, 19f
Muscular function 130
Musculocutaneous nerve 230, 230f
entrapment 309, 309f
Musculoskeletal dysfunction
diagnosis of 48
management of 5
Musculoskeletal red flag assessment 65
Musculoskeletal system 5, 326
Myofascial dysfunction 240, 242
Myofascial points 155f
Myofascial tender points 88, 88f, 123, 124f, 144, 144f, 152, 155, 184, 184f, 195, 196f, 211, 212f
Myofasical dysfunction 242
Myotomes 237

N

Navicular talus dorsal glide 138, 140, 140f
Neck side flexion away, release of 243
Nerve 45, 47, 161
cell 218
compression 149
dysfunction
  hypothetical somatic concept of 47
  mechanical 232
entrapment 172, 202, 285, 288
irritation 133, 160
law of 10
mediated pain 265
mediation 266
mobility 233
palsy 160
root 219
  irritation 253, 269, 270
vascularity 218
Nervous system 217
Neural mobilization 15
Neuralgia, intercostal 79, 90, 262
Neurapraxia 215
Neurodynamics 47
Neurokinematic restriction 47, 245-250
Neuromas 133
Neuromuscular therapies 14, 15
Neurotmesis 215
Non-neutral dysfunction, correction of 123

Notalgia paresthetica 230
Nuchal line 329

O

Obliquus capitis
inferior 57
superior 57, 57f, 73f
Obturator 160, 240, 248, 285
nerve 222, 222f
  entrapment, sites of 285f
Occipitalis 338
Occipitoatlantal ligament
anterior 55
lateral 55
Occipitoaxial ligament 55
Olecranon 29
bursitis 189
local tenderness over medial aspect of 317
Opponens digiti minimi 228
Opponens pollicis 227
Orbit distraction 339, 340f
Orthopedic manual physical therapy 6
Osteitis pubis 286
Osteoarthritis 158, 283, 287, 306
hip 160, 283f
knee 295
Osteokinematic movements 232
Osteopathy 9, 10
Osteoporosis 50, 127

P

Pain 285, 302
chronic 23
knife-like 69
mechanism of 335
reproduction 288
sciatic 20
Palmar glide 210
Palmaris longus 227
Palpation 25, 36, 38
Paraspinals 270, 277
Passive movement tests 65
Passive neck flexion 232
Patella
compression 148, 290, 293, 347
inferior glide 152, 291, 292, 296
medial tilt 291, 292, 294-296
superior lateral position of 150f
superolateral 150, 151
tendinitis 291

tendon 32, 291
tracking 148, 290, 347
    dysfunction 290
    lateral 291f
Patellofemoral dysfunction 240
Patellofemoral joint 146
Pectoralis
    major 28, 169, 241, 248
    minor 28, 78, 90, 168, 244, 308, 328, 329
Pelvic
    complex 105
        dysfunctions of 114
        somatic diagnosis 115
    dysfunction 112
    floor 123
        muscles 123
    inlet, superior view of 224f
Pelvis 30, 36, 131
    downslip of 109
    dysfunctions of 110
    mechanics of 110
Perineurium 218
Peripheral nerve 219, 232, 237
    injury 215
    structure of 218
Peroneal dysfunction 294, 302f
Peroneal nerve 226f
    entrapment 225, 293, 294f
Peroneal tears 302
Peroneal tendon 32
    injury 301
        types of 301
Peroneus longus, tenderness over 295
Peroneus tertius 226
Pes anserine bursitis 148, 292, 293, 347
Phalen's test 322
Phasic muscles 123
Piriformis 30, 107, 109, 123, 160, 161, 224f, 246, 270, 277, 285
    local tenderness over 288
    muscle 115
    syndrome 224, 280, 288
Pisiform 206, 207
Pisohamate ligament 198, 201
Plantar
    calcaneonavicular ligament 130
    fascia 33, 297, 297f
    fasciitis 132, 297
    flexion 134, 138
    glide 139, 142, 142f, 143
    nerve 224, 225, 247, 298f
        entrapment 298
        lateral 133, 225

    neural mobilization of 299
Plantarflexed talus 134f
    correction of 136f
Popliteus injury 295
Positive sitting flexion test 118
Posterior impingement elbow, site for 318f
Posterior sacrum, torsional positions of 113f
Postlaminectomy syndrome 279
Postural muscles 123
Pronated foot 134
Pronator
    quadratus 227
    syndrome 188, 320
    teres 29, 187, 211, 227, 241
Prone hip flexor tightness 344
Prone knee
    band 233
    flexion 118f
Prone leg length
    assessment 118f
Prone lying technique 103, 103f
Prone passive lag test 348
Prone prop up test 116
Proprioceptive neuromuscular facilitation 11, 14, 15, 110
Psoas major 240, 246
Pubic dysfunctions 112, 285, 286
    manipulation of 285, 287
Pubic tubercle 30, 115, 116f
Pubis
    dysfunction, diagnosis of 116
    inferior 163
    superior 112, 120, 162, 163
Pump handle, depiction of 89f
Pupil light reflex 68
Pupillary reflex testing 68f

Q

Q-angle 148
Quadratus lumborum 107, 109, 123, 239, 270, 277
    syndrome 223
Quadriceps 107, 108, 123
    strength 108
Quadrilateral space 28, 311f
    syndrome 173, 244, 311

R

Raccoon sign 69
Radial glide, proximal row 208f
Radial groove 29, 242

Radial head 29, 319, 320
  anterior glide of 193
  compression 189, 319
  dysfunctions 190
  inferior 190, 191, 202, 204
    glide 192f
  posterior glide of 193, 194
  superior 190, 191, 202, 204
    glide 192f
Radial nerve 228, 228f, 229f, 249, 311
  entrapment 173, 309
  neural mobilization of 319, 320
  neuritis 202
  tension test 241, 243f
Radial styloid 29, 242
Radial tunnel syndrome 189, 191, 319
Radicular pain 253, 269
  lower extremity mechanical 245
  mechanical 246, 247, 249, 250
Radiculopathy 20, 270f
Radiocapitellar chondromalacia 319
Radiocarpal
  distraction 205, 206, 206f
  dorsal glide 205, 206, 207f
  joint 205, 206
  retraction 193, 195, 195f
  ulnar glide 206f
  volar glide 206, 207, 207f
Radius
  anterior posterior glide 195f
  caudal movement of 205
  cephalad movement of 206, 207
  inferior glide 192f, 194, 194f, 204, 205f
  moves cephalad 44
  superior glide 192f, 193, 194, 204, 204f
Ramus
  anterior primary 217
  posterior primary 217
Range of motion 138, 139, 152, 163, 179, 193
Rearfoot 129
Rectus capitis posterior
  major 57, 57f, 73f
  minor 57, 57f
Rectus femoris 108, 123
Reflexes 237
Restriction, capsular pattern of 265
Retinacular nerve 149
  entrapment 294
Retinaculum, lateral 32
Retrocalcaneal bursitis 303, 303f
Rheumatoid arthritis 50, 91, 127
Rhomboid 79, 168, 328, 330
  major 78

  minor 78
  strain 266
Ribs 77, 88
  anterior slipping of 89
  dysfunction
    anterior 93
    superior 92
Roos test 90
Rotation 35, 42, 59, 62, 65, 152
  MTP joint 142f
  restriction 71
  side bending 75
Rotator cuff
  impingement 312
  strains 171
  syndrome 229, 310
  tendinitis 171

S

Sacral dysfunctions 115, 271
  manipulation of 284-288
  presence of 285
Sacral extension 123
Sacral flexion 123
Sacral torsion 161, 163
  left on left 113, 117, 120
  left on right 113, 118, 120
Sacroiliac dysfunction 289
Sacroiliac joint 31, 111
  anterior 239, 246
  dysfunction 223
Sacroiliac ligament
  anterior 106
  posterior 31, 106
Sacroiliac pain 20
Sacrum 36, 105f
  base of 30
  dysfunction 112
    diagnosis of 116
    treatment of 120
  inferior lateral angle of 30
  locating inferior aspect of 117f
Saphenous nerve 149, 221, 222f, 240, 246, 247, 292
  irritation 292
    sites of 292f
Sartorius, soft tissue mobilization of 154, 154f
Scalenes 90, 75, 241, 244, 248
  anterior 53
  lateral 53
  posterior 53
  stretch 75f

Index

Scaphoid 29, 206
Scapholunate ligament 212*f*
Scapula 78, 175, 327
    and humeral dysfunction 265
    backward tipping test 330
    direction of 332*f*
    distraction 179, 180, 181*f*
    downward rotation 175*f*, 180
    dysfunctional states of 328
    inferior angle of 28
    protracted 184
    retraction 179*f*, 307-310, 312-315
    spine of 28
    superolateral border of 310
    upward rotation 178*f*, 179-181, 181*f*, 307-310, 312-315
Scapular protraction 176*f*
Scapulothoracic articulation 167
Scapulothoracic joint 168, 170
Schwann cells 218
Sciatic nerve 222, 223*f*, 238, 245, 246
    entrapment sites 224*f*
Sciatic notch 30
Segmental ligaments 99
Semispinalis 53, 78
    stretch 338*f*
Sensation 227
Serratus
    anterior 78, 79, 168, 328
        strengthening 94, 94*f*, 331*f*
    posterior superior 78, 267
Seventh thoracic spine, spinous process of 28
Sharpey's fibers 335
Shotgun technique 120, 120*f*
Shoulder 28, 167, 249
    abduction 242
        release of 243
    depression 242
        release of 242, 243
    elevation 170*f*, 333*f*
    external rotation 333*f*
    girdle depression 240, 241
    internal rotation arm behind back 333*f*
    joint 167
        somatic diagnosis 173
    medial rotation 241
        release of 242
    pain
        anterior 307
        lateral 309
        posterior 310
        superior 306

    pathology 265
    region 306
Side bending 59, 62, 62*f*, 73
    mobilization 103*f*
    restriction 71
Side lying
    knee bend test 239, 240*f*
    technique 103, 103*f*
Sinus tarsi 32, 301, 301*f*
    syndrome 301
Sitting flexion test 115, 115*f*
Slacken musculature 63*f*
Slipping rib syndrome 92
Slump 233, 238
    test 239*f*
Snapping scapula 172, 264
Soft tissue 25, 174-176, 286, 287
    dysfunction 189
    inhibition 71, 74, 101, 119
    irritability 46
    mobilization 15, 82, 83*f*, 101*f*, 180*f*, 259, 291, 292, 302, 337, 338, 350*f*
        mid-thoracic paraspinals 82*f*
        myofascial release 14
    strains 160
Specific somatic dysfunction, treatment for 136, 150, 162, 177, 191, 204
Spinal anomalies, congenital 50
Spinal column 98
Spinal cord 218*f*, 219
Spinal joint motion 63
Spinal nerve 217, 218*f*
Spine 34
Spinoglenoid ligament 229, 310
Spinous process
    deviation 38*f*
    palpation of 37*f*
Splenius 53
    capitis 78
    cervicis 78
Spondylolisthesis 50, 223, 276
    causes of 277
Spondylolysis 50, 276
Sporadic pain behind outside ankle bone 302
Squamous suture stretch 339, 339*f*
Standing flexion test 118
Stenosis 273
Sternoclavicular inferior anterior glide 179-181
Sternoclavicular joint 28, 167, 170, 177
    inferior anterior glide of 179*f*
    posterior glide of 179*f*
    superior glide of 179*f*

Sternoclavicular mobility 177*f*
Sternoclavicular superior posterior glide 179-181
Sternomastoid 53
Stork test 115, 116*f*
Straight-leg raise 47, 232, 233, 271
Strain counterstrain 14, 16, 211
    methods 123, 155, 184, 195
Stress fractures 133
Stretch
    anterior capsule 308
    hamstrings 123
    hip flexors 284-288
    iliopsoas 123
    inferior capsule 308
    internal rotators 284, 286, 287
    piriformis 123
    posterior capsule 308, 313-315
    quadratus lumborum 123
Strongly supports test 6
Subacromial bursa, location of 310*f*
Subacromial bursitis 172, 310
Subclavius 78
Subcoracoid impingement 314
Subcranial dysfunction 266
Subcranial spine 36, 50, 54, 64, 177
    facet joint of 61
    inhibitive distraction of 72
    somatic diagnosis 69
Suboccipital release 254-257, 259, 260, 266, 267, 306
Suboccipital stretch 337*f*
Suboccipital triangle 57
Subscapularis 169, 313
    dysfunction 312
Subtalar neutral assessment 134*f*
Superficial peroneal nerve 32, 133, 149, 226, 226*f*, 247
Superior tibiofibular dysfunction, management of 350
Superolateral patella 291
Supinator brevis 187
Supinator hypertrophy 242
Suprascapular nerve 229, 229*f*
    entrapment sites 310, 310*f*
    impingement 172
Supraspinatus 168, 169, 229, 312, 328
    weakness of 174
Swelling 302
Symphysis pubis
    dysfunction 111
        treatment of 120
    joint 112
    shotgun for 286
Symphysitis 286
Systemic lupus erythematosis 66

T

Talocrural anterior glide 301-304
Talocrural distraction 298-305
Talocrural joint 138, 139
Talocrural posterior glide 298, 300, 304, 305
Talofibular ligament, anterior 32, 130, 301
Talus 32
    anterior medial glide of 139, 140*f*
    lateral glide of 138, 142
    medial glide of 138, 142
    plantar flexed 134, 136
    posterior lateral glide of 136*f*, 139
Tarsal tunnel 239, 247, 299*f*
    syndrome 133, 299, 300
Tectorial membrane 52
Temporomandibular joint 60
Tendinitis 132, 285-287, 301
Tendoachilles 304
    tear 304*f*
    tendon degeneration 303*f*
Tendon 45, 200, 320
    calcification 303
Tendonitis, impingement 266
Tennis elbow 46, 189, 318
Tensor fascia lata 31, 286, 293, 343
Teres
    major 28, 169, 242, 311, 328, 329, 331*f*
    minor 28, 168, 169, 174, 311, 313, 328
Thenar eminence 227
Third thoracic spine, spinous process of 28
Thomas test 285, 288
Thoracic
    disk herniation 264
    dorsal ramus 230, 244, 249
    dysfunction 92, 330
    kyphosis 314
    outlet 28, 173, 244
        syndrome 90, 258, 307, 308
    region 262
    spinal nerves
        anterior rami of 79
        posterior rami of 79
        ventral rami of 91
    spine 27, 36, 77, 167, 177
        lower 81, 84, 85
        mechanical dysfunctions of 77, 177
        spine somatic diagnosis 80
    vertebra, typical 77, 77*f*
Thoracolumbar junction 269
    dysfunction 286
    syndrome 104, 278

Throwing 188
Thrust 15
Thumb
    reinforcement 101*f*
    ulnar collateral ligament of 198, 201
Thunderclap 337
Thyroid gland 27
Tibia
    anterior glide 154*f*
        medial condyle 152, 350, 351*f*
    distraction 152, 153, 153*f*, 296
    external rotation 150
    glides 296
    internal rotation of 150, 151*f*
    posteriomedial glide 294
    posterior glide 152, 154*f*
    superomedial aspect of 292
Tibial condyle, lateral 31
Tibial external rotation 295, 349*f*
Tibial internal rotation 291, 292, 350*f*
Tibial nerve 298
    posterior 224, 247
Tibial rotation 149, 346, 348
Tibialis anterior 226
    tendon 32
Tibialis posterior 32, 224
    tendinitis 300
Tibiofibular anterior glide, superior 352*f*
Tibiofibular joint, superior 150*f*, 239, 247, 294-296, 346, 348, 350*f*, 351
Tibiofibular posterior glide, superior 351*f*
Tinel's sign 317
Tissue
    mobility 26, 41, 47
    tenderness 71
    tension testing 46
        selective 46
Torsion
    anterior 113
    posterior 113
Torsional dysfunctions 113, 117
Traction and passive gliding 138, 193, 205
Transverse arch 131
Transverse carpal ligament, contracture of 322
Transverse ligament 55, 66
    compromise and consequence 56*f*
    integrity in sitting 66*f*, 67*f*
Transversospinalis 79, 107, 109
Transversus abdominis 107, 123
    strengthen 123
    tenderness of 286
Trapezius 27, 29, 53, 74, 78, 168, 207, 327, 330
    strain 306

stretch 74*f*
Trapezoid 207
Trauma 61
Trendelenburg gait 108, 159, 284
Triangular fibrocartilage complex 197, 200
Triangular interval syndrome 173, 309, 311
Triceps brachii 211
Triceps strain 189
Trigger point compression 285, 287, 288
Trochanteric bursitis 159, 284, 284*f*, 286
Tumors 50, 127

U

Ulna
    anterior glide 193*f*
    distraction 193, 194*f*
    styloid
        anterior glide 195*f*, 205*f*
        posterior glide 195*f*
Ulnar 250
    deviation 200, 204-206, 242
    glide, proximal row 208*f*
    nerve 29, 227, 228*f*, 248, 249
        neural mobilization of 318, 321
        tension test 242, 243*f*
    styloid 29
        anterior glide of 193
        posterior 191, 193, 204
            glide of 193, 195
    traction spur 188
    variance 191, 191*f*, 193, 202, 203*f*
Upper extremity mechanical radicular pain 248
Upper limb 227, 237
    tension tests 90, 232, 233, 250, 255
Upper quarter dysfunction 329, 332
Upper thoracic facet dysfunction 231
Upper thoracic region 83*f*, 84*f*
    general mobilization of 83
Upper thoracic spine 80, 84, 85*f*
    closing restriction of 85*f*
    opening restriction of 84*f*
Upper trapezius 53
    stretch 307, 308, 310, 312

V

Valgus stress 317
Varus stress test 295
Vastus medialis obliquus 155, 221, 247, 290-293
Vertebral artery 56, 56*f*, 67
    insufficiency 50
    testing 67*f*

Vertex compression 68, 68f
Viral infections 91
Volar glide 206, 208, 209
    radiocarpal 316, 317-320
von Luschka joints 52

W

Weight bearing arches 131
Whiplash injury 257, 277
    mechanism 257f
Wrist 250, 316
    and hand 29, 197
        somatic diagnosis 202
    drop 215
    extension 189, 206
        radial deviation 203, 205, 242
        release of 243
    flexion 188, 200, 204, 205, 242
    pain
        lateral 318
        medial 316
    radial deviation of 44

Z

Zygoapophyseal joints 51
Zygoma depression 339, 339f
Zygomatic arch 339
    soft tissue kneading 339f